# Cognitive Rehabilitation
# Therapy for Traumatic Brain Injury

*A Guide for Speech-Language Pathologists*

# Cognitive Rehabilitation Therapy for Traumatic Brain Injury

## A Guide for Speech-Language Pathologists

Jennifer A. Ostergren, PhD, CCC-SLP

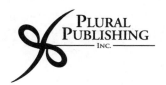

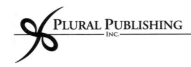

5521 Ruffin Road
San Diego, CA 92123

e-mail: info@pluralpublishing.com
website: http://www.pluralpublishing.com

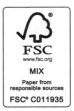

Copyright © 2018 by Plural Publishing, Inc.

Typeset in 10.5/13 Minion Pro by Flanagan's Publishing Services, Inc.
Printed in the United States of America by McNaughton & Gunn, Inc.

Library of Congress Cataloging-in-Publication Data

Names: Ostergren, Jennifer A., author.
Title: Cognitive rehabilitation therapy for traumatic brain injury : a guide
  for speech-language pathologists / Jennifer A. Ostergren.
Description: San Diego, CA : Plural, [2018] | Includes bibliographical
  references and index.
Identifiers: LCCN 2017047091| ISBN 9781597567893 (alk. paper) | ISBN
  1597567892 (alk. paper)
Subjects: | MESH: Brain Injuries, Traumatic—rehabilitation | Brain Injuries,
  Traumatic--complications | Language Disorders—therapy | Cognition
  Disorders--therapy | Cognitive Therapy—methods | Speech-Language
  Pathology—methods
Classification: LCC RC451.4.B73 | NLM WL 354 | DDC 617.4/81044—dc23
LC record available at https://lccn.loc.gov/2017047091

# Contents

## SECTION I
## Foundational Knowledge

## SECTION II
## Treatment in Action

# Introduction

As the title suggests, this book is about cognitive rehabilitation therapy (CRT) after traumatic brain injury (TBI). Its emphasis is on TBI in adults, written specifically for use by speech-language pathologists (SLPs). This is not to suggest that this is the sole area of rehabilitation needs of individuals with TBI. To the contrary, SLPs who have worked with individuals with TBI understand that there are many facets of rehabilitation following TBI (not solely CRT), and several parallel roles of SLPs who work with individuals with TBI. This includes rehabilitation guided by SLPs in the areas of speech, swallowing, and alternative and augmentative communication (AAC), to name a few. There are many helpful resources in each of these areas. This book is specific to CRT, given the growing (but still limited) research evidence in this area, as well as the cardinal role cognition plays in communication, daily activities, and the rehabilitation process after a TBI.

This book is limited to CRT for adults, as the research evidence for CRT in adults and children are distinctly different. Children with TBI and their families are also in need of helpful and evidence-based resources in this area, but collapsing these two distinct evidence foundations is neither simplistic nor conducive to the format of this text, as an applied resource for SLPs. The approaches described in this book are drawn directly from the research studies in the area of CRT for adults following TBI.

Section I of this book (Foundational Knowledge) includes information on the mechanisms of injury and neuropathology of TBI (Chapter 1: Mechanisms of Injury and Neuropathology), and recovery patterns and applicable classification/outcome measures following TBI (Chapter 2: Classification and Recovery). These two chapters are followed by a description of common compounding and concomitant conditions that impact individuals with TBI and the rehabilitation process (Chapter 3: Compounding and Concomitant Conditions), and of course a description of the nature of cognition and communication following TBI (Chapter 4: Cognition and Communication). The final two chapters in Section I focus on general rehabilitation practices and principles, including the concept of CRT within the broader landscape of interdisciplinary and patient-centered rehabilitation (Chapter 5: Coordinated Care) and general CRT treatment principles (Chapter 6: Cognitive Rehabilitation Therapy Principles), which will serve as the foundation for the CRT approaches discussed in Section II.

Section II (Treatment in Action) is devoted to describing clinically relevant information about CRT approaches with demonstrated efficacy and effectiveness for adults following TBI. There are four chapters in Section II, structured around the categorical nature of descriptions of cognitive impairments following TBI. They include a chapter on approaches for attention and information processing speed impairments (Chapter 7: Attention and Information Processing Speed), one on memory impairments

(Chapter 8: Memory), a chapter on deficits in the area of executive function and awareness (Chapter 9: Executive Function and Awareness), and a chapter devoted specifically to *social* communication (Chapter 10: Social Communication). The format of these Section II chapters includes first an introduction to the landscape of CRT evidence in that specific area, followed by sub-chapters that address a specific evidence-based treatment approach *in detail*, including: (1) recommended candidates, (2) theoretical foundations, (3) relevant background information, and (4) a section titled, "Treatment in Action." In this Treatment in Action section, the research evidence available on a specific approach is distilled into applicable steps, procedures, and needed materials for implementation. In each of these sections, the applied nature

of this text for SLPs was given special attention. Where possible, charts, figures, tables, and appendices are included to facilitate the use of these approaches tailored by an SLP for a wide variety of individuals with TBI. Although this later section is more formulaic in nature, throughout this text the reader is encouraged to view each individual with TBI as unique. The one undeniably true fact about TBI is that there are no two individuals with TBI who are alike. As such, their rehabilitation (and the use of these techniques) is never the same. This text will serve as a guide only, offering descriptions of approaches supported by research evidence. As is consistent with our training, it is then the job of the SLP to individualize each approach to the unique needs and desires of a specific individual with TBI.

# Acknowledgments

Thank you to my wonderful husband, Scott, and lovely daughter, Gwen, for your tireless support and endless patience. Without your gifts of love and time, this book would have not been possible. Thank you as well to the many individuals with TBI (and their families) whom I have had the great pleasure of serving throughout my many years as a speech-language pathologist. You have informed the content of this book with your experiences and inspired me with your grace, humor, creativity, and courage in the face of traumatic brain injury (TBI). My deepest wish is that this book will be a helpful resource to speech-language pathologists in offering cognitive rehabilitation therapy that meets the unique needs of each individual with TBI (and his/her family).

# Contributor

Carley B. Crandall is a graduate student at California State University, Long Beach (CSULB). She earned her BA Communicative Disorders from CSULB and is pursuing her Master's degree with a keen interest in traumatic brain injury–related communicative disorders, as well as the application of treatment within group settings. Carley has held research assistant positions in the area of evidence-based practice in traumatic brain injury (TBI) and augmentative and alternative communication (AAC). Carley is a licensed speech-language pathology assistant and looks forward to furthering her education of, and contributing to, the field of speech-language pathology.

# Reviewers

Plural Publishing, Inc. and the author would like to thank the following reviewers for taking the time to provide their valuable feedback during the development process:

**Kathryn Atkinson, MA, CCC-SLP, BC-ANCDS**
Clinical Instructor
Central Michigan University
Board Certification in Neurologic Communication Disorders in Adults
Mount Pleasant, Michigan

**Rebecca D. Eberle, MA, CCC-SLP, BC-ANCDS**
Clinical Professor
Department of Speech and Hearing Sciences
Indiana University
Bloomington, Indiana

**Yolanda T. Evans, MA, CCC/SLP**
Clinical Instructor
Communication Sciences and Disorders
Saint Louis University
St. Louis, Missouri

**Dana Hanifan, MA, CCC**
Senior Speech-Language Pathologist
Michigan Medicine
University of Michigan Health System
Ann Arbor, Michigan

**Lisa Schoenbrodt, EdD, CCC-SLP**
Professor and Chair
Department of Speech-Language-Hearing Sciences
Loyola University Maryland
Baltimore, Maryland

# SECTION I

## Foundational Knowledge

# 1 Mechanisms of Injury and Neuropathology

*In examining disease, we gain wisdom about anatomy and physiology and biology. In examining the person with disease, we gain wisdom about life.*

—Oliver Sacks

Author Stephen Shore once said about individuals with autism, "If you've met one person with autism—you've met one person with autism" (as cited in Kolarik, 2016, p. 479). The same is true for individuals with traumatic brain injury (TBI). Diversity among individuals who experience a TBI is infinite, as are the ways in which the trauma associated with TBI can occur. No two individuals or their injuries are exactly alike. It is nonetheless important for those who want to be of assistance to individuals with TBI (and their families) to consider both general trends in the nature of TBI, as well as its potential neurologic impact. This chapter will discuss important terms and definitions, the distribution and determinants of TBI (epidemiology), and the neuropathology associated with TBI.

## Defining TBI

To define something is the act of making it clear or distinct. This is an important first step in understanding TBI. The Centers for Disease Control and Prevention (CDC) defines TBI as "a disruption in the normal function of the brain that can be caused by a bump, blow, or jolt to the head or a pene-

trating head injury" (CDC, 2015, p. 15). An explosive blast can also cause a TBI (CDC, 2015). The World Health Organization (WHO) uses the term "neurotrauma" to highlight the acquired and traumatic nature of this type of injury. TBI can result when the head suddenly and violently hits an object, or when an object pierces the skull and enters brain tissue (National Institute of Neurologic Disorders and Stroke [NINDS], n.d.).

The presence of any of the following clinical signs constitutes a disruption in normal brain function after a TBI (Menon, Schwab, Wright, & Maas, 2010):

1. Any period of loss of or decreased consciousness
2. Any loss of memory for events immediately before (retrograde amnesia) or after the injury (posttraumatic amnesia)
3. Neurologic deficits such as muscle weakness, loss of balance and coordination, disruption of vision, change in speech and language, or sensory loss
4. Any alteration in mental state at the time of the injury such as confusion, disorientation, slowed thinking, or difficulty with concentration.

TBI ranges in severity (from mild to severe), but according to the *Diagnostic*

3

*and Statistical Manual of Mental Disorders,* 5th edition (DSM-5; American Psychiatric Association, 2013), after an injury, the characteristics of TBI include one or more of the following:

1. Changes in levels of consciousness
2. Memory disturbances
3. Confusion associated with deficits in orientation
4. Neurological signs such as brain injury observable on neuroimaging, new onset or worsening of seizure disorder, visual field deficits, hemiparesis, and so forth.

A concussion is also a form of TBI, defined by McCrory et al. (2013, pp. 1–2) as:

1. Caused either by a direct blow to the head, face, neck, or elsewhere on the body with an "impulsive" force transmitted to the head.
2. Typically resulting in the rapid onset of short-lived impairment of neurological function that resolves spontaneously. However, in some cases, symptoms and signs may evolve over a number of minutes to hours.
3. May result in neuropathological changes, but the acute clinical symptoms largely reflect a functional disturbance rather than a structural injury, and as such no abnormality is seen on standard structural neuroimaging studies.
4. Results in a graded set of clinical symptoms that may or may not involve loss of consciousness.

## Epidemiology of TBI

Incidence is the occurrence, rate, or frequency of a disease, while prevalence is the percentage of a population affected by that disease. These are both important factors to consider in understanding TBI, particularly since TBI has often been described as a silent epidemic. Worldwide, TBI is a major cause of death, especially among young people, and a significant source of lifelong disability (CDC, 2015; Roozenbeek, Maas, & Menon, 2013). Unfortunately, the incidence of TBI is on the rise globally (CDC, 2015).

Each year in the United States, 1.7 million people sustain a TBI (CDC, n.d.-a). Every day, 138 people die from injuries related to TBI (CDC, n.d.-c). In the European Union, estimates suggest that approximately 7.7 million people are living with TBI-related disabilities, while in the United States this number is estimated to be 5.3 million people (Roozenbeek, Maas, & Menon, 2013). Globally, the incidence of TBI varies (Figure 1–1). The WHO estimates that TBI will surpass many diseases as the major cause of death and disability by the year 2020 (Hyder, Wunderlich, Pucanachandra, Gururaj, & Kobusingye, 2007).

Common causes of TBI vary globally as well. Figure 1–2 represents the leading causes of TBI in the United States, with falls currently reported as the most prevalent (CDC, n.d.-a). Worldwide, motor vehicle accidents are the most prevalent cause of TBI (Roozenbeek, Maas, & Menon, 2013). Figure 1–3 contains the distribution of types of injury within specific age groups.

## Risk Factors

Risk factors associated with TBI are multiple, complex, and interdependent (Coronado, McGuire, Faul, Sugerman, & Pearson, 2012). Table 1–1 contains a summary of several risk factors in the United States associated with TBI, including age, sex, race/ethnicity, socioeconomic status, recurrent TBI, comorbid factors, and prescription drug and alcohol use.

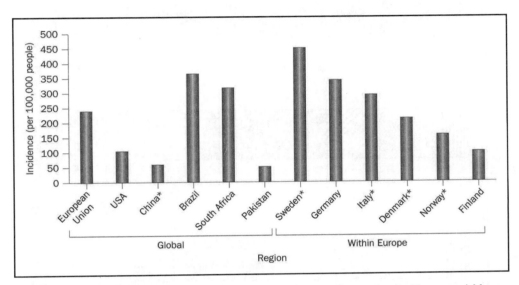

**Figure 1–1.** Estimates of global incidence of TBI. *Source:* Roozenbeek, Maas, and Menon (2013). Copyright © Macmillan Publishers Limited, part of Springer Nature. Used with permission.

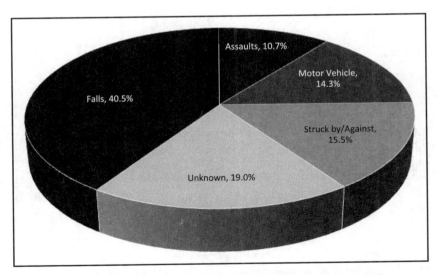

**Figure 1–2.** Leading causes of TBI in the United States. *Source:* CDC (n.d.-a, Leading Causes of TBI).

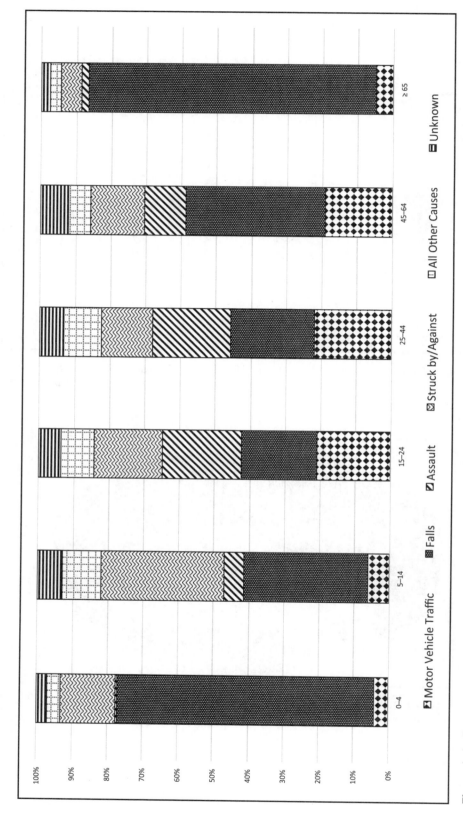

**Figure 1–3.** Percent distributions of TBI-related emergency department visits by age group and injury mechanism. *Source:* CDC (n.d.-c, Percent Distributions).

| **Table 1–1.** Risk Factors Associated with TBI | |
|---|---|
| *Demographic Feature* | *Risk Factor* |
| Age | Children ages 0–4, adolescents ages 15–24, and adults ages 65 and older are at greater risk of TBI. This risk of TBI for older adults increases with age. |
| Sex | TBI rates are higher among males than females (across all age groups). |
| Ethnicity | Emergency room visits for TBIs are highest among African Americans and Caucasians, followed by American Indian, Alaska Native, Asian, or Pacific Islanders. |
| Socioeconomic status | Higher rates of TBI are seen in geographical areas with lower mean incomes and in metropolitan areas. |
| Recurrent TBI | The risk of a TBI progressively increases after a first or second brain injury, with the risk of experiencing a second TBI three times as great in those with a previous TBI than those in the general population. |
| Comorbidity and prescription drug use | Prescription drug use (especially in older adults) increases the risk of TBI, as does the comorbidities of diabetes mellitus, cardiac arrhythmias, dementias, depression, and Parkinson disease. |
| Alcohol use | Alcohol use increases the risk of TBI, with one quarter to one half of all adults with acute TBI being intoxicated at the time of injury. |

*Source:* Coronado, McGuire, Faul, Sugerman, & Pearson (2012, pp. 91–92).

## Neuropathology of TBI

When studying how a TBI may impact an individual who experiences one, it is important to understand the neuropathology of the injury. To view TBI from this perspective is to understand how a TBI impacts the brain and its structures and functions. This is a critical foundation for speech-language pathologists providing rehabilitation services, as it shapes an understanding of the nature of recovery and rehabilitation approaches after a TBI.

As was mentioned at the start of this chapter, the ways in which TBI can occur are infinite. As such, it is helpful to have a method for categorizing TBI according to shared qualities or characteristics. This is also known as classification. To date, there is no one classification system that encompasses all clinical and pathological features of TBI (Koehler & Wilhelm, 2011; Langlois Orman, Kraus, Zaloshnja, & Miller, 2011; Saatman, Duhaime, Bullock, Maas, Valadka, & Manley, 2008). Classification of TBI from a clinical or symptom perspective includes descriptions of TBI given severity and those variables associated with prognosis and outcome following a TBI. These aspects of TBI will be discussed in Chapter 2 (Classification and Recovery). TBI can also be classified given pathological classifications, including anatomical (diffuse versus focal) or physiological (primary versus secondary injuries). Pathological classifications can be further extended to descriptions of TBI as a result of penetrating versus non-penetrating injuries (primary brain injury) and extra-cranial and intracranial injuries (secondary brain injury). Figure 1–4 contains a representation of this method of classification. The section that follows will discuss each of these in greater detail.

## Primary Brain Injury

Primary brain injury is the result of the initial mechanical forces of the trauma (Greve & Zink, 2009). Primary injuries are classified into those that are caused by penetrating forces (also known as open-head injuries) and those caused by non-penetrating forces (also known as closed-head injuries). More recently, blast injuries have also been discussed as a unique form of primary brain injury (Kocsis & Tessler, 2009; Magnuson, Leonessa, & Ling, 2012).

### Penetrating (Open) Head Injury

A penetrating injury (also known as an open-head injury) occurs when the skull is pierced by an object (NINDS, n.d.). This could be from a bullet, shrapnel, bone fragment, or a weapon such as a baseball bat, hammer, or knife. With this type of injury the meninges are ruptured, with cerebral tissue that is torn or cut (also known as laceration) (Smith, 2011). This type of injury is less common than non-penetrating injuries (Kazim et al., 2011). Brain tissue is damaged along the route of the penetrating object, as well as in surrounding areas (Kazim et al., 2011; Young et al., 2015). The trajectory and location of the wound and

the speed and velocity of the object both play a significant role in the outcome after a penetrating brain injury (Greve & Zink, 2009; Kazim et al., 2010; Young et al., 2015). Penetrating brain injuries are commonly classified as high-velocity or low-velocity, as follows.

**High-Velocity Penetrating Brain Injury.** High-velocity penetrating brain injuries are most commonly from high-velocity objects, such as rifle bullets, artillery shells, and shell fragments traveling at a high speed (Kazim et al., 2011; Young et al., 2015). High-velocity penetrating brain injuries result in more complex injuries and a higher mortality rate than low-velocity penetrating brain injuries (Kazim et al., 2011; Young et al., 2015). They are characterized by high levels of kinetic energy and an accompanying shock wave (Young et al., 2015). This shock wave creates three distinct areas of tissue damage: (1) crushing and cutting of brain tissue along the path of the projectile, (2) an adjacent area of tissue damage due to shearing and stretching of brain tissue, and (3) a surrounding area of tissue damage as a result of a lack of filling of small blood vessels and leakage of blood into brain tissue.

**Low-Velocity Penetrating Brain Injury.** Low-velocity penetrating brain injuries result from a penetrating object traveling at a lower rate of speed (compared with high velocity projectiles), such as clubs, baseball bats, and knives (Kazim et al., 2011; Young et al., 2015). Low-velocity penetrating brain injuries are rarer and are commonly associated with a better outcome than high-velocity penetrating injuries (Kazim et al., 2011; Young et al., 2015). Low-velocity penetrating wounds cause lacerations to the scalp, depressed skull fractures, and localized brain tissue damage along the object's path within the brain (Smith, 2011; Young et al.,

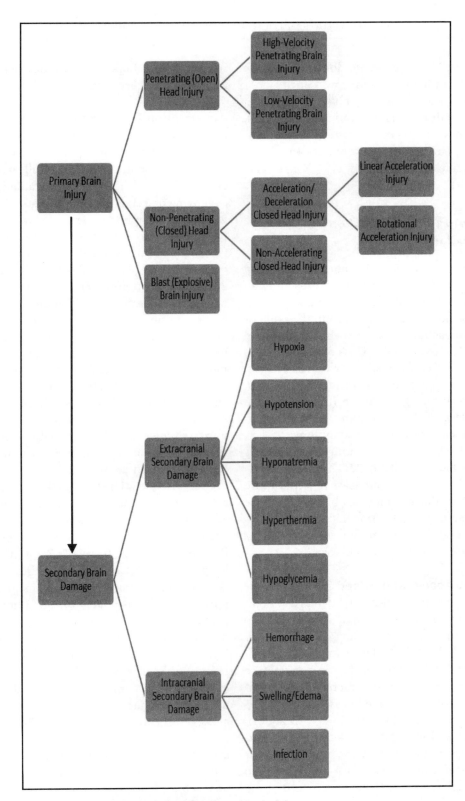

**Figure 1–4.** Pathological classification of brain injury.

2015). If the projectile does not exit the skull, individuals with low-velocity penetrating brain injuries are at risk for infection and/or hematoma (Young et al., 2015). In these instances, neurosurgical intervention may be needed to remove the debris (Mendelow & Crawford, 1997; Young et al., 2015).

### Non-Penetrating (Closed) Head Injury

Non-penetrating brain injuries (also known as closed-head injuries) are caused by an external force that produces rapid rotation or shaking of the brain within the skull, or an impact to the skull (Koehler & Wilhelm, 2011; NINDS, n.d.). This could occur from causes such as falls, motor vehicle crashes, sports injuries, or being struck by an object. Axonal injury, contusion (bruising on the surface of the brain), and subdural hemorrhage are common symptoms associated with non-penetrating head injuries (Koehler & Wilhelm, 2011). Non-penetrating brain injuries are classified into those that are due to a moving object striking the brain (non-acceleration injury) or the moving brain striking an object (acceleration/deceleration injury), as follows.

**Non-Acceleration Head Injuries.** Non-acceleration injuries cause damage to brain tissue primarily from a moving object striking the skull, causing deformation of the skull at the point of impact (McLean & Anderson, 1997). If the force and nature of the object create a fracture to the skull and rupture of the meninges, this is referred to as a penetrating head injury (as above). The skull is slightly elastic, however, and can press inward to some degree, without a penetrating injury. When this occurs, the underlying brain tissue is damaged at the point of deformation (compression). This is referred to as an impression trauma (Ylvisaker, Szekeres, & Feeney, 2008).

**Acceleration/Deceleration Head Injuries.** Acceleration/deceleration injuries cause brain tissue damage due to movement of the brain within the skull, from either the moving head striking a stationary or moving object or the head being shaken violently. Two important factors play a role in injury due to acceleration/deceleration: (1) pressure changes and (2) shearing forces on brain tissue (King et al., 2003; Kleiven, 2013). Although both can occur simultaneously, acceleration/deceleration injuries are commonly described in relation to type of movement associated with the injury: linear or rotational (angular) acceleration movement (Greve & Zink, 2009; King et al., 2003). Linear acceleration injury occurs with movement in a linear fashion from the vertical axis (such as in a forward and backward movement), while rotational acceleration occurs when the brain rotates around the axis point in an angular fashion (Figure 1–5). Acceleration/deceleration injuries associated with linear acceleration motion are thought to result primarily in pressure changes that create focal and more superficial tissue damage (Greve & Zink, 2009; King et al., 2003), while rotational (angular) motion is thought to result in more diffuse axonal injury due to the additional shearing forces associated with rotational movement (Greve & Zink, 2009; King et al., 2003; Kleiven, 2013). Due to bony protrusions and the irregular surface of the interior of the skull, damage from acceleration/deceleration injury is common in prefrontal areas and the anterior portion of the temporal lobes (Figure 1–6). Also common to acceleration/deceleration injury is *coupcontrecoup injury*, in which contusion is evident at the site of impact and at the opposite side of the injury (Figure 1–7).

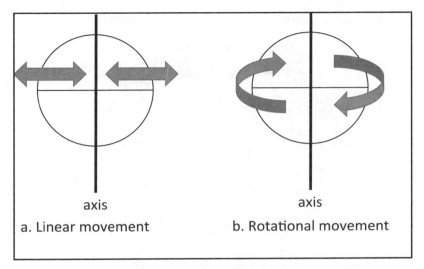

**Figure 1–5.** Acceleration/deceleration brain injury. Movement associated with acceleration/deceleration injury: linear and rotational (angular) movement.

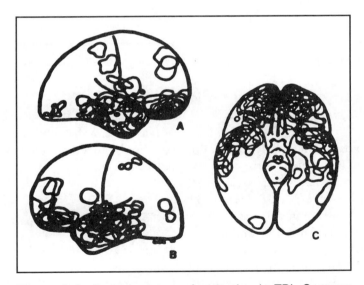

**Figure 1–6.** Common areas of contusion in TBI. Common pathology in the orbital frontal temporal regions of the brain due to TBI. *Source*: Courville (1937). Copyright © Pacific Press Publishing Association. Used with permission.

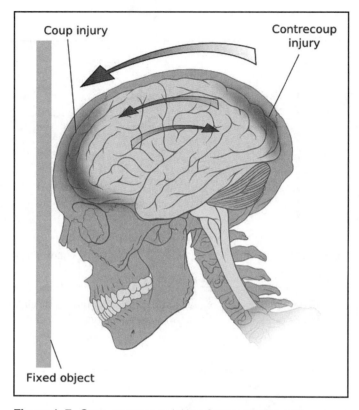

**Figure 1–7.** Coup-contrecoup injury. *Source:* Creative Commons.

### Blast (Explosive) Brain Injury

Blast or explosive injuries to the brain are thought to be a unique form of injury (Magnuson, Leonessa, & Ling, 2012). Blast injuries (also known as blast-induced neurotrauma) are most commonly seen in military personnel, as a result of improvised explosive devices (IEDs) (Koehler & Wilhelm, 2011; Magnuson, Leonessa, & Ling, 2012). The nature and severity of blast injuries on the brain are predicated both by the energy of the blast and by an individual's proximity to the blast epicenter (CDC, NIH, DoD, & VA Leadership Panel, 2013). Blast injuries are commonly described relative to the primary, secondary, tertiary, and quaternary injuries (Magnuson, Leonessa, &

Ling, 2012). Table 1–2 contains a summary of blast injury characteristics, body parts commonly affected, and types of injury (CDC, n.d.-b).

## Secondary Injury

Secondary injuries result from biologic changes that can occur minutes to days after the primary injury (CDC, NIH, DoD, & VA Leadership Panel, 2013). If an individual survives that neurodestructive process of the primary injury, morbidity (disease) and mortality (death) are influenced greatly by the secondary injury processes (Greve & Zink, 2009). Traditional classification of secondary brain damage includes those

**Table 1–2.** Mechanisms of Blast Injury

| Category | Characteristics | Body Part Affected | Types of Injuries |
|---|---|---|---|
| Primary injury | Unique to high order explosives,[a] resulting from the impact of an overpressurization wave on the brain and body | Gas-filled structures are most susceptible, such as the lungs, gastrointestinal tract, and middle ear | – Blast lung (injury to the lungs from changes in air pressure)<br>– Tympanic membrane rupture and middle ear damage<br>– Abdominal hemorrhage and perforation<br>– Eye rupture<br>– Concussion |
| Secondary injury | Results from flying debris and bomb fragments | Any body part may be affected | – Penetrating blast fragmentation or blunt injuries<br>–Eye penetration |
| Tertiary injury | Results from individuals being thrown by the blast wind[b] | Any body part may be affected | – Fracture and traumatic amputation<br>– Closed and open brain injury |
| Quaternary | All explosion-related injuries, illnesses, or diseases *not* due to primary, secondary, or tertiary mechanisms | Any body part may be affected | – Burns<br>– Crushing injuries<br>– Closed and open brain injury<br>– Asthma, chronic obstructive pulmonary disease, or other breathing problems from dust, smoke, or toxic fumes<br>– Angina<br>– Hyperglycemia, hypertension |

*Note.* [a]Explosives are classified into high order and low order explosives. High order explosives produce a supersonic overpressurization shock wave, while low order explosives create a subsonic explosion, without an overpressurization wave. [b]A blast wind is a forced superheated air flow, which can occur in both high and low order explosives.

*Source:* CDC (n.d.-b).

that are extracranial (outside the cranium) and those that are intracranial (within the cranium) (Table 1–3; Mendelow & Crawford, 1997). Each of these will be described briefly in the section that follows.

### *Extracranial Secondary Brain Damage*

Generally speaking, extracranial causes of secondary brain injury result from processes

**Table 1–3.** Extracranial and Intracranial Causes of Secondary Brain Damage

| Extracranial Causes | Intracranial Causes |
|---|---|
| • Hypoxia | • Hemorrhage |
| • Hypotension | ○ Extradural |
| • Hyponatremia | ○ Subdural |
| • Hyperthermia | ○ Intracerebral |
| • Hypoglycemia | ○ Intraventricular |
| | ○ Subarachnoid |
| | • Swelling |
| | ○ Venous congestion/ hyperemia |
| | ○ Edema |
| | ▪ Vasogenic |
| | ▪ Cytotoxic |
| | ▪ Interstitial |
| | • Infection |
| | ○ Meningitis |
| | ○ Brain abscess |

*Source:* Mendelow & Crawford (1997, p. 73).

outside the brain, which cause brain cells to either die or become swollen (also known as cytotoxic edema) (Mendelow & Crawford, 1997). This occurs in the form of under-activation or low (hypo-) levels of oxygen in the blood (hypoxia), low blood pressure (hypotension), low sodium concentrations in the blood (hyponatremia), or low blood glucose (hypoglycemia). Elevated (hyper-) body temperature (hyperthermia) can also result in damage to brain cells.

### Intracranial Secondary Brain Damage

Intracranial causes of secondary injury results from either bleeding, swelling, or infection that impacts brain cells (Mendelow & Crawford, 1997). Hemorrhage (bleeding) after a brain injury can occur in various locations, based on the nature of injury, including between the dura mater and the skull (extradural), between the dura mater and the brain (subdural), and between the arachnoid mater and the pia mater (subarachnoid). Each of these occurs within the skull, but outside the brain tissue, within the outer covering of the brain. Hemorrhage can also occur within the brain tissue (intracerebral) and within the ventricle (intraventricular). Hemorrhage is one of the most common causes of clinical deterioration after an injury (Smith, 2011).

Swelling after a brain injury can also occur, due to an increase in cerebral blood volume (venous congestion/hyperemia) or an increase in water content of the brain tissue (edema). Cerebral edema can be specific to a certain area of the brain, commonly adjacent to contusions, or more widespread.

Cerebral edema can take many forms, including vasogenic, in which changes in the blood–brain barrier create water accumulation between the cells, and cyctotoxic, in which the cells themselves swell. Although rarer, hydrocephalic (or interstitial) edema can occur as a result of obstruction of the cerebral spinal fluid (Unterberg, Stover, Kress, & Kiening, 2004). Widespread swelling is referred to as diffuse swelling. This can occur within one hemisphere of the brain, typically associated with a hematoma, or within both cerebral hemispheres. Diffuse and widespread swelling within both cerebral hemispheres is a common cause of fatal TBI (Smith, 2011). Any expansion of brain volume related to swelling can have a critical and negative impact on both morbidity and mortality, as it increases intracranial pressure, which can lead to impaired cerebral blood flow and oxygenation (Unterberg, Stover, Kress, & Kiening, 2004). One such potentially deadly side effect of increased intracranial pressure is brain herniation, in which the brain is pressed against and squeezed across structures within the skull or through the opening in the skull that connects the brain to the spinal cord (foramen magnum) (Ylvisaker, Szekeres, & Feeney, 2008). When this occurs, emergency medical management is needed.

Infection following brain injury, particularly a penetrating TBI, can also occur, in the form of either meningitis (inflammation of the meninges) or brain abscess (collection of pus, immune cells, or other material in the brain). This source of infection after TBI is most commonly bacterial (Mendelow & Crawford, 1997).

## Diffuse Versus Focal Injury

In addition to viewing TBI from the lens of primary versus secondary injury, pathological classification given diffuse versus focal injury is also helpful in fully understanding TBI and an individual's presenting neurologic deficits. Table 1–4 provides an example of injuries considered to be diffuse versus focal in nature (Smith, 2011). As can be seen, these are each aspects of brain injury discussed above but categorized to suggest the nature of injury: localized to a specific region or area (focal), or injury that crosses multiple regions of the brain (diffuse).

In focal injuries, functions that take place in the damaged region are impacted, while in diffuse brain injury, the axons connecting brain structures are subject to damage (CDC, NIH, DoD, & VA Leadership Panel, 2013). If you visualize the brain as a map of highly connected and interdependent cities, linked by crucial and numerous roads and highways, then focal damage represents a city or group of cities that have

| Table 1–4. Classification of Traumatic Brain Injury | |
|---|---|
| *Focal* | *Diffuse* |
| Scalp lacerations | Global ischemic injury |
| Skull fractures | Traumatic axonal injury/ diffuse vascular injury |
| Contusions/lacerations | |
| Intracranial hemorrhage | Brain swelling |

*Source:* Smith (2011, p. 24).

become dysfunctional, while their connecting highways and roads remain more intact. In contrast, diffuse damage can be thought of as a distribution to the highways and interconnecting roads. It is important, however, to recognize that some individuals with TBI may present with both diffuse and focal injuries.

## Additional Pathological Considerations

In the past 10 years, researchers have turned their attention to an additional pathological presentation related to TBI: chronic traumatic encephalopathy (CTE). CTE has since received national recognition specific to sports-related injury, including repeated concussive injury. In general terms, CTE is a progressive neurodegenerative process associated with one or multiple blows to the head, resulting in mood, cognitive, and behavioral changes later in life (Love & Solomon, 2014). CTE was first described in boxers as early as the 1920s. At that time, it was referred to as dementia pugilistica, with reference to individuals who years to decades after cessation of boxing presented with tremors, slowed motor movements, speech problems, and confusion (Roberts, Allsop, & Burton, 1990).

CTE is the modern iteration of this disorder, described as a syndrome that manifests within one to two decades after repeated head trauma, resulting in a constellation of neuropsychiatric, motor, behavioral, and cognitive signs and symptoms (Baugh et al., 2012). CTE is considered to be a distinct neuropathological process which manifests in gross and microscopic neuropathology. Gross neuropathological changes observed in the later stages of CTE include generalized atrophy, most prominent in the frontal and medial temporal lobes, as well

as enlargement of the lateral and third ventricles, and cavum septum pellucidum with fenestration (Lakhan & Kirchgessner, 2012). Microscopically, individuals with CTE present with tau-positive neurofibrillary tangles in the frontal and temporal areas of the brain and widespread proteinopathology (Lakhan & Kirchgessner, 2012).

Early symptoms of CTE are cognitive, mood, and behavioral (Baugh et al., 2012, p. 6). Cognitive symptoms reported are impairments in the area of memory and executive function, such as poor planning, organization, multitasking, and judgement. In the area of mood disturbances, there have been reported depression, apathy, irritability, and suicidality. Behavioral symptoms reported include impulse control problems, disinhibition, substance abuse/addiction, and aggression or violent behavior. Dizziness and headaches have also been reported in early stages of CTE (Lakhan & Kirchgessner, 2012; McKee et al., 2009). As CTE progresses, individuals experience additional symptoms, including social instability, erratic behaviors, additional memory loss, and the initial signs of Parkinson's disease (McKee et al., 2009). In the later stages, deterioration results in overt dementia, speech and gait abnormality, dysarthria, dysphagia, and ocular issues, such as ptosis (McKee et al., 2009).

Confirmed cases of CTE to date have reported a history of progressive brain trauma (Lakhan & Kirchgessner, 2012); however, the exact incidence of CTE is as yet unknown across a variety of professional and non-professional contact sports and in non-athletic repeated head trauma. Historical studies on dementia pugilistica estimated that between 17% and 20% of professional boxers would develop dementia pugilistica later in life (Jordan, 2000; McCrory, 2007; Robert, Allsop, & Burton, 1990). Researchers have also suggested that at least 3.7% of National Football League players will develop CTE in their lifetimes (Gavett, Stern, & McKee, 2011). More research is needed in this area, particularly relative to risk factors and the incidence in children and adolescents who experience repeated head trauma during sports and non-related sports activities.

## References

American Psychiatric Association. (2013). *Diagnostic and statistical manual of mental disorders* (5th ed.). Washington, DC: Author.

Baugh, C. M., Stamm, J. M., Riley, D. O., Gavett, B. E., Shenton, M. E., Lin, A., . . . Stern, R. A. (2012). Chronic traumatic encephalopathy: Neurodegeneration following repetitive concussive and subconcussive brain trauma. *Brain Imaging and Behavior, 6*(2), 244–254.

Centers for Disease Control and Prevention (CDC). (n.d.-a). *TBI: Get the facts.* Retrieved from http://www.cdc.gov/traumaticbraininjury/get_the_facts.html

Centers for Disease Control and Prevention (CDC). (n.d.-b). *Explosion and blast injuries: A primer for clinicians.* Retrieved from: http://www.cdc.gov/masstrauma/preparedness/primer.pdf

Centers for Disease Control and Prevention (CDC). (n.d.-c). *Percent distributions of TBI-related emergency department visits by age group and injury mechanism: United States, 2006–2010.* Retrieved from http://www.cdc.gov/traumaticbraininjury/data/dist_ed.html

Centers for Disease Control and Prevention (CDC). (2015). *Report to Congress on traumatic brain injury in the United States: Epidemiology and rehabilitation.* National Center for Injury Prevention and Control; Division of Unintentional Injury Prevention, Atlanta, GA. Retrieved from http://www.cdc.gov/traumaticbraininjury/pdf/tbi_report_to_congress_epi_and_rehab-a.pdf

CDC, NIH, DoD, & VA Leadership Panel. (2013). *Report to Congress on traumatic brain injury in the United States: Understanding the public health problem among current and former military personnel.* Centers for Disease Control and Prevention (CDC), the National Institutes of Health (NIH), the Department of Defense (DoD), and the Department of Veterans Affairs (VA). Retrieved from http://www.cdc.gov/traumaticbraininjury/pdf/report_to_congress_on_traumatic_brain_injury_2013-a.pdf

Coronado, V. G., McGuire, L. C., Faul, M., Sugerman, D. E., & Pearson, W. S. (2012). Traumatic brain injury: Epidemiology and public health issues. In N. D. Zasler, D. I. Katz, & R. D. Zafonte (Eds.), *Brain injury medicine: Principles and practice* (pp. 84–100). New York, NY: Demos Medical.

Gavett, A., Stern, R., & McKee, A. (2011). Chronic traumatic encephalopathy: A potential late effect of sport-related concussive and subconcussive head trauma. *Clinical Sports Medicine, 30*(1), 179–188.

Greve, M. W., & Zink, B. J. (2009). Pathophysiology of traumatic brain injury. *Mount Sinai Journal of Medicine, 76*(2), 97–104.

Hyder, A., Wunderlich, C., Puvanachandra, P., Gururaj, G., & Kobusingye, O. (2007). The impact of traumatic brain injuries: A global perspective. *NeuroRehabilitation, 22*(5), 341–353.

Kazim, S. F., Shamim, M. S., Tahir, M. Z., Enam, S. A., & Waheed, S. (2011). Management of penetrating brain injury. *Journal of Emergencies, Trauma, and Shock, 4*(3), 395–402.

King, A. I., Yang, K. H., Zhang, L., & Hardy, W. (2003, September). *Is head injury caused by linear or angular acceleration?* Paper presented at the IRCOBI Conference, Lisbon, Portugal.

Kleiven, S. (2013). Why most traumatic brain injuries are not caused by linear acceleration but skull fractures are. *Frontiers in Bioengineering and Biotechnology, 1*(15), 1–5.

Kocsis, J. D., & Tessler, A. (2009). Pathology of blast-related brain injury. *Journal of Rehabilitation Research and Development, 46*(6), 667–672.

Koehler, R., & Wilhelm, E. (2011). Traumatic brain injury. In R. Koehler, E. E. Wilhelm,

& I. Shoulson (Eds.), *Cognitive rehabilitation therapy for traumatic brain injury: Evaluating the evidence* (pp. 37–58). Washington, DC: The National Academies Press. Retrieved from http://www.ebrary.com

Kolarik, J. (2016). In their own words: Stories from CIP. In M. P. McManmon (Author), *Autism and learning differences: An active learning teaching toolkit* (pp. 455–482). Philadelphia, PA: Jessica Kingsley.

Lakhan, S. E., & Kirchgessner, A. (2012). Chronic traumatic encephalopathy: The dangers of getting "dinged." *SpringerPlus, 1*(2), 2–14.

Langlois Orman, J. A., Kraus, J. F., Zaloshnja, E., & Miller, T. (2011). Epidemiology. In J. M. Silver, T. W. McAllister, & S. C. Yodofksy (Eds.), *Textbook of traumatic brain injury* (2nd ed). Washington, DC: American Psychiatric Association

Love, S., & Solomon, G. (2015). Talking with parents of high school football players about chronic traumatic encephalopathy. *American Journal of Sports Medicine, 43*(5), 1260–1264.

Magnuson, J., Leonessa, F., & Ling, G. (2012). Neuropathology of explosive blast traumatic brain injury. *Current Neurology and Neuroscience Reports, 12*(5), 570–579.

McCrory, P. (2007). Boxing and the brain. Revisiting chronic traumatic encephalopathy. *British Journal of Sports Medicine, 36*, 2.

McCrory, P., Meeuwisse, W. H., Aubry, M., Cantu, B., Dvořák, J., Echemendia, Ruben J., . . . Turner, M. (2013). Consensus statement on concussion in sport: The 4th International Conference on Concussion in Sport held in Zurich, November 2012. *British Journal of Sports Medicine, 47*, 250–258.

Mckee, A. C., Cantu, R. C., Nowinski, C. J., Hedley-Whyte, E. T., Gavett, B. E., Budson, A. E., . . . Stern, R. A. (2009). Chronic traumatic encephalopathy in athletes: Progressive tauopathy after repetitive head injury. *Journal of Neuropathology and Experimental Neurology, 68*(7), 709–735. doi:10.1097/nen.0b013 e3181a9d503.

McLean, A. J., & Anderson, R.W. (1997). Biomechanics of closed head injury. In P. Reilly & R. Bullock (Eds.), *Head injury: Pathophysiology and management of severe closed head injury.* London, UK: Chapman & Hall.

Kolarik, J. (2016). In their own words: Stories from CIP. In M. P. McManmon (Author), *Autism and learning differences: An active learning teaching toolkit* (pp. 455–482). Philadelphia, PA: Jessica Kingsley.

Mendelow, D. A., & Crawford, P. J. (1997). Primary and secondary brain injury. In P. Reilly & R. Bullock (Eds.), *Head injury: Pathophysiology and management of severe closed head injury* (pp. 71–88). London, UK: Chapman & Hall

Menon, D. K., Schwab, K., Wright, D. W., Maas, A. I., & Demographics and Clinical Assessment Working Group of the International and Interagency Initiative toward Common Data Elements for Research on Traumatic Brain Injury and Psychological Health. (2010). Position statement: Definition of traumatic brain injury. *Archives of Physical Medicine and Rehabilitation, 91*(11), 1637–1640.

National Institute of Neurologic Disorders and Stroke (NINDS). (n.d.). *Traumatic brain injury: Hope through research.* Retrieved from http://www.ninds.nih.gov/disorders/tbi/detail_tbi.htm

Roberts, G. W., Allsop, D., & Burton, C. (1990). The occult aftermath of boxing. *Journal of Neurology, Neurosurgery, and Psychiatry, 53*(5), 373–378.

Roozenbeek, B., Maas, A. I., & Menon, D. (2013). Changing patterns in epidemiology of traumatic brain injury. *Nature Reviews: Neurology, 9*, 231–236.

Saatman, K. E., Duhaime, A., Bullock, R., Maas, A. I., Valadka, A., & Manley, G. (2008). Classification of traumatic brain injury for targeted therapies. *Journal of Neurotrauma, 25*, 719–738.

Smith, C. (2011). Neuropathology. In J. M. Silver, T. W. McAllister, & S. C. Yodofsky (Eds.), *Textbook of traumatic brain injury* (2nd ed., pp. 23–35). Washington, DC: American Psychiatric Association.

Unterberg, A. W., Stover, J., Kress, B., & Kiening, K. L. (2004). Edema and brain trauma. *Neuroscience, 129*, 1021–1029.

Ylivisaker, M., Szekeres, S., & Fenney, T. (2008). Communication disorders associated with traumatic brain injury. In R. Chapey (Ed.), *Language intervention strategies in aphasia and related communication disorders* (pp. 879–962). Baltimore, MD: Lippincott Williams & Wilkins.

Young, L., Rule, G. T., Bocchieri, R. T., Walilko, T. J., Burns, J. M., & Ling, G. (2015). When physics meets biology: Low and high-velocity penetration, blunt impact, and blast injuries to the brain. *Frontiers in Neurology*, 6(89), 1–19.

# 2 Classification and Recovery

*The uncertainty that exists about the likely outcome after traumatic brain injury (TBI) is encapsulated in the Hippocratic aphorism: 'No head injury is so serious that it should be despaired of nor so trivial that it can be ignored.'*

—Chestnut et al. (n.d.)

A perfectly normal and expected question often asked by an individual who has experienced a TBI (or his/her family) is, "How serious is it?" or "Will I (he/she) recover?" As many individuals with TBI (and those that seek to help them) quickly learn, these are impossible questions to answer with any degree of certainty. Many chapters can be written on this topic alone and how best to help individuals with TBI and their families navigate the difficult process of recovering from a TBI, when there is rarely a clear roadmap as to the path ahead. As the topic of this book is that of treatment, this chapter addresses the recovery process after a TBI from the perspective of the processes at work neurologically during recovery, prognostic indicators that may suggest patterns of recovery, and outcome measures to track recovery and response to treatment after a TBI.

## Recovery and Neuroplasticity

Individuals with TBI and families often ask team members about the process of recovery, from the perspectives of both *if* recovery will occur but also *how quickly* it will occur. As the start of this chapter suggests, these are questions that are impossible to answer with exact precision, but there are areas of research that can be of value in having a meaningful discussion with an individual with TBI and family members on this topic.

Most neurologic recovery after TBI occurs gradually and is largely dependent on the severity of TBI, though even individuals with similarly described severity levels often vary considerably (Koehler, Wilhelm, & Shoulson, 2012). For those with mild (single concussive) injury, many will be symptom free within several weeks, while those with more severe TBI have more prolonged recovery, with the resolution of some symptoms occurring as late as 1 to 2 years post injury (Koehler et al., 2012).

To date, the exact mechanisms of neurologic recovery after a brain injury remain as yet to be fully defined, but newer research which focuses on neuroplasticity has begun to offer additional insight into this area (Stein, 2000). In general, the term "plasticity" refers to the ability to change. Hence, *neuro*plasticity refers to the the ability of the nervous system to change and more specifically to change and adapt in response to environmental cues, experience, behavior, injury or disease (Ludlow et al., 2008). These changes can occur in the cognitive, sensory, and motor systems of the central nervous system (CNS) (Moucha & Kilgard, 2006). After an injury, neuroplasticity occurs in response to the injury itself (injury induced) and in response to activity and the environment (activity induced and environment induced) (Overman & Carmichael, 2014). Although the capacity for neuroplasticity is greatest during development in the immature brain, there is now overwhelming evidence that robust neuroplasticity also occurs in injured and non-injured adult brains (Kleim & Jones, 2008). This is good news for individuals who experience a TBI and is information that clinicians can use in tailoring treatment to maximize recovery.

What is measured as "change" after a brain injury is different depending on who is studying the topic (Stein & Hoffman, 2003). For example, molecular biologists measure neuroplastic change structurally, often at a cellular level, such as alterations in the numbers of neurotransmitter receptors post injury, decreases or increases in dendritic branching after a brain injury, or the regeneration of axons post neurologic trauma (Stein & Hoffman, 2003). Professionals providing behavioral intervention and rehabilitation often measure neuroplastic change functionally, sometimes as changes seen in the areas of the brain active during tasks, or as measures of behavioral change, such as cognitive, sensory, or motor impairments that gradually diminish or are eliminated over time (Stein & Hoffman, 2003).

Both views of neuroplasticity are in fact interrelated to that actual neuroplastic process that occurs post injury. This is conceptually represented by the analogy introduced in Chapter 1 of the CNS and its workings as a massive and dense cityscape of millions of interconnecting highways, bridges, roads, and streets formed by the brain's neurons (soma, axons, and dendrites) and their massive synaptic connections with one another. These massive connections are in turn the "roadways" of human behavior. Structurally, neuroplastic changes of the CNS restructure the roadways and communication networks of the brain, through mechanisms such as axonal sprouting, changes in dendritic structures, alterations in the synaptic connectivity, and neurogenesis and cell death (Brosh & Barkai, 2004; Overman & Carmichael, 2014). Functionally, these structural changes can alter behavior. New learning, experience, change in use, or even the injury itself and neurologic responses to injury can also further alter the structure of neural roadways through unmasking of surrounding structures or recruitment of new neural systems (Kou & Iraji, 2014; Lundlow et al., 2008).

Neuroscience approaches to brain injury ultimately seek to enhance these processes of neuroplasticity and thereby improve recovery. This is done given efforts that both minimize the impairments of the initial injury and loss of function, and those that seek to reorganize the brain and restore and compensate for function that has been compromised or lost due to an injury (Klein & Jones, 2008). Table 2–1 describes four broad methods to enhance recovery after a brain injury.

For speech-language pathologists (SLP), *rehabilitation techniques* have direct relevance. These are discussed in greater details below and throughout this textbook. Chapter 5 (Coordinated Care) provides a general description of some medical interventions (which occur prior to or simultaneously with rehabilitation services), including *neuroprotective* and *pharmacotherapy* rehabilitation methods. Although *regeneration* techniques are beyond the scope of this textbook, interested readers are referred to *Brain Damage, Brain Repair* by Fawcett, Rosser, and Dunnett (2001) for a comprehensive review of this and other related topics.

**Table 2–1.** Current Methods to Enhance Recovery of Function

| Method to Enhance Recovery | Description |
|---|---|
| Neuroprotection | Administration of compounds that protect neural tissue from the effects of the injury due to either cytotoxicity (substances that cause living cells to die) or excitotoxicity (processes that result in cell death due to overstimulation of neurotransmitters) |
| Regeneration | Administration of neurotrophic factors (substances that support growth, development, and survival of neural tissue) or transplantation of cells to re-establish normal neural structures |
| Rehabilitation | Use of behavioral training or manipulation to stimulate the brain to relearn various tasks |
| Pharmacotherapy | Administration of pharmacological agents to enhance the effects of rehabilitation |

*Source:* Stein & Hoffman (2003, p. 329). Adapted with permission.

In the area of rehabilitation and neuroplasticity, the body of research in this area has expanded rapidly in recent years. One such expansion has been the translation of experience-dependent learning principles to an understanding of neuroplasticity. Kleim and Jones (2008) described 10 principles guided by these concepts which offer excellent insight into recovery for adults after TBI (Table 2–2). These principles can and should help guide treatment decisions following a TBI. These are also principles that can and should be shared directly with individuals with TBI and their families to assist them in understanding the process of neurologic recovery after TBI.

## Prognosis Indicators

A prognosis is a forecast of the likely course of a disease or ailment. As the introduction to this chapter highlights, predicting or anticipating the likely outcome of TBI remains very difficult and subject to multiple factors. It is nonetheless a relevant discussion to the topic of treatment to have at least foundational knowledge about factors that *may* serve as prognostic indicators following a TBI.

One of the most frequently cited prognostic indicators of increased mortality and long-term disability is the severity of a TBI (mild, moderate, or severe) (Maas et al., 2010). Classification of severity is often discussed given the length of loss of consciousness (LOC), alterations in consciousness (AOC), and posttraumatic amnesia (PTA) (CDC, NIH, DoD, and VA Leadership Panel, 2013). Structural or neuroimaging (ranging from normal to abnormal) can also play a role in classification of severity after a TBI (CDC, NIH, DoD, & VA Leadership Panel, 2013; Saatman et al., 2008). Table 2–3 describes these factors and their application to classifying a TBI as mild, moderate, or severe. It is important to note, however, that while establishment of initial severity using these factors may have prognostic value, it does not automatically reflect an ultimate or final level of functioning after a TBI.

**Table 2–2.** Experience-Dependent Principles of Neuroplasticity

| Principle | Description |
|---|---|
| Use It and Improve It | Training that drives a specific brain function can lead to enhancement of that function. |
| Use It or Lose It | Failure to drive specific brain functions can lead to functional degradations. |
| Specificity | The nature of training experience dictates the nature of the plasticity. |
| Repetition Matters | Induction of plasticity requires sufficient repetition. |
| Intensity Matters | Induction of plasticity requires sufficient training intensity. |
| Time Matters | Different forms of plasticity occur at different times during training. |
| Salience Matters | The training experience must be sufficiently salient to induce plasticity. |
| Age Matters | Training-induced plasticity occurs more readily in younger brains. |
| Transference | Plasticity in response to one training experience can enhance the acquisition of similar behaviors. |
| Interference | Plasticity response to one experience can interfere with the acquisition of other behaviors. |

*Source:* Kleim & Jones (2008, p. s227).

**Table 2–3.** DoD/VA Severity Stratification for Non-Penetrating TBI

| Criteria | Severity | | |
| | Mild | Moderate | Severe |
|---|---|---|---|
| Length of time of loss of consciousness | 0–30 min | >30 min and <24 hr | >24 hr |
| Glasgow Coma Scale | 13–15 | 9–12 | 3–8 |
| Structure imaging | Normal | Normal or abnormal | Normal or abnormal |
| Posttraumatic amnesia | 0–1 day | >1 and <7 days | >7 days |
| Alteration of consciousness/ mental state | A moment up to 24 hr | >24 hr severity based on other criteria | >24 hr severity based on other criteria |

*Source:* Centers for Disease Control and Prevention (CDC), National Institutes of Health (NIH), Department of Defense (DOD), & Department of Veterans Affairs (VA) (2013, p. 18).

## Loss of Consciousness

LOC is frequently utilized in establishing severity level associated with TBI, particularly for moderate to severe TBI (CDC, NIH, DoD, & VA Leadership Panel, 2013). The most widely utilized tool in assessing LOC is the Glasgow Coma Scale (GCS; Table 2–4; Teasdale & Jennett, 1974). The GCS measures coma and impaired consciousness, given eye opening (none to spontaneous), motor function (normal to abnormal flexion or extension), and verbal responses (normal conversation to none). Twenty-four hours post injury, persons with total GCS scores of 3 to 8 are classified as having a *severe* TBI, those with scores of 9 to 12 as having a *moderate* TBI, and those with scores of 13 to 15 as having a *mild* TBI (Teasdale & Jennett, 1974).

## Posttraumatic Amnesia

The term "amnesia" is derived from the Latin *a-*, meaning without, and *mnesia*,

| Table 2–4. Glasgow Coma Scale (GCS) | |
| :--- | ---: |
| **Ability** | **Score** |
| Eye Opening (E) | |
| Spontaneous | 4 |
| To voice | 3 |
| To pain | 2 |
| None | 1 |
| Motor Response (M) | |
| Normal | 6 |
| Localized to pain | 5 |
| Withdraws to pain | 4 |
| Flexion (an abnormal posture that can include rigidity, clenched fists, legs held straight out, and arms bent inward toward the body with the wrists and fingers bent and held on the chest) | 3 |
| Extension (an abnormal posture that can include rigidity, arms and legs held straight out, toes pointed downward, head and neck arched backward) | 2 |
| None | 1 |
| Verbal Response (V) | |
| Normal conversation | 5 |
| Disoriented conversation | 4 |
| Words, but not coherent | 3 |
| No words, only sounds | 2 |
| None | 1 |

*Source:* Teasdale & Jennett (1974, pp. 82–83).

meaning memory. As such, amnesia is loss of memory. Memory loss after a TBI is referred to as posttraumatic amnesia (Kosch, Browne, King, Fitzgerald, & Cameron, 2010). A common definition for PTA is "an interval during which the patient is confused, amnesic for ongoing events, and likely to evidence behavioral disturbances" (Levin, O'Donnell, & Grossman, 1979, p. 675). PTA is divided into two types of memory loss: retrograde amnesia and anterograde amnesia (Cantu, 2001). Retrograde amnesia is a loss of the ability to recall events immediately preceding brain injury, whereas anterograde amnesia is a deficit in forming new memory after the injury.

Similar to LOC, the duration of PTA after a TBI is used as a factor in suggesting severity of injury. Some studies have suggested that duration of PTA is superior to the GCS and neuroimaging in predicting functional outcomes and cognitive recovery following TBI (Katz & Alexander, 1994; Kosch et al., 2010; Levin, Benton, & Grossman, 1982). A frequently utilized assessment tool in the measurement of PTA is the Galveston Orientation and Amnesia Test (GOAT; Table 2–5). Persons with

| Table 2–5. Galveston Orientation and Amnesia Test (GOAT) | |
|---|---|
| *Questions* | *Point Value* |
| What is your name? | 2 |
| When were you born? | 4 |
| Where do you live? | 4 |
| Where are you now? (City) | 5 |
| What are you now? (Hospital) | 5 |
| On what date were you admitted to the hospital? | 5 |
| How did you get here? | 5 |
| What is the first event you remember after the injury? | 5 |
| Can you describe in detail (e.g., date, time, companions) the first event you recall before the accident? | 5 |
| What time is it now? | 1 point for each ½ hour removed from the correct time to a maximum of 5 points |
| What day of the week is it? | 1 point for each day removed from the correct one |
| What day of the month is it? | 1 point for each day removed from the correct date to a maximum of 5 points |
| What is the year? | 10 points for each year removed from the correct one to a maximum of 30 points |

*Source:* Levin, O'Donnell, & Grossman (1979, p. 677).

PTA of 0–1 day are classified as having a *mild* TBI, greater than 1 day but less than 7 days as having *moderate* TBI, and greater than 7 days as having *severe* TBI (CDC, NIH, DoD, & VA Leadership Panel, 2013; Levin, O'Donnell, & Grossman, 1979; Levin et al., 1982).

## Outcome Measures

TBI outcome measures are scales or tools that measure physical, cognitive, and/or psychological functioning after an injury. The terms "outcome(s)," "outcome research," "efficacy research," and the like are used to reflect the change(s) that occur (either positive or negative) in relation to intervention. As such, a discussion of common tools used in the measurement of outcomes after a TBI has direct relevance to speech-language pathologists in understanding recovery and potential impacts of TBI, as well as potential benchmarks for use in measuring the intervention provided to individuals with TBI. It is important to note, however, that there is not one universally accepted measure for outcome following TBI. Further, outcome measurements are not without significant limitations, including "poor operational definitions, lack of sensitivity or low ceiling effects, inability to evaluate patients who cannot report, lack of integration of morbidity and mortality categories, and limited domains of functioning assessed" (Shukla, Devi, & Agrawal, 2011, p. 435).

At present, there are a variety of tools which address outcomes after a TBI. Some are more general, designed to provide a global index of outcome, while others are designed to measure functional abilities in daily activities and community integration after a TBI (Shukla et al., 2011). Others are targeted to specific populations, such as mild TBI (Shukla et al., 2011).

The World Health Organization (WHO) International Classification of Functioning, Disability and Health (ICF) is integral to understanding this complex dynamic of recovery and outcome after a TBI. The ICF is "biopsychosocial," as it integrates medical and social perspective of disability and function (WHO, 2002, pp. 9, 19). Importantly, it acknowledges the concept of "disability" as something every human being may experience in their lives, through a change in health or environment. ICF frames disability as "a universal human experience, sometimes permanent, sometimes transient and not restricted to a small part of the population" (WHO, n.d., para. 3). This important framework is also present in the American Speech-Language-Hearing Association's *Scope of Practice for Speech-Language Pathology* (ASHA, 2007).

Figure 2–1 is a representation of the ICF model. As can be seen, disability and functioning are viewed as outcomes of the interactions between health conditions (diseases, disorders, and injuries) and contextual factors (personal and environmental). Personal contextual factors are independent of the health condition but may have an influence on how a person functions, such as gender, race, education, coping strategies, and so forth. Environmental contextual factors are those things outside of the person's control, such as family, work, laws, cultural norms. There is a synergy and interrelationship among health conditions and contextual factors which influence three levels of human functioning: impairments at the level of body or body part (Body Structure/Function), limitations of the whole person in execution of a task or action (Activity), and restrictions on the whole person during involvement in life situations (Participation).

In 2010, the ICF Research Branch, in collaboration with WHO and the International Society of Physical and Rehabilitation

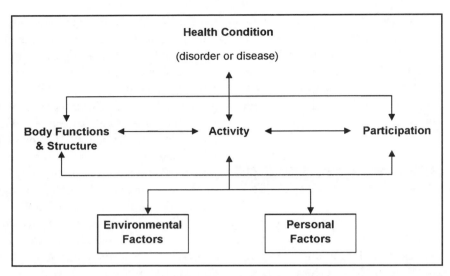

**Figure 2–1.** World Health Organization (WHO) International Classification of Functioning, Disability and Health (ICF). *Source:* WHO and IFC (2002)

Medicine (ISPRM), identified relevant ICF categories to comprehensively describe and measure the spectrum of potential limitations in functioning by persons with TBI. These included the *Brief ICF Core Set for TBI* (Table 2–6), recommended for use in settings in which a brief description and assessment of functioning of a person with TBI is sufficient (e.g., primary care, research) and the *Comprehensive ICF Core for TBI* for conducting a comprehensive, multidisciplinary assessment (Appendix 2–1).

ICF categories are also useful for classifying other traditional outcome measures utilized with individuals with TBI. The sections that follow will discuss several common outcome measures in greater detail.

## Glasgow Coma Scale

The GCS is the most frequently utilized outcome measure relative to the ICF's category of Body Structure/Function.

## Functional Independence Measure (FIM)

The FIM is widely utilized in rehabilitation settings (particularly inpatient settings) as a measure of functional progress (Shukla et al., 2011). Although not specifically for TBI, it consists of a motor domain (containing 13 items) and a cognitive domain (containing 5 items) applicable to individuals with TBI (Linacre, Heinemann, Wright, Granger, & Hamilton, 1994). Scoring is based on a 7-point scale, from "complete independence" (7 points) to "total assistance" (1 point), and a total possible independence rating score ranging from 18 (lowest) to 126 (highest). It is designed to be administered upon admission to rehabilitation, at discharge, and post discharge. The FIM-annex (or Functional Assessment Measure, FAM) was created to extend the areas covered by the FIM to an additional 12 items in the domains of communication, cognition, and behavioral disturbances (Hall, 1997). Combined, these

| **Table 2–6.** Brief ICF Core Set for TBI |
| --- |
| *ICF Category Title* |
| Body Functions |
|    Higher-level cognitive functions |
|    Emotional functions |
|    Energy and drive functions |
|    Control of voluntary movement functions |
|    Memory functions |
|    Sensation of pain |
|    Attention functions |
|    Consciousness functions |
| Body Structures |
|    Structure of brain |
| Activities & Participation |
|    Carrying out daily routine |
|    Conversation |
|    Walking |
|    Complex interpersonal interactions |
|    Acquiring, keeping, and terminating a job |
|    Self-care |
|    Recreation and leisure |
|    Family relationships |
| Environmental Factors |
|    Immediate family |
|    Health services, systems, and policies |
|    Products and technology for personal use in daily living |
|    Friends |
|    Social security services, systems, and policies |
|    Products and technology for personal indoor and outdoor mobility and transportation |

*Source:* ICF Research Branch (2013).

scales are referred to as the FIM + FAM (Wright, 2000a; Appendix 2–2).

# Functional Communication Measure

Similar to the FIM, the American Speech-Language-Hearing Association (ASHA) has an outcome measurement specific to adults in health care settings, but unique to the services provided by speech-language pathologists: the Functional Communication Measure (FCM) (ASHA, 2011a, b, c, d). Scoring is based on a 7-point scale, ranging from least functional (level 1) to most functional (level 7), given any of the 15 applicable FCM categories (Table 2–7; ASHA 2011a, p. 46).

| **Table 2–7.** Functional Communication Measure (FCM) |
| --- |
| Alaryngeal Communication |
| Attention |
| Augmentative-Alternative Communication |
| Fluency |
| Memory |
| Motor Speech |
| Pragmatics |
| Problem Solving |
| Reading |
| Spoken Language Comprehension |
| Spoken Language Expression |
| Swallowing |
| Voice |
| Voice Following Tracheostomy |
| Writing |

*Source:* American Speech-Language-Hearing Association (2011a).

Trained clinicians use observation to rank an individual's applicable communication and/or swallowing abilities upon admission and again at discharge from speech-language pathology services.

## Craig Handicap Assessment and Reporting Technique (CHART)

CHART was designed to measure the degree to which impairments and disabilities result in handicaps years after initial rehabilitation (Whiteneck, Charlifue, Gerhart, Overholser, & Richardson, 1992). The *revised* CHART contains 32 questions, with up to 7 questions in each of the following domains: physical independence, cognitive independence, mobility, social integration, occupation, and economic self-sufficiency (Whiteneck et al., n.d.). Each of the subscales for each of these domains has a maximum score of 100 points (considered normative for an able-bodied person). It can be administered by interview (either in person or via telephone). A short-form of the CHART (CHART-SF) is also available, using 19 items (Appendix 2–3).

## Community Integration Questionnaire (CIQ)

The CIQ measures community integration after a TBI, using 15 questions in the domains of home integration (H), social integration (S), and productive activities (P) (Table 2–8; Callaway et al., 2014). The CIQ can be administered in person or over the phone, either with the person with TBI or his/her proxy (Dijkers, 2000). Subtotals in each of the above domains are obtained, as is a total CIQ score.

## Rancho Los Amigos Scale of Cognitive Levels (RLAS)

The RLAS (also known as the Rancho Los Amigos Levels of Cognitive Functioning Scale) is a widely utilized tool in rehabilitation settings, developed by Hagen, Malkmus, and Durham (1972) and later revised by Hagen in 1979 (RLAS-R). The RLAS-R (Table 2–9) contains 10 classifications of performance/assistance used for "planning of treatment, tracking of recovery, and classifying of outcome levels" after TBI (Sander, 2002).

## Disability Rating Scale (DRS)

The DRS was designed to track the progress of individuals with head injury from "coma to community" (Rappaport, Hall, Hopkins, Belleza, & Cope, 1982). A summary of the DRS is displayed in Table 2–10. The full scale is in Appendix 2–4. The DRS comprises categories which encompass all three WHO ICF domains (Wright, 2000b). The first three categories (Eye Opening, Communication Ability, and Motor Response) reflect the Body Structure/Function domain of the ICF. These categories are similar to those assessed within the GCS specific to an individual's level of consciousness. The categories of Cognitive Ability, Feeding, Toileting, and Grooming on the DRS address the Activity domain of the ICF. Lastly, the categories of Level of Functioning and Employability are within the Participation domain of the ICF. Items on the DRS are rated using scales ranging from 0 to 3 to 0 to 5, with lower scores associated with less disability. The overall DRS score can be used to assign a specific disability outcome category, ranging from no disability to extreme vegetative state and death.

**Table 2–8.** Community Integration Questionnaire–Revised

| Items | Response Categories |
|---|---|
| **Home Integration Subscale** | |
| 1. Who usually does the shopping for groceries or other necessities in your household? | ○ Yourself alone<br>○ Yourself and someone else<br>○ Someone else |
| 2. Who usually prepares meals in your household? | ○ Yourself alone<br>○ Yourself and someone else<br>○ Someone else |
| 3. In your home who usually does normal everyday housework? | ○ Yourself alone<br>○ Yourself and someone else<br>○ Someone else |
| 4. Who usually cares for the children in your home? | ○ Yourself alone<br>○ Yourself and someone else<br>○ Someone else<br>○ Not applicable (no children under 17 yr in the home) |
| 5. Who usually plans social arrangements such as get-togethers with family and friends? | ○ Yourself alone<br>○ Yourself and someone else<br>○ Someone else |
| 6. Who usually looks after your personal finances, such as banking or paying bills? | ○ Yourself alone<br>○ Yourself and someone else<br>○ Someone else |
| **Social Integration Subscale** | |
| 7. Approximately how many times a month do you usually participate in shopping outside your home? | ○ 5 or more<br>○ 1–4 times<br>○ Never |
| 8. Approximately how many times a month do you usually participate in leisure activities such as movies, sports, restaurants, etc.? | ○ 5 or more<br>○ 1–4 times<br>○ Never |
| 9. Approximately how many times a month do you usually visit friends or relatives? | ○ 5 or more<br>○ 1–4 times<br>○ Never |
| 10. When you participate in leisure activities do you usually do this alone or with others? | ○ Mostly alone<br>○ Mostly with family members<br>○ Mostly with friends who have a disability<br>○ Mostly with friends who do not have disability<br>○ With a combination of friends and family |

*continues*

**Table 2–8.** *continued*

| Items | Response Categories |
|---|---|
| 11. Do you have a best friend in whom you confide? | ○ Yes<br>○ No |
| *Productivity Subscale* | |
| 12. How often do you travel outside the home? | ○ Almost every day<br>○ Almost every week<br>○ Seldom/never (less than once per week) |
| 13. Please check the answer that best corresponds to your current (during the past month) work situation: | ○ Full-time (more than 20 hours per week)<br>○ Part-time (less than or equal to 20 hours per week)<br>○ Not working, but actively looking for work<br>○ Not working, not looking for work<br>○ Not applicable, retired due to age |
| 14. Please check the answers that best corresponds to your current (during the past month) school or training program situation: | ○ Full-time<br>○ Part-time<br>○ Not attending school or training program<br>○ Not applicable, retired due to age |
| 15. In the past month, how often did you engage in volunteer activities? | ○ 5 or more<br>○ 1–4 times<br>○ Never |
| *Electronic Social Networking (ETS) Subscale* | |
| 16. How often do you write to people for social contact using the Internet (e.g., email, social networking sites such as Facebook)? | ○ Every day/most days<br>○ Almost every week<br>○ Seldom/never |
| 17. How often do you talk to people for social contact using an online video link (e.g., Skype, FaceTime)? | ○ Every day/most days<br>○ Almost every week<br>○ Seldom/ never |
| 18. How often do you make social contact with people by talking or text messaging using your phone? | ○ Every day/most days<br>○ Almost every week<br>○ Seldom/never |
| Comments: | |

*Source:* Callaway, Winkler, Tippett, Migliorini, Herd, & Willer (2014). Copyright protected. Used with permission. Permission to use the CIQ-R should be requested by contacting Libby Callaway via email at libby.callaway@ summerfoundation.org.au or Barry Willer at bswiller@buffalo.edu.

**Table 2–9.** Rancho Los Amigos Scale of Cognitive Levels–Revised

| Level | Specification(s)/Description |
|-------|------------------------------|
| Level I—No Response: Total Assistance | • Complete absence of observable change in behavior when presented visual, auditory, tactile, proprioceptive, vestibular, or painful stimuli. |
| Level II—Generalized Response: Total Assistance | • Demonstrates generalized reflex response to painful stimuli.<br>• Responds to repeated auditory stimuli with increased or decreased activity.<br>• Responds to external stimuli with physiological changes generalized, gross body movement and/or not purposeful vocalization.<br>• Responses noted above may be same regardless of type and location of stimulation.<br>• Responses may be significantly delayed. |
| Level III—Localized Response: Total Assistance | • Demonstrates withdrawal or vocalization to painful stimuli.<br>• Turns toward or away from auditory stimuli.<br>• Blinks when strong light crosses visual field.<br>• Follows moving object passed within visual field.<br>• Responds to discomfort by pulling tubes or restraints.<br>• Responds inconsistently to simple commands.<br>• Responses directly related to type of stimulus.<br>• May respond to some persons (especially family and friends) but not to others. |
| Level IV—Confused/ Agitated: Maximal Assistance | • Alert and in heightened state of activity.<br>• Purposeful attempts to remove restraints or tubes or crawl out of bed.<br>• May perform motor activities such as sitting, reaching, and walking but without any apparent purpose or upon another's request.<br>• Very brief and usually non-purposeful moments of sustained alternatives and divided attention.<br>• Absent short-term memory.<br>• May cry out or scream out of proportion to stimulus even after its removal.<br>• May exhibit aggressive or flight behavior.<br>• Mood may swing from euphoric to hostile with no apparent relationship to environmental events.<br>• Unable to cooperate with treatment efforts.<br>• Verbalizations are frequently incoherent and/or inappropriate to activity or environment. |

*continues*

| Table 2–9. *continued* | |
| --- | --- |
| *Level* | *Specification(s)/Description* |
| Level V—Confused, Inappropriate Non-Agitated: Maximal Assistance | • Alert, not agitated but may wander randomly or with a vague intention of going home.<br>• May become agitated in response to external stimulation, and/or lack of environmental structure.<br>• Not oriented to person, place, or time.<br>• Frequent brief periods, non-purposeful sustained attention.<br>• Severely impaired recent memory, with confusion of past and present in reaction to ongoing activity.<br>• Absent goal directed, problem solving, self-monitoring behavior.<br>• Often demonstrates inappropriate use of objects without external direction.<br>• May be able to perform previously learned tasks when structured and cues provided.<br>• Unable to learn new information.<br>• Able to respond appropriately to simple commands fairly consistently with external structures and cues.<br>• Responses to simple commands without external structure are random and non-purposeful in relation to command.<br>• Able to converse on a social, automatic level for brief periods of time when provided external structure and cues.<br>• Verbalizations about present events become inappropriate and confabulatory when external structure and cues are not provided. |
| Level VI—Confused, Appropriate: Moderate Assistance | • Inconsistently oriented to person, time and place.<br>• Able to attend to highly familiar tasks in non-distracting environment for 30 minutes with moderate redirection.<br>• Remote memory has more depth and detail than recent memory.<br>• Vague recognition of some staff.<br>• Able to use assistive memory aide with maximum assistance.<br>• Emerging awareness of appropriate response to self, family and basic needs.<br>• Moderate assist to problem solve barriers to task completion.<br>• Supervised for old learning (e.g. self-care).<br>• Shows carry over for relearned familiar tasks (e.g. self-care).<br>• Maximum assistance for new learning with little or nor carry over.<br>• Unaware of impairments, disabilities, and safety risks.<br>• Consistently follows simple directions.<br>• Verbal expressions are appropriate in highly familiar and structured situations. |

**Table 2–9.** *continued*

| Level | Specification(s)/Description |
|---|---|
| Level VII—Automatic, Appropriate: Minimal Assistance for Daily Living Skills | • Consistently oriented to person and place, within highly familiar environments. Moderate assistance for orientation to time. |
| | • Able to attend to highly familiar tasks in a non-distraction environment for at least 30 minutes with minimal assist to complete tasks. |
| | • Minimal supervision for new learning. |
| | • Demonstrates carry over of new learning. |
| | • Initiates and carries out steps to complete familiar personal and household routine but has shallow recall of what he/she has been doing. |
| | • Able to monitor accuracy and completeness of each step in routine personal and household ADLs and modify plan with minimal assistance. |
| | • Superficial awareness of his/her condition but unaware of specific impairments and disabilities and the limits they place on his/her ability to safely, accurately and completely carry out his/her household, community, work, and leisure ADLs. |
| | • Minimal supervision for safety in routine home and community activities. |
| | • Unrealistic planning for the future. |
| | • Unable to think about consequences of a decision or action. |
| | • Overestimates abilities. |
| | • Unaware of others' needs and feelings. |
| | • Oppositional/uncooperative. |
| | • Unable to recognize inappropriate social interaction behavior. |
| Level VIII—Purposeful, Appropriate: Standby Assistance | • Consistently oriented to person, place, and time. |
| | • Independently attends to and completes familiar tasks for 1 hour in distracting environments. |
| | • Able to recall and integrate past and recent events. |
| | • Uses assistive memory devices to recall daily schedule, "to do" lists and record critical information for later use with standby assistance. |
| | • Initiates and carries out steps to complete familiar personal, household, community, work, and leisure routines with standby assistance and can modify the plan when needed with minimal assistance. |
| | • Requires no assistance once new tasks/activities are learned. |
| | • Aware of and acknowledges impairments and disabilities when they interfere with task completion but requires standby assistance to take appropriate corrective action. |
| | • Thinks about consequences of a decision or action with minimal assistance. |

*continues*

| Table 2–9. *continued* | |
|---|---|
| *Level* | *Specification(s)/Description* |
| Level VIII *continued* | • Overestimates or underestimates abilities. |
| | • Acknowledges others' needs and feelings and responds appropriately with minimal assistance. |
| | • Depressed. |
| | • Irritable. |
| | • Low frustration tolerance/easily angered. |
| | • Argumentative. |
| | • Self-centered. |
| | • Uncharacteristically dependent/independent. |
| | • Able to recognize and acknowledge inappropriate social interaction behavior while it is occurring and takes corrective action with minimal assistance. |
| Level IX—Purposeful, Appropriate: Standby Assistance on Request | • Independently shifts back and forth between tasks and completes them accurately for at least two consecutive hours. |
| | • Uses assistive memory devices to recall daily schedule, "to do" lists and record critical information for later use with assistance when requested. |
| | • Initiates and carries out steps to complete familiar personal, household, work and leisure tasks independently and unfamiliar personal, household, work, and leisure tasks with assistance when requested. |
| | • Aware of and acknowledges impairments and disabilities when they interfere with task completion and takes appropriate corrective action but requires standby assist to anticipate a problem before it occurs and take action to avoid it. |
| | • Able to think about consequences of decisions or actions with assistance when requested. |
| | • Accurately estimates abilities but requires standby assistance to adjust to task demands. |
| | • Acknowledges others' needs and feelings and responds appropriately with standby assistance. |
| | • Depression may continue. |
| | • May be easily irritable. |
| | • May have low frustration tolerance. |
| | • Able to self-monitor appropriateness of social interaction with standby assistance. |

| Level | Specification(s)/Description |
|---|---|
| **Table 2–9.** *continued* | |
| *Level* | *Specification(s)/Description* |
| Level X—Purposeful, Appropriate: Modified Independent | • Able to handle multiple tasks simultaneously in all environments but may require periodic breaks. |
| | • Able to independently procure, create, and maintain own assistive memory devices. |
| | • Independently initiates and carries out steps to complete familiar and unfamiliar personal, household, community, work, and leisure tasks but may require more than usual amount of time and/or compensatory strategies to complete them. |
| | • Anticipates impact of impairments and disabilities on ability to complete daily living tasks and takes action to avoid problems before they occur but may require more than usual amount of time and/or compensatory strategies. |
| | • Able to independently think about consequences of decisions or actions but may require more than usual amount of time and/or compensatory strategies to select the appropriate decision or action. |
| | • Accurately estimates abilities and independently adjusts to task demands. |
| | • Able to recognize the needs and feelings of others and automatically respond in appropriate manner. |
| | • Periodic periods of depression may occur. |
| | • Irritability and low frustration tolerance when sick, fatigued, and/or under emotional stress. |
| | • Social interaction behavior is consistently appropriate. |

*Note.* Original scale co-authored by Chris Hagen, Ph.D., Danese Malkmus, M.A., Patricia Durham, M.A. Communication Disorders Service, Rancho Los Amigos Hospital, 1972. Revised 11/15/74 by Danese Malkmus, M.A., and Kathryn Stenderup, O.T.R. Revised scale 1997 by Chris Hagen.

**Table 2–10.** Disability Rating Scale (DRS)

| Item/Ability | Score | Item/Ability | Score |
|---|---|---|---|
| **Eye Opening** | | **Grooming (Cognitive ability only)** | |
| Spontaneous | 0 | Complete | 0 |
| To speech | 1 | Partial | 1 |
| To pain | 2 | Minimal | 2 |
| None | 3 | None | 3 |
| **Communication Ability** | | **Level of Functioning (Physical, mental, emotional, or social functioning)** | |
| Oriented | 0 | | |
| Confused | 1 | Completely independent | 0 |
| Inappropriate | 2 | Independent in special environment | 1 |
| Incomprehensible | 3 | | |
| None | 4 | Mildly dependent—limited assistance (non-resident-helper) | 2 |
| **Motor Response** | | Moderately dependent—moderate assistance (person in home) | 3 |
| Obeying | 0 | | |
| Localizing | 1 | | |
| Withdrawing | 2 | Markedly dependent—assistance all major activities, all times | 4 |
| Flexing | 3 | | |
| Extending | 4 | | |
| None | 5 | Totally dependent—24-hour nursing care | 5 |
| **Feeding (Cognitive ability only)** | | **"Employability" (As a full-time worker, homemaker, or student)** | |
| Complete | 0 | | |
| Partial | 1 | Not restricted | 0 |
| Minimal | 2 | Selected jobs, competitive | 1 |
| None | 3 | Sheltered workshop, non-competitive | 2 |
| **Toileting (Cognitive ability only)** | | Not employable | 3 |
| Complete | 0 | | |
| Partial | 1 | | |
| Minimal | 2 | | |
| None | 3 | | |

*Note.* This information is from Wright (2000b), available at: http://www.tbims.org/combi/drs. Copyright 2000 by The Center for Outcome Measurement in Brain Injury. Wright is not the scale author for the DRS.

## Functional Status Examination (FSE)

The FSE (Dikmen, Machamer, Miller, Doctor, & Temkin, 2001) evaluates change in activities of daily life due to a sudden event or illness, such as TBI, using comparisons between current functional status and that of pre-injury, in the following domains:

- Executive functioning (cognitive competency)
- Social integration (behavioral competency)
- Personal care
- Ambulation
- Standard of living
- Home management
- Travel
- Financial independence
- Major activity involving work or school
- Leisure and recreation

The FSE is administered via interview with either the individual with TBI or a familiar significant other. Scores in each domain are totaled, providing a range of 0 to 30.

## Glasgow Outcome Scale (GOS)

The GOS and the Extended Glasgow Outcome Scale (GOSE) are indices of social outcome following head injury, designed as a complement to the GCS. The GOS consists of a hierarchical rating scale in which individuals are assigned to one of five possible outcome categories: Dead, Vegetative State, Severe Disability, Moderate Disability, and Good Recovery (Jennett & Bond 1975). The GOSE is a modified version of the GOS (Wilson, Pettigrew, & Teasdale, 1997) which includes a structured interview addressing social and personal functional ability (Appendix 2–5) and the subdivision of outcome categories of severe disability, moderate disability, and good recovery, into a lower and upper category (Table 2–11).

## Quality of Life after Brain Injury (QOLIBRI)

The QOLIBRI assesses *health-related* quality of life after a TBI (HRQoL), (Shukla, Devi, & Agrawal, 2011). Scale content (Table 2–12)

| Table 2–11. Extended Glasgow Outcome Scale (GOSE) | | |
|---|---|---|
| *Score* | *Category* | *Symbol* |
| 1 | Death | D |
| 2 | Vegetative state | VS |
| 3 | Lower severe disability | SD– |
| 4 | Upper severe disability | SD + |
| 5 | Lower moderate disability | MD– |
| 6 | Upper moderate disability | MD + |
| 7 | Lower good recovery | GR– |
| 8 | Upper good recovery | GR + |

*Source:* Wilson, Pettigrew, & Teasdale (1997). Used with permission.

**Table 2–12.** Quality of Life after Brain Injury (QOLIBRI) Scale Content

| QOLIBRI Scale | Number of Items | Content |
|---|---|---|
| | | **"Satisfaction" Items** |
| Cognition | 7 | Cognitive problems such as memory, attention, expressive speech, and decision making |
| Self | 7 | Aspects of self, including energy, motivation, physical appearance, and self-esteem |
| Daily life & autonomy | 7 | Independence, activities of daily life, and participation in social roles |
| Social relationships | 6 | Relationships with friends, family, and partner |
| | | **"Bothered" Items** |
| Emotions | 5 | Feelings of depression, anxiety, loneliness, boredom, and anger |
| Physical problems | 5 | Physical problems, such as slowness, pain, sensory impairment, or other consequences of injury |

*Source:* von Steinbüchel, Wilson, Gibbons, Hawthorne, Höfer, Schmidt, et al. (2010a, b).

comprises six scales: Cognition, Self, Daily life and Autonomy, Social Relationships, Emotions, and Physical Problems. The first four scales assess "satisfaction," while the final two scales assess "feeling bothered" with key aspects of life (von Steinbüchel et al., 2010a). Individuals with TBI are asked to rate their satisfaction or level of feeling bothered on a 5-point scale from "Not at all" (satisfied/bothered) to "Very" (satisfied/bothered), given responses to QOLIBRI questions in each category.

## References

American Speech-Language-Hearing Association. (2007). *Scope of practice in speech-language pathology* [Scope of practice]. Retrieved from http://www.asha.org/policy

American Speech-Language-Hearing Association. (2011a). *National outcomes measurement system: Adults in healthcare—Acute Hospital National Data Report 2011*. Rockville, MD: National Center for Evidence-Based Practice in Communication Disorders.

American Speech-Language-Hearing Association. (2011b). *National outcomes measurement system: Adults in healthcare—Inpatient National Data Report 2011*. Rockville, MD: National Center for Evidence-Based Practice in Communication Disorders.

American Speech-Language-Hearing Association. (2011c). *National outcomes measurement system: Adults in healthcare—Outpatient National Data Report 2011*. Rockville, MD: National Center for Evidence-Based Practice in Communication Disorders.

American Speech-Language-Hearing Association. (2011d). *National outcomes measurement system: Adults in healthcare—Skilled Nursing Facility National Data Report 2011*.

Rockville, MD: National Center for Evidence-Based Practice in Communication Disorders.

Brosh, I., & Barkai, E. (2004). Learning-induced long-term synaptic modification in the olfactory cortex. *Current Neurovascular Research, 1*(4), 389–395.

Callaway, L., Winkler, D., Tippett, A., Migliorini, C., Herd, N., & Willer, B. (2014). *The Community Integration Questionnaire–Revised (CIQ-R).* Melbourne, Australia: Summer Foundation.

Cantu, R. C. (2001). Postraumatic retrograde and anterograde amnesia: Pathophysiology and implications in grading and safe return to play. *Journal of Athletic Training, 36*(3), 244–248.

CDC, NIH, DoD, & VA Leadership Panel. (2013). *Report to Congress on traumatic brain injury in the united states: understanding the public health problem among current and former military personnel.* Centers for Disease Control and Prevention (CDC), the National Institutes of Health (NIH), the Department of Defense (DoD), and the Department of Veterans Affairs (VA). Retrieved from http://www.cdc.gov/traumaticbraininjury/pdf/report_to_congress_on_traumatic_brain_injury_2013-a.pdf

Dijkers, M. (2000). The Community Integration Questionnaire. *The Center for Outcome Measurement in Brain Injury.* Retrieved from http://www.tbims.org/combi/ciq

Dikmen, S., Machamer, J., Miller, B., Doctor, J., & Temkin, N. (2001). Functional status examination: A new instrument for assessing outcome in traumatic brain injury. *Journal of Neurotrauma, 18*(2), 127–140.

Fawcett, J. W., Rosser, A. E., & Dunnett, S. B. (2001). *Brain damage, brain repair.* Oxford, UK: Oxford University Press.

Hagen, C., Malkmus, D., & Durham, P. (1972). *Levels of cognitive functioning.* Downey, CA: Rancho Los Amigos Hospital.

Hall, K. M. (1997). The functional assessment measure. *Journal of Rehabilitation Outcomes Measures, 1,* 63–65.

ICF Research Branch. (2013). *Development of ICF core sets for traumatic brain injury (TBI).* Retrieved from https://www.icf-research-branch.org/icf-core-sets-projects2/neurological-conditions/development-of-icf-core-sets-for-traumatic-brain-injury-tbi

Jennett, B., & Bond, M. (1975). Assessment of outcome after severe brain damage: A practical scale. *Lancet, 1,* 480–484.

Katz, D. I., & Alexander, M. P. (1994). Traumatic brain injury: Predicting the course of recovery and outcome of patients admitted to rehabilitation. *Archives of Neurology, 51,* 661–670.

Kleim, J. A., & Jones, T. A. (2008). Principles of experience-dependent neural plasticity: Implications for rehabilitation after brain damage. *Journal of Speech, Language, and Hearing Research, 51*(1), S225–S239.

Koehler, R., Wilhelm, E. E., & Shoulson, I. (2012). *Cognitive rehabilitation therapy for traumatic brain injury: Evaluating the evidence.* Washington, DC: National Academies Press.

Kosch, Y., Browne, S., King, C., Fitzgerald, J., & Cameron, I. (2010). Post-traumatic amnesia and its relationship to the functional outcome of people with severe traumatic brain injury. *Brain Injury, 24*(3), 479–485.

Kou, Z., & Iraji, A. (2014). Imaging brain plasticity after trauma. *Neural Regeneration Research, 9*(7), 693–700.

Levin, H. S., Benton, A. L., & Grossman, R. G. (1982). *Neurobehavioral consequences of traumatic brain injury.* New York, NY: Oxford University Press.

Levin, H. S., O'Donnell, V. M., & Grossman, R. G. (1979). The Galveston Orientation and Amnesia Test: A practical scale to assess cognition after head injury. *Journal of Nervous Mental Disease, 167*(11), 675–684.

Linacre, J. M., Heinemann, A. W., Wright, B. D., Granger, C. V., & Hamilton, B. B. (1994). The structure and stability of the functional independence measure. *Archives of Physical Rehabilitation, 75,* 127–132.

Ludlow, C. L., Hoit, J., Kent, R., Ramig, L. O., Shrivastav, R., Strand, E., . . . Sapienza, C. (2008). Translating principles of neural plasticity into research on speech motor control recovery and rehabilitation. *Journal of Speech, Language, and Hearing Research: JSLHR, 51*(1), S240–S258.

Maas, A. I., Harrison-Felix, C. L., Menon, D., Adelson, D., Balkin, T., Bullock, R., . . . Schwab, K. (2010). Common data elements for traumatic brain injury: Recommendations from the interagency working group on demographics and clinical assessment. *Archives of Physical Medicine and Rehabilitation, 91*(11), 1641–1649.

Moucha, R., & Kilgard, M. P. (2006). Cortical plasticity and rehabilitation. *Progressive Brain Research, 57*, 111–389.

Overman, J., & Carmichael, S. (2014). Plasticity in the injured brain. *The Neuroscientist, 20*(1), 15–28.

Rappaport, M., Hall, K. M., Hopkins, K., Belleza, T., & Cope, D. N. (1982). Disability rating scale for severe head trauma: Coma to community. *Archives of Physical Medicine Rehabilitation, 63*(3), 118– 123.

Saatman, K. E., Duhaime, A., Bullock, R., Mass, A. I., Valadka, A., & Manley, G. (2008). Classification of traumatic brain injury for targeted therapies. *Journal of Neurotrauma, 25*, 719–738.

Sander, A. (2002). The Level of Cognitive Functioning Scale. *The Center for Outcome Measurement in Brain Injury.* Retrieved from http://www.tbims.org/combi/lcfs

Shukla, D., Devi, B. I., & Agrawal, A. (2011). Outcome measures for traumatic brain injury. *Clinical Neurology and Neurosurgery, 113*, 435–441.

Stein, D. G., & Hoffman, S. W. (2003). Concepts of CNS plasticity in the context of brain damage and repair. *Journal of Head Trauma Rehabilitation, 18*(4), 317–341.

Teasdale, G., & Jennett, B. (1974). Assessment of coma and impaired consciousness. A practical scale. *Lancet, 2*(7872), 81–84.

von Steinbüchel, N., Wilson, L., Gibbons, H., Hawthorne, G., Höfer, S., Schmidt, S., . . . the QOLIBRI Task Force. (2010a). Quality of Life after Brain Injury (QOLIBRI): Scale validity

and correlates of quality of life. *Journal of Neurotrauma, 27*(7), 1157–1165.

von Steinbüchel, N., Wilson, L., Gibbons, H., Hawthorne, G., Höfer, S., Schmidt, S., . . . the QOLIBRI Task Force. (2010b). Quality of Life after Brain Injury (QOLIBRI): Scale development and metric properties. *Journal of Neurotrauma, 27*(7), 1167–1185.

Whiteneck, G. G., Brooks, C. A., Charlifue, S., Gerhart, K. A., Mellick, D., Overholser, D., & Richardson, G. N. (n.d.). *Guide for use of the CHART: Craig Handicap Assessment and Reporting Technique.* Retrieved from https://craighospital.org/uploads/CraigHospital.CHARTManual.pdf

Whiteneck, G. G., Charlifue, S. W., Gerhart, K. A., Overholser, J. D., & Richardson, G. N. (1992). Quantifying handicap: A new measure of long-term rehabilitation outcomes. *Archives of Physical Medicine Rehabilitation, 73*, 519–526.

Wilson, J. T. L., Pettigrew, L. E. L., & Teasdale, G. M. (1997). Structured interviews for the Glasgow Outcome Scale and the Extended Glasgow Outcome Scale: Guidelines for their use. *Journal of Neurotrauma, 15*, 573–585.

World Health Organization (WHO). (n.d.). *International Classification of Functioning, Disability and Health (ICF).* World Health Organization. Retrieved from http://www.who.int/classifications/icf/icf_more/en/

World Health Organization (WHO). (2002). *Towards a Common Language for Functioning, Disability and Health: ICF.* Geneva: Author. Retrieved from http://www.who.int/classifications/icf/training/icfbeginnersguide.pdf

Wright, J. (2000a). The Functional Assessment Measure. *The Center for Outcome Measurement in Brain Injury.* Retrieved from http://www.tbims.org/combi/FAM

Wright, J. (2000b). The Disability Rating Scale. *The Center for Outcome Measurement in Brain Injury.* Retrieved from http://www.tbims.org/combi/drs

APPENDIX 2–1

# Comprehensive ICF Core Set for Traumatic Brain Injury (TBI)

**ICF Category Title**

*Body Functions*

Consciousness functions

Orientation functions

Temperament and personality functions

Energy and drive functions

Sleep functions

Attention functions

Memory functions

Psychomotor functions

Emotional functions

Perceptual functions

Thought functions

Higher-level cognitive functions

Mental functions of language

Seeing functions

Functions of structures adjoining the eye

Vestibular functions

Sensations associated with hearing and vestibular function

Smell function

Proprioceptive function

Sensation of pain

Voice functions

Articulation functions

Fluency and rhythm of speech functions

Blood pressure functions

Exercise tolerance functions

Ingestion functions

Defecation functions

Endocrine gland functions

Urination functions

Sexual functions

Mobility of joint functions

Muscle power functions

Muscle tone functions

Involuntary movement reaction functions

Control of voluntary movement functions

Involuntary movement functions

Gait pattern functions

*Body Structures*

Structure of brain

Structure of head and neck regions

*Activities & Participation*

Watching

Listening

Acquiring skills

Focusing attention

Thinking

Reading

Writing

Solving problems

Making decisions

Undertaking a single task

Undertaking multiple tasks

Carrying out daily routine

Handling stress and other psychological demands

Communicating with—receiving—spoken messages

Communicating with—receiving—nonverbal messages

Speaking

Producing nonverbal messages

Writing messages

Conversation

Using communication devices and techniques

Changing basic body position

Maintaining a body position

Transferring oneself

Lifting and carrying objects

Fine hand use

Hand and arm use

Walking

Moving around

Moving around using equipment

Using transportation

Driving

Washing oneself

Caring for body parts

Toileting

Dressing

Eating

Drinking

Looking after one's health

Acquisition of goods and services

Preparing meals

Doing housework

Assisting others

Basic interpersonal interactions

Complex interpersonal interactions

Relating with strangers

Formal relationships

Informal social relationships

Family relationships

Intimate relationships

Vocational training

Higher education

Apprenticeship (work preparation)

Acquiring, keeping and terminating a job

Remunerative employment

Non-remunerative employment

Basic economic transactions

Complex economic transactions

Economic self-sufficiency

Community life

Recreation and leisure

Religion and spirituality

*Environmental Factors*

Food

Drugs

Non-medicinal drugs and alcohol

Products and technology for personal use in daily living

Products and technology for personal indoor and outdoor mobility and transportation

Products and technology for communication

Products and technology for employment

Design, construction, and building products and technology of buildings for public use

Design, construction and building products and technology of buildings for private use

Products and technology of land development

Assets

Physical geography

Sound

Immediate family

Extended family

Friends

Acquaintances, peers, colleagues, neighbors, and community members

People in positions of authority

Personal care providers and personal assistant

Health professionals

Other professionals

Individual attitudes of immediate family members

Individual attitudes of extended family members

Individual attitudes of friends

Individual attitudes of acquaintances, peers, colleagues, neighbors, and community members

Individual attitudes of personal care providers and personal assistants

Individual attitudes of health professionals

Individual attitudes of other professionals

Societal attitudes

Architecture and construction services, systems and policies

Housing, services, systems and policies

Communication services, systems, and policies

Transportation services, systems, and policies

Legal services, systems, and policies

Social security services, systems, and policies

General social support services, systems, and policies

Health services, systems, and policies

Education and training services, systems, and policies

Labor and employment services, systems, and policies

*Source:* ICF Research Branch (2013).

## APPENDIX 2-2

# Functional Independence Measure™ and Functional Assessment Measure: Brain Injury

Scale:

| | |
|---|---|
| 7 | Complete Independence (timely, safely) |
| 6 | Modified Independence (extra time, devices) |
| 5 | Supervision (cuing, coaxing, prompting) |
| 4 | Minimal Assist (performs 75% or more of task) |
| 3 | Moderate Assist (performs 50%–74% of task) |
| 2 | Maximal Assist (performs 25%–49% of task) |
| 1 | Total Assist (performs less than 25% of task) |

*(Patient Stamp)*

| SELF-CARE ITEMS | Adm | Goal | D/C | F/U |
|---|---|---|---|---|
| 1. Feeding | | | | |
| 2. Grooming | | | | |
| 3. Bathing | | | | |
| 4. Dressing Upper Body | | | | |
| 5. Dressing Lower Body | | | | |
| 6. Toileting | | | | |
| 7. Swallowing* | | | | |
| SPHINCTER CONTROL | | | | |
| 8. Bladder Management | | | | |
| 9. Bowel Management | | | | |
| MOBILITY ITEMS (Type of Transfer) | | | | |
| 10. Bed, Chair, Wheelchair _____ | | | | |
| 11. Toilet _____ | | | | |
| 12. Tub or Shower _____ | | | | |
| 13. Car Transfer* _____ | | | | |
| LOCOMOTION | | | | |
| 14. Walking/Wheelchair (circle) | | | | |
| 15. Stairs | | | | |
| 16. Community Access* | | | | |
| COMMUNICATION ITEMS | | | | |
| 17. Comprehension-Audio/Visual (circle) | | | | |
| 18. Expression-Verbal/Non-Verbal (circle) | | | | |
| 19. Reading* | | | | |
| 20. Writing* | | | | |
| 21. Speech Intelligibility* | | | | |

| PSYCHOSOCIAL ADJUSTMENT | Adm | Goal | D/C | F/U |
|---|---|---|---|---|
| 22. Social Interaction | | | | |
| 23. Emotional Status* | | | | |
| 24. Adjustment to Limitations* | | | | |
| 25. Employability* | | | | |
| COGNITIVE FUNCTION | | | | |
| 26. Problem Solving | | | | |
| 27. Memory | | | | |
| 28. Orientation* | | | | |
| 29. Attention* | | | | |
| 30. Safety Judgment* | | | | |

*FAM items

| | Admt | Date | D/C | Date |
|---|---|---|---|---|
| RN | _____ | _____ | _____ | _____ |
| PT | _____ | _____ | _____ | _____ |
| OT | _____ | _____ | _____ | _____ |
| ST | _____ | _____ | _____ | _____ |
| PSY | _____ | _____ | _____ | _____ |
| REC | _____ | _____ | _____ | _____ |

*Source:* The Functional Independence Measure (FIM) is a registered trademark. This information is from Wright (2000a), available at: http://www.tbims.org/combi/FAM. Copyright 2000 by The Center for Outcome Measurement in Brain Injury. Wright is not the scale author for the FAM.

# Craig Handicap Assessment and Reporting Technique: Short Form (CHART-SF)

**WHAT ASSISTANCE DO YOU NEED?**

*People with disabilities often need assistance. We would like to differentiate between personal care for physical disabilities and supervision for cognitive problems. First, focus on physical "hands on" assistance: This includes help with eating, grooming, bathing, dressing, management of a ventilator or other equipment, transfers, etc. Keeping in mind these daily activities . . .*

1. How many hours in a typical 24-hour day do you have someone with you to provide physical assistance for personal care activities such as eating, bathing, dressing, toileting, and mobility?

   _____ hours paid assistance

   _____ hours unpaid (family, others)

*Now, focus on supervision for cognitive problems instead of physical assistance. This includes remembering, decision making, judgment, etc. . . .*

2. How much time is someone with you in your home to assist you with activities that require remembering, decision making, or judgment?

   (1) _____ Someone else is always with me to observe or supervise.

   (2) _____ Someone else is always around, but they only check on me now and then.

   (3) _____ Sometimes I am left alone for an hour or two.

   (4) _____ Sometimes I am left alone for most of the day.

   (5) _____ I have been left alone all day and all night, but someone checks in on me.

   (6) _____ I am left alone without anyone checking on me.

3. How much of the time is someone with you to help you with remembering, decision making, or judgment when you go away from your home?

   (1) _____ I am restricted from leaving, even with someone else.

   (2) _____ Someone is always with me to help with remembering, decision making, or judgment when I go anywhere.

   (3) _____ I go to places on my own as long as they are familiar.

   (4) _____ I do not need help going anywhere.

*Now, I have a series of questions about your typical activities.*

## ARE YOU UP AND ABOUT REGULARLY?

4. On a <u>typical day</u>, how many hours are you out of bed?

    _____ hours

5. In a <u>typical week</u>, how many days do you get out of your house and go somewhere?

    _____ days

6. In the <u>last year</u>, how many nights have you spent away from your home (excluding hospitalizations)?

    (0) _____ none

    (1) _____ 1–2

    (3) _____ 3–4

    (5) _____ 5 or more

## HOW DO YOU SPEND YOUR TIME?

7. How many hours per week do you spend working in a job for which you get paid?

    _____ hours

    (occupation: _____ )

8. How many hours per week do you spend in school working toward a degree or in an accredited technical training program (including hours in class and studying)?

    _____ hours

9. How many hours per week do you spend in active homemaking including parenting, housekeeping, and food preparation?

    _____ hours

10. How many hours per week do you spend in home maintenance activities such as gardening, house repairs, or home improvement?

    _____ hours

11. How many hours per week do you spend in recreational activities such as sports, exercise, playing cards, or going to movies? Please do not include time spent watching TV or listening to the radio.

    _____ hours

## WITH WHOM DO YOU SPEND TIME?

12. How many people do you live with?

    _____ people

*continues*

13. Is one of them your spouse or significant other?

    (1) _____ Yes

    (0) _____ No

    (9) _____ Not applicable (subject lives alone)

14. Of the people you live with how many are relatives?

    _____ relatives

15. How many business or organizational associates do you visit, phone, or write to at least once a month?

    _____ associates

16. How many friends (non-relatives contacted outside business or organizational settings) do you visit, phone, or write to as least once a month?

    _____ friends

17. With how many strangers have you initiated a conversation in the last month (for example, to ask information or place an order)?

    (0) _____none

    (1) _____ 1–2

    (3) _____ 3–5

    (6) _____ 6 or more

## WHAT FINANCIAL RESOURCES DO YOU HAVE?

18. Approximately what was the combined annual income, in the last year, of all family members in your household? (Consider all sources including wages and earnings, disability benefits, pensions and retirement income, income from court settlements, investments and trust funds, child support and alimony, contributions from relatives, and any other source.)

    a. Less than 25,000—If no ask e; if yes ask b

    b. Less than 20,000—If no code 22500; if yes ask c

    c. Less than 15,000—If no code 17500; if yes ask d

    d. Less than 10,000—If no code 12500; if yes code 5000

    e. Less than 35,000—If no ask f; if yes code 30000

    f. Less than 50,000—If no ask g; if yes code 42500

    g. Less than 75,000—If no code h; if yes code 62500

    h. 75,000 or more code 80000

19. Approximately how much did you pay last year for medical care expenses? (Consider any amounts paid by yourself or by the family members in your household and not reimbursed by insurance or benefits.)

"Would you say your unreimbursed medical expenses are . . . "

a. Less than 1000—If no ask b; if yes code 500.

b. Less than 2500—If no ask c; if yes code 1750

c. Less than 5000—If no ask d; if yes code 3750

d. Less than 10000—If no ask e; if yes code 7500

e. 10000 or more code 15000

For information regarding CHART please contact:
Craig Hospital
Research Department
3425 S. Clarkson Street
Englewood, Colorado 80110
(303) 789-8202

*Source:* Whiteneck, Brooks, Charlifue, Gerhart, Mellick, Overholser, & Richardson (n.d.).

# Disability Rating Scale (DRS)

| Item/Ability | Score | Specification |
|---|---|---|
| *Eye Opening* | | |
| Spontaneous | 0 | Eyes open with sleep/wake rhythms indicating active arousal mechanisms, does not assume awareness. |
| To speech | 1 | A response to any verbal approach, whether spoken or shouted, not necessarily the command to open the eyes. Also, response to touch, mild pressure. |
| To pain | 2 | Tested by a painful stimulus. |
| None | 3 | No eye opening even to painful stimulation. |
| *Communication Ability* | | |
| Oriented | 0 | Implies awareness of self and the environment. Patient able to tell you (a) who he is; (b) where he is; (c) why he is there; (d) year; (e) season; (f) month; (g) day; (h) time of day. |
| Confused | 1 | Attention can be held and patient responds to questions but responses are delayed and/or indicate varying degrees of disorientation and confusion. |
| Inappropriate | 2 | Intelligible articulation but speech is used only in an exclamatory or random way (such as shouting and swearing); no sustained communication exchange is possible. |
| Incomprehensible | 3 | Moaning, groaning, or sounds without recognizable words, no consistent communication signs. |
| None | 4 | No sounds or communications signs from patient. |
| *Motor Response* | | |
| Obeying | 0 | Obeying command to move finger on best side. If no response or not suitable, try another command such as "move lips," "blink eyes," etc. Do not include grasp or other reflex responses. |
| Localizing | 1 | A painful stimulus at more than one site causes limb to move (even slightly) in an attempt to remove it. It is a deliberate motor act to move away from or remove the source of noxious stimulation. If there is doubt as to whether withdrawal or localization has occurred after 3 or 4 painful stimulations, rate as localization. |
| Withdrawing | 2 | Any generalized movement away from a noxious stimulus that is more than a simple reflex response. |

| Item/Ability | Score | Specification |
|---|---|---|
| Flexing | 3 | Painful stimulation results in either flexion at the elbow, rapid withdrawal with abduction of the shoulder or a slow withdrawal with adduction of the shoulder. If there is confusion between flexing and withdrawing, then use pinprick on hands. |
| Extending | 4 | Painful stimulation results in extension of the limb. |
| None | 5 | No response can be elicited. Usually associated with hypotonia. Exclude spinal transection as an explanation of lack of response; be satisfied that an adequate stimulus has been applied. |

*Feeding (Cognitive ability only)*

Does the patient show awareness of how and when to perform this activity? Ignore motor disabilities that interfere with carrying out this function.

| Complete | 0 | Continuously shows awareness that he knows how to feed and can convey unambiguous information that he knows when this activity should occur. |
|---|---|---|
| Partial | 1 | Intermittently shows awareness that he knows how to feed and/or can intermittently convey reasonably clearly information that he knows when the activity should occur. |
| Minimal | 2 | Shows questionable or infrequent awareness that he knows in a primitive way how to feed and/or shows infrequently by certain signs, sounds, or activities that he is vaguely aware when the activity should occur. |
| None | 3 | Shows virtually no awareness at any time that he knows how to feed and cannot convey information by signs, sounds, or activity that he knows when the activity should occur. |

*Toileting (Cognitive ability only)*

Does the patient show awareness of how and when to perform this activity? Ignore motor disabilities that interfere with carrying out this function. Rate best response for toileting based on bowel and bladder behavior.

| Complete | 0 | Continuously shows awareness that he knows how to toilet and can convey unambiguous information that he knows when this activity should occur. |
|---|---|---|
| Partial | 1 | Intermittently shows awareness that he knows how to toilet and/or can intermittently convey reasonably clearly information that he knows when the activity should occur. |
| Minimal | 2 | Shows questionable or infrequent awareness that he knows in a primitive way how to toilet and/or shows infrequently by certain signs, sounds, or activities that he is vaguely aware when the activity should occur. |

*continues*

| Item/Ability | Score | Specification |
|---|---|---|
| None | 3 | Shows virtually no awareness at any time that he knows how to toilet and cannot convey information by signs, sounds, or activity that he knows when the activity should occur. |

*Grooming (Cognitive ability only)*

Does the patient show awareness of how and when to perform this activity? Ignore motor disabilities that interfere with carrying out this function. (This is rated under Level of Functioning described below.) Grooming refers to bathing, washing, brushing of teeth, shaving, combing or brushing of hair, and dressing.

| Item/Ability | Score | Specification |
|---|---|---|
| Complete | 0 | Continuously shows awareness that he knows how to groom self and can convey unambiguous information that he knows when this activity should occur. |
| Partial | 1 | Intermittently shows awareness that he knows how to groom self and/or can intermittently convey reasonably clearly information that he knows when the activity should occur. |
| Minimal | 2 | Shows questionable or infrequent awareness that he knows in a primitive way how to groom self and/or shows infrequently by certain signs, sounds, or activities that he is vaguely aware when the activity should occur. |
| None | 3 | Shows virtually no awareness at any time that he knows how to groom self and cannot convey information by signs, sounds, or activity that he knows when the activity should occur. |

*Level of Functioning (Physical, mental, emotional, or social function)*

| Item/Ability | Score | Specification |
|---|---|---|
| Completely independent | 0 | Able to live as he wishes, requiring no restriction due to physical, mental, emotional, or social problems. |
| Independent in special environment | 1 | Capable of functioning independently when needed requirements are met (mechanical aids). |
| Mildly dependent— limited assistance (non-residential helper) | 2 | Able to care for most of own needs but requires limited assistance due to physical, cognitive, and/or emotional problems (e.g., needs non-resident helper). |
| Moderately dependent— moderate assistance (person in home) | 3 | Able to care for self partially but needs another person at all times. (Person in home) |

| Item/Ability | Score | Specification |
|---|---|---|
| Markedly dependent— assistance all major activities, all times | 4 | Needs help with all major activities and the assistance of another person at all times. |
| Totally dependent—24-hour nursing care | 5 | Not able to assist in own care and requires 24-hour nursing care. |
| *"Employability" (As a full-time worker, homemaker, or student)* | | |
| Not restricted | 0 | Can compete in the open market for a relatively wide range of jobs commensurate with existing skills; or can initiate, plan, execute, and assume responsibilities associated with homemaking; or can understand and carry out most age-relevant school assignments. |
| Selected jobs, competitive | 1 | Can compete in a limited job market for a relatively narrow range of jobs because of limitations of the type described above and/or because of some physical limitations; or can initiate, plan, execute, and assume many but not all responsibilities associated with homemaking; or can understand and carry out many but not all school assignments. |
| Sheltered workshop, non-competitive | 2 | Cannot compete successfully in a job market because of limitations described above and/or because of moderate or severe physical limitations; or cannot without major assistance initiate, plan, execute, and assume responsibilities for homemaking; or cannot understand and carry out even relatively simple school assignments without assistance. |
| Not employable | 3 | Completely unemployable because of extreme psychosocial limitations of the type described above, or completely unable to initiate, plan, execute, and assume any responsibilities associated with homemaking; or cannot understand or carry out any school assignments. |

*Source:* Adapted from Wright (2000b), available at: http://www.tbims.org/combi/drs. Copyright 2000 by The Center for Outcome Measurement in Brain Injury. Wright is not the scale author for the DRS.

# Extended Glasgow Outcome Scale: Structured Interview

Patient's name: _____ Date of interview: _____

Date of birth: _____ Date of injury: _____ Gender: M/F

Age at injury: _____ Interval post-injury: _____

Respondent:
Patient alone _____ Relative/friend/carer alone _____ Patient + relative/friend/carer _____

Interviewer: _____

## CONSCIOUSNESS

1. Is the head-injured person able to obey simple commands or say any words?

   1 = No (VS)

   2 = Yes

Anyone who shows ability to obey even simple commands or utter any word or communicate specifically in any other way is no longer considered to be in the vegetative state. Eye movements are not reliable evidence or meaningful responsiveness. Corroborate with nursing staff. Confirmation of VS requires full assessment as in the Royal College of Physician Guidelines.

## INDEPENDENCE IN THE HOME

2a. Is the assistance of another person at home essential every day for some activities of daily living?

   1 = No

   2 = Yes

   If "No" go to question 3a.

For a "No" answer they should be able to look after themselves at home for 24 hours if necessary, though they need not actually look after themselves. Independence includes the ability to plan for and carry out the following activities: getting washed, putting on clean clothes without prompting, preparing food for themselves, dealing with callers, and handling minor domestic crises. The person should be able to carry out activities without needing prompting or reminding, and should be capable of being left alone overnight.

2b. Do they need frequent help or someone to be around at home most of the time?

   1 = No (Upper SD)

   2 = Yes (Lower SD)

For a "No" answer they should be able to look after themselves at home for up to 8 hours during the day if necessary, though they need not actually look after themselves.

2c. Was assistance at home essential before the injury?

    1 = No

    2 = Yes

## INDEPENDENCE OUTSIDE THE HOME

3a. Are they able to shop without assistance?

    1 = No (Upper SD)

    2 = Yes

This includes being able to plan what to buy, take care of money themselves, and behave appropriately in public. They need not normally shop, but must be able to do so.

3b. Were they able to shop without assistance before the injury?

    1 = No

    2 = Yes

4a. Are they able to travel locally without assistance?

    1 = No (Upper SD)

    2 = Yes

They may drive or use public transport to get around. Ability to use a taxi is sufficient, provided the person can phone for it themselves and instruct the driver.

4b. Were they able to travel without assistance before the injury?

    1 = No

    2 = Yes

## WORK

5a. Are they currently able to work to their previous capacity?

    1 = No

    2 = Yes

If they were working before, then their current capacity for work should be at the same level. If they were seeking work before, then the injury should not have adversely affected their chances of obtaining work or the level or work for which they are eligible. If the patient was a student before the injury then their capacity for study should not have been adversely affected.

5b. How restricted are they?

    a) Reduced work capacity.

    b) Able to work only in a sheltered workshop or non-competitive job, or currently unable to work.

    1 = a (Upper MD)

    2 = b (Lower MD)

*continues*

5c. Were they either working or seeking employment before the injury (answer "yes") or were they doing neither (answer "no")?

1 = No

2 = Yes

## SOCIAL & LEISURE ACTIVITIES

6a. Are they able to resume regular social and leisure activities outside home?

1 = No

2 = Yes

They need not have resumed all their previous leisure activities, but should not be prevented by physical or mental impairment. If they have stopped the majority of activities because of loss of interest or motivation then this is also considered a disability.

6b. What is the extent or restriction on their social and leisure activities?
   a) Participate a bit less: at least half as often as before injury.
   b) Participate much less: less than half as often.
   c) Unable to participate: rarely, if ever, take part.

1 = a (Lower GR)

2 = b (Upper MD)

3 = c (Lower MD)

6c. Did they engage in regular social and leisure activities outside home before the injury?

1 = No

2 = Yes

## FAMILY & FRIENDSHIPS

7a. Have there been psychological problems which have resulted in ongoing family disruption or disruption to friendships?

1 = No

2 = Yes

Typical post-traumatic personality changes: quick temper, irritability, anxiety, insensitivity to others, mood swings, depression, and unreasonable or childish behavior.

7b. What has been the extent of disruption or strain?
   a) Occasional: less then weekly.
   b) Frequent: once a week or more, but tolerable.
   c) Constant: daily and intolerable

1 = a (Lower GR)

2 = b (Upper MD)

3 = c (Lower MD)

7c. Were there problems with family or friends before the injury?

    1 = No

    2 = Yes

If there were some problems before the injury, but these have become markedly worse since injury then answer "no" to Q7c.

## RETURN TO NORMAL LIFE

8a. Are there any other current problems relating to the injury which affect daily life?

    1 = No (Upper GR)

    2 = Yes (Lower GR)

Other typical problems reported after head injury: headaches, dizziness, tiredness, sensitivity to noise or light, slowness, memory failures, and concentration problems.

8b. Were similar problems present before the injury?

    1 = No

    2 = Yes

If there were some problems before the injury, but these have become markedly worse since injury then answer "no" to Q8b.

Epilepsy:

Since the injury has the head injured person had any epileptic fits?    No/Yes

Have they been told that they are currently at risk of developing epilepsy?    No/Yes

What is the most important factor in outcome?

_____ Effects of head injury

_____ Effects of illness or injury to another part of the body

_____ A mixture of these

Scoring: The patient's overall rating is based on the lowest outcome category indicated on the scale. Refer to Guidelines for further information concerning administration and scoring.

1    Dead
2    Vegetative State (VS)
3    Lower Severe Disability (Lower SD)
4    Upper Severe Disability (Upper SD)
5    Lower Moderate Disability (Lower MD)
6    Upper Moderate Disability (Upper MD)
7    Lower Good Recovery (Lower GR)
8    Upper Good Recovery (Upper GR)

*Source:* Lindsay Wilson, Laura Pettigrew, Graham Teasdale 1998. Used with permission.

# 3 Compounding and Concomitant Conditions

As the name *traumatic* brain injury suggests, the physical trauma associated with TBI can have far-reaching negative impacts beyond those of cognitive-communication disorders (American Speech-Language-Hearing Association, n.d.). Those who seek to be of service to individuals with TBI (and their families) must be well versed in the potential domains of impact associated with TBI and their influence on treatment and recovery. The purpose of this chapter is to provide an overview of some primary compounding and concomitant domains of impact from TBI relevant to the role of the speech-language pathologist, including hearing, neurobehavioral, physical, speech, swallowing, and vision concerns. This is meant to serve as a primer, not a comprehensive review. There are many excellent sources on each of these topics specific to TBI and treatment. Although this text is devoted to cognitive rehabilitation therapy (CRT), it warrants emphasizing that those serving individuals with TBI must view each individual with TBI as unique and from a holistic perspective, including careful reflection and discussion about each of the concerns noted in this chapter, their presence and impact on the individual with TBI, and their influence on CRT.

As discussed in Chapter 1 (Mechanisms of Injury and Neuropathology), there are two main forms of TBI: open-head injury, which generally results in neurologic injury of a more focal nature, and closed-head injury, which results in neurologic injury of a more diffuse nature. These are important distinctions to consider when discussing compounding and concomitant conditions in TBI. The nature of compounding and concomitant conditions will be closely tied to the particular pathophysiology of injury (closed-head injury, open-head injury, or both), as well as other premorbid and demographic factors. Much of the research in this area has been conducted on closed-head injury. In some cases relative to open-head injury, researchers refer to studies on other types of more focal neurologic disorders, such as the focal lesions associated with stroke and tumor. It is therefore important when investigating treatment options in the areas of compounding and concomitant conditions to have a clear understanding of: (1) the neurologic nature of injury of the individual with TBI and (2) the foundation of the research used to guide decisions in terms of the participants studied and the nature of their injuries.

## Hearing Concerns

Estimates suggest that between 48% and 74% of individuals who experience a TBI will exhibit some type of hearing loss (Bergemalm, 2003; Coelho & Hoffer, 2013;

Zimmerman, Ganzel, Windmill, Nazar, & Phillips, 1993). How this loss manifests and its severity will vary based on the severity and nature of the TBI. Table 3–1 contains a list of common auditory (hearing) and vestibular (balance) effects of TBI.

Hearing loss following TBI can originate from either peripheral or central auditory system dysfunction (Vander Werff, 2012). Peripheral auditory system injury can occur when the temporal bone receives direct impact or as a result of blast injury or explosion. These mechanisms can impact the external, middle, and inner ear. The central auditory system is also susceptible to injury due to TBI, including damage to any part of the brain and cranial nerves associated with hearing. Treatment for hearing loss after TBI can encompass medical, surgical, behavioral, or supportive approaches, or combinations of each (Coelho & Hoffer, 2013). Given the critical relationship between hearing and communication, involvement of an audiologist in evaluation and treatment of hearing loss after a TBI is critical. Of note, blast injury and its unique impact on the ear and hearing has also received recent investigation given the numbers of military service members exposed to improvised explosive devices (IEDs) in recent military conflicts.

## Neurobehavioral Concerns

As the term "neurobehavioral" suggests, deficits in this area relate to neurologic impacts of a TBI on behavior. Table 3–2 includes a general overview of some common neurobehavioral effects of TBI (ASHA, n.d.).

## Personality Changes

Changes in emotional and behavioral regulation after a brain injury are common and often described by individuals with TBI and their families as changes in personality (McAllister, 2011). These can be changes that are exaggerations of pre-injury traits or behaviors that are fundamentally different from pre-injury responses (McAllister, 2011). They can also be due to psychiatric disorders or secondary to cognitive deficits or medical or structural lesions (Riggio & Wong, 2009, p. 165). They can manifest as an emotional response to the TBI and the resulting functional and physical limitations (Riggio & Wong, 2009). Table 3–3 includes a sample of behavioral presentations related to injury in specific brain regions. It is important to note that neurobehavioral changes after TBI are influenced by many factors, including the nature and location of injury, but also the environment, social support systems, and personal factors such as premorbid personality (Figure 3–1).

It is also helpful to conceptualize behavioral changes after a TBI given outcomes,

**Table 3–1.** Common Auditory and Vestibular Effects of TBI

Auditory dysfunction stemming from mechanical injuries to the outer ear, middle ear, and/or inner ear and temporal lobe lesions

Central auditory dysfunction

Difficulty hearing speech in noise

Hearing loss that may be transient or permanent

Hypersensitivity to sounds (hyperacusis)

Tinnitus

Dizziness, vertigo, and/or imbalance

Source: ASHA (n.d., Auditory and Vestibular Effects).

**Table 3–2.** Common Neurobehavioral Effects of TBI

Affective changes, including overemotional or overreactive affect or flat (i.e., emotionless) affect

Agitation and/or combativeness

Anxiety disorder

Depression

Difficulty identifying emotions in others (alexithymia)

Emotional lability and mood changes or mood swings

Excessive drowsiness and change in sleep patterns, including difficulty falling or staying asleep (insomnia), excessive sleepiness (hypersomnia)

Feeling of disorientation or fogginess

Increased state of sensory sensitivity accompanied by exaggerated response to perceived threats (hypervigilance)

Impulsivity

Irritability and reduced frustration tolerance

Stress disorders

*Source:* ASHA (n.d., Neurobehavioral Effects).

**Table 3–3.** Behavior and Corresponding Brain Region

| Behavior | Brain Region |
|---|---|
| Difficulties switching parameters and planning<br>Mental inflexibility<br>Irritability<br>Slowed performance<br>Low frustration tolerance | Dorsolateral frontal region |
| Agitation<br>Disinhibition<br>Poor impulse control | Orbitofrontal region |
| Apathy (potentially misdiagnosed as depression) | Medial frontal region |
| Memory disturbance<br>Emotional lability | Temporal region |
| Mood symptoms | Basal ganglia (or dorsolateral frontal region) |
| Mania<br>Psychotic symptoms (with lesions to right and left hemispheres) | Right hemisphere limbic area |

*Source:* Riggio & Wong (2009, p. 164).

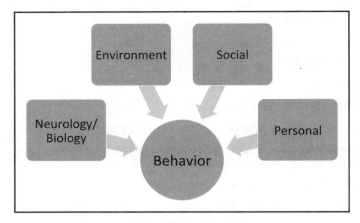

**Figure 3–1.** Factors that can influence behavior after TBI.

etiology, and noted behavioral problems (Garcia, 1994). As can be seen in Figure 3–2, transient behaviors develop due to temporary changes in neuropathology. Typically, transient behaviors resolve with little or no behavioral intervention. Modifiable behaviors are those that have a strong environmental component and may manifest as the individual with TBI faces new demands in his/her environment. Unlike transient behaviors, modifiable behaviors do not disappear spontaneously but are amenable to change via applied behavioral analysis and behavioral intervention techniques. Lastly, chronic behaviors are those that are resistant to change, despite behavioral intervention. The numbers and severity of chronic behaviors are believed to be correlated with more permanent neuropathology, and in particular significant frontal impairment (Garcia, 1994).

Common clusters of behavioral changes after a TBI include impulsivity, irritability, affective instability, and apathy (McAllister, 2011). Aggression and emotional instability after TBI have also been reported (Riggio & Wong, 2009), as has lack of awareness (McAllister, 2011). Both apathy and impulsivity are discussed in further detail below.

## Apathy

Apathy is a frequent symptom following TBI, with prevalence rates in individuals with TBI ranging from 20% to 72% (Arnould, Rochat, Azouvi, & Linden, 2013). When apathy is present, it can have negative consequences on family life, social reintegration, and participation in rehabilitation after TBI (Gray, Shepherd, & McKinley, 1994). As with impulsivity, apathy is multifaceted, comprising dimensions of cognition, motivation, affect, and personal identity, values, and beliefs (Arnould et al., 2013). There exists varying definitions and terminology used to define apathy, but it is essentially a deficit in motivated behavior (McAllister, 2011). Mulin and colleagues proposed definitions given the core feature of loss of motivation that persists for four weeks or more (compared with the individual's previous level of functioning), with at least one symptom in at least two of the following domains: (1) diminished goal-directed behavior; (2) diminished goal-directed cognitive activity; and (3) diminished emotions (Mulin et al., 2011). Four subtypes of apathy have also been described, including: (1) cognitive apathy related to executive function

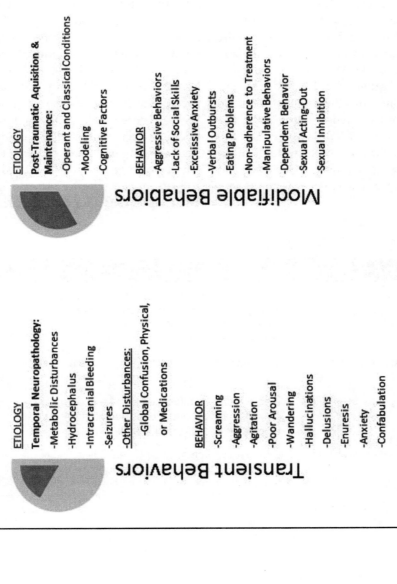

**Figure 3–2.** Behavioral changes after a TBI, given outcomes, etiology, and noted behavioral problems. *Source:* Garcia (1994, p. 263).

impairment, (2) motor apathy associated with extrapyramidal motor dysfunction, (3) sensory apathy following cortical sensory impairment, and (4) affective apathy occurring in the absence of the three other forms of apathy (Lane-Brown & Tate, 2011).

Apathy is more common in individuals with TBI who also have a diagnosis of depression (Andersson, Krogstad, & Finset, 1999; Lengenfelder, Goverover, Cagna, Smith, & Chiaravalloti, 2016). Most studies do not report a correlation between apathy and the severity of the brain injury (Andersson & Bergedalen, 2002; Glenn et al., 2002). Apathy is associated with a variety of cortical and subcortical regions of the brain, including areas in the ventral medial and lateral prefrontal cortex, anterior cingulate cortex, basil ganglia, insula, and white matter tracts connecting these regions (Arnould et al., 2013). Treatment research in the area of apathy following TBI is limited but can include medications or behavioral intervention such as external compensation and structure treatment activities (Lane-Brown & Tate, 2011).

## Impulsivity

Impulsivity (or poor impulse control) is common in individuals after a TBI (Kocka & Gagnon, 2014; Rochat et al., 2010). Impulsivity after TBI is an area closely related to negative social and professional outcomes. A pattern of impulsivity after TBI can manifest in "increased irritability, verbal or physical aggression, loss of temper, impatience and poor decision making or judgment abilities" (Rochat et al., 2010, p. 779). Although the outward aspects of impulsivity, acting without forethought, may appear similar, Whiteside and Lynam (2001) offer a description of four facets of impulsivity in the general population that serve as a helpful framework when considering impulsivity after TBI (urgency, perseverance, premeditation, and sensation seeking, UPPS). These are described in Table 3–4. Rochat and colleagues studied these domains of impulsivity in individuals with TBI and found that urgency, lack of premeditation, and lack of perseverance increase after the TBI, while sensation seeking decreases

**Table 3–4.** Domains of Impulsivity

| | |
|---|---|
| Urgency | A tendency to experience strong impulses and engage in impulsive behaviors in order to alleviate negative emotions, despite the long-term harmful consequences of these actions |
| Lack of premeditation | The tendency to act on the spur of the moment and without regard to the consequences |
| Lack of perseverance | Inability to remain focused on a task, complete projects, or work under conditions that require resistance to distracting stimuli |
| Sensation seeking | A tendency to enjoy and pursue activities that are exciting and an openness to trying new experiences that may or may not be dangerous |

*Source:* Whiteside & Lynam (2001, pp. 685–687).

(Rochat et al, 2010; Rochat, Beni, Annoni, Vuadens, & Van der Linden, 2013).

Several authors have suggested that additional specificity is needed in the terms and corresponding definitions used relative to impulsivity in general, but also given impulsivity noted after TBI. This is particularly true because impulsivity has been conceptually linked to models of executive function deficits after TBI (Arnould, Dromer, Rochat, Van der Linden, & Azouvi, 2016; Sohlberg & Mateer, 2001). There also remains an unclear distinction between attention impairment after TBI and impulsivity (Kocka & Gagnon, 2014).

## Psychiatric Disorder

TBI can also result in an increased risk for developing various psychiatric disorders. After a TBI, the rate for developing a new psychiatric disorder is almost half (48%) (Kopenen et al., 2002). Common psychiatric disorders after a TBI include mood and anxiety disorders, sleep disorders, and psychotic syndromes (McAllister, 2011). Substance abuse after TBI can also occur, with prevalence ranging from 12% to 22%, in contrast to a 15% lifetime prevalence in the general population (Rogers & Read, 2007; van Reekum, Cohen, & Wong, 2000). Although psychiatric disorders after TBI are treated by team members who are specialists in this area, it is important that SLPs recognize both the increased presence of these concerns after TBI and, as applicable, their impact on treatment. Depression and posttraumatic stress disorder (PTSD) are described briefly below.

### Depression

The most commonly diagnosed psychiatric disorder after TBI is depression (Kennedy et al., 2005). The lifetime prevalence of depression in individuals with TBI is much higher than that in the general population (Rogers & Read, 2007). Excluding individuals with depression at the time of injury, the rate of depression one year after injury is estimated to be 49% of individuals with TBI (Bombardier et al., 2010). Both major depression disorder (MDD) and minor depression (considered a risk factor for MDD) occur at high rates in individuals after TBI (Hart et al., 2012). Depression after a TBI can be due to a variety of factors, including premorbid personality, psychiatric history, social support, reaction to injury and disability, and organic changes (Griffen & Hanks, 2014). Depression has been linked to poor quality of life in individuals who experience TBI (Diaz et al., 2012). Numerous negative societal outcomes have also been shown to be related to depression after TBI, including decreased social activity and unemployment and suicide (Hart et al., 2012; Kennedy et al., 2005).

The presence of depression can also impact specific aspects of treatment for TBI, such as self-assessment (Goverover & Chiaravalloti, 2014). For example, depression has been shown to be strongly related to an individual's perceptions about his/her level of impairment after a TBI, regardless of injury type or severity (Malec, Testa, Rush, Brown, & Moessner, 2007), such that individuals with TBI who were depressed underestimate their level of function via self-report measures (Chamelian & Feinstein, 2006). This is an important factor to consider in provision of treatment services by an SLP. In addition, although SLPs do not assess or treat depression, it is imperative that all team members offering services to individuals with TBI and their families have an awareness of the signs and symptoms of depression (and the high risk of its occurrence in individuals with TBI) so the individuals can be referred promptly to a mental health professional. Table 3–5 contains a list of common signs and symptoms of depression.

### Posttraumatic Stress Disorder

The topic of PTSD and TBI has received recent attention given the high incidence of both in military personnel serving in the wars in Iraq and Afghanistan (Hoge & Castro, 2014). According to the *Diagnostic and Statistical Manual of Mental Disorders*, Fifth edition (DSM-5) (American Psychiatric Association, 2013), a diagnosis of PTSD is appropriate in individuals who had been exposed to or threatened with death, serious injury, or sexual violence. These traumatic events are persistently re-experienced by individuals with PTSD, through intrusive thoughts, nightmares, flashback, emotional

distress, or physical reactivity after exposure to traumatic reminders. An individual with PTSD avoids trauma-related thoughts or feelings and trauma-related reminders. He/she also has negative thoughts or feelings that began (or worsened) after the trauma and trauma-related arousal and reactivity that began (or worsened) after the trauma. These symptoms of PTSD last for more than one month, impact functional abilities, and create significant distress for the individual with PTSD.

PTSD has been noted after mild, moderate, and severe TBI (Greenspan, Stringer, Phillips, Hammond, & Goldstein, 2006; Harvey & Bryant, 2000; McMillan, 1991, 1996). This is despite initial assumptions that individuals with significant retrograde and anterograde amnesia associated with severe TBI would not experience recall of the event and thereby not experience PTSD.

PTSD occurs in both military and civilian populations. Estimates of the prevalence of PTSD in Iraq and Afghanistan veterans range from 5% to 20% (Ramchand et al., 2010). Among military personnel with PTSD, the occurrence of mild TBI increases the risk of developing PTSD more than twofold (Schneiderman, Braver, & Kang, 2008). Military blast-type TBI (as compared with non-blast injury) also increases the rate of re-experiencing trauma symptoms (Kennedy, Leal, Lewis, Cullen, & Amador, 2010). In civilian populations, the prevalence of PTSD from any type of trauma (TBI and non-TBI-related) is between 6% and 8% (Kessler et al., 2005). When the trauma is TBI, the presence of PTSD ranges from 14% to 56% (Carlson et al., 2011).

Treatment for PTSD can include prescription of specific medications and/or specific types of psychotherapies (Howlett & Stein, 2016). A compounding factor in assessment and treatment of TBI with concomitant PTSD is the presence of over-

| Table 3–5. Signs and Symptoms of Depression |
| --- |
| Persistent sad, anxious, or "empty" mood |
| Feelings of hopelessness, pessimism |
| Feelings of guilt, worthlessness, helplessness |
| Loss of interest or pleasure in hobbies and activities |
| Decreased energy, fatigue, being "slowed down" |
| Difficulty concentrating, remembering, making decisions |
| Difficulty sleeping, early-morning awakening, or oversleeping |
| Appetite and/or weight changes |
| Thoughts of death or suicide, suicide attempts |
| Restlessness, irritability |
| Persistent physical symptoms |

*Source:* National Institute of Mental Health (2016).

lapping symptoms, including irritability, concentration deficits, amnesia for the traumatic event, impairments in cognitive skills, and sleep disturbances (Glaesser, Neuner, Lütgehetmann, Schmidt, & Elbert, 2004, p. 5). This is also true for postconcussive symptoms which overlap with PTSD symptoms in the areas of "depressed mood, anxiety, insomnia, irritability, difficulty concentrating, fatigue, hyperarousal, and avoidance" (Howlett & Stein, 2016, Diagnosis of PTSD and TBI, para. 2). The role of influencing factors of these two diagnoses also needs careful attention in treatment decisions for either TBI or PTSD.

## Physical (Somatic) Concerns

The term "somatic" refers to that which is of or related to the body. Individuals with TBI can have a variety of somatic (physical) concerns after a TBI. These can be temporary or more long term (chronic) in nature. These are important areas of consideration in recovery, as research suggests that the presence and nature of these physical concerns after a TBI can have a negative impact on recovery and functional status (Riggio & Wong, 2009).

Physical trauma to the cranial nerves (CN) can occur with TBI, including associate paresis or paralysis. The facial (CN VII) and vestibulocochlear (CN VIII) cranial nerves are said to be the second most commonly occurring cranial nerve injury after a TBI (Hammon & Masel, 2013). Damage to CN VII can impact facial sensation and facial expression, while damage to CN VIII can impact hearing and balance. Table 3–6 contains a list of additional physical effects resulting from TBI (ASHA, n.d.). Headache, fatigue, seizures, and sleep disturbance will be discussed briefly below.

**Table 3–6.** Common Physical Effects of TBI

Changes in level of consciousness (ranging from brief loss of consciousness to coma)

Seizures

Headaches

Dizziness

Nausea

Fatigue

Reduced muscle strength (paresis/paralysis)

Impairment in movement, balance, and/or coordination, apraxia, and dyspraxia

Motor planning deficits (apraxia and dyspraxia)

*Source:* ASHA (n.d., Physical Effects).

## Headache

Headache after TBI is one of the most commonly reported somatic symptoms (Riggio & Wong, 2009; Riggio, 2010). A premorbid history of headaches increases risk of headaches after TBI. Headaches after TBI range in prevalence from 25% to 90% of individuals who experience a TBI (Baandrup & Jensen, 2005; Paniak et al., 2002). At one year post injury, the cumulative incidence of headaches is 71% after moderate or severe TBI and 91% after mild TBI (Lucas, Hoffman, Bell, Walker, & Dikmen, 2012). Two forms of headache after a TBI have been reported: posttraumatic headache (PTHA), defined as a headache that develops within 7 days after head trauma, and chronic posttraumatic headache (CPTHA), encompassing PTHA that continues for more than 2 months after injury (Defrin, 2014). The frequency of headaches after TBI varies, but many individuals report experiencing daily or weekly headaches which last from a few minutes to a few hours each time (Defrin, 2014). The majority of those with headache after TBI present with symptoms classified as either migraine or probable migraine headaches (Lucas et al., 2012). Treatment for headache after TBI will depend on several factors but can include medications, physical therapy, and manual medicine to the upper cervical spine, and adjunct interventions of cognitive-behavioral therapy and biofeedback (Horn, Siebert, Patel, & Zasler, 2012).

## Fatigue

Fatigue is generally defined as extreme tiredness, resulting from mental or physical exertion. Posttraumatic fatigue (PTF) is common after TBI, ranging from 50% to 80% of individuals with a TBI who report experiencing fatigue (Bushnik, Englander, & Wright, 2008). Two types of fatigue have been described: (1) central fatigue, which impacts primarily mental processes, and (2) peripheral fatigue, which impacts physical, metabolic, and muscular processes (Henrie & Elovic, 2013). Both forms of fatigue are important to consider post trauma, as they stand to impair functional recovery, but central fatigue in particular has relevance to treatment and the role of the SLP and cognitive rehabilitation therapy. PTF is likely related to a combination of factors, such as pain, sleep disorders, cognitive deficits, depression, and anxiety (Riggio & Wong, 2009; Riggio, 2010). Medications and factors such as vertigo, diplopia, and neuroendocrine abnormalities can also play a role in fatigue after TBI. When present, fatigue has been shown to be associated with negative outcomes such as poorer social integration, decreased activity levels, and overall poorer quality of life (Cantor et al. 2008). Manage-

ment of PTF is interdisciplinary in nature and includes approaches such as activity/routine modification, dietary adjustments, and weight loss (Henrie & Elovic, 2013). Adjustments to medications may also be pursued in addressing PTF.

## Seizures

Posttraumatic seizures (PTS) are a common complication of TBI. Estimates suggest that 1 to 5 of every 10 people who have had a TBI will experience a seizure (Englander, Cifu, Diaz-Arrastia, & Model Systems Knowledge Translation Center, 2014, p. 1). These incidence rates vary given the nature of TBI, with markedly higher rates noted for those with open-head/penetrating TBI (35%–65% of individuals) compared with those with closed-head/non-penetrating injury (4%–7% of individuals) (Yablon & Towne, 2013, p. 653). Seizures are caused by abnormal patterns of neuronal discharge in the brain, resulting in sudden, transitory, and abnormal alterations in consciousness, motor, sensory, autonomic, or psychic processes (Yablon & Towne, 2013). After a TBI, seizures can result from the mechanisms of injury itself or other "precipitants," such as hydrocephalus (abnormal buildup of cerebrospinal fluid in the ventricles of the brain), sepsis (presence in tissues of harmful bacteria and their toxins), hypoxia (lack of oxygen to tissues), metabolic abnormalities, or occupying lesions (Yablon & Towne, 2013, p. 636). The use of drugs, alcohol, and prescription medications can also be a seizure precipitant after TBI (Yablon & Towne, 2012). Table 3–7 contains a list of common symptoms of a seizure.

In general, the term "epilepsy" refers to a condition in which seizures recur and are unprovoked by an immediate or identifiable cause. In individuals with TBI, recurrent

| Table 3–7. Common Symptoms of a Seizure |
| --- |
| Strange movement of your head, body, arms, legs, or eyes, such as stiffening or shaking |
| Unresponsiveness and staring |
| Chewing, lip smacking, or fumbling movements |
| Strange smell, sound, feeling, taste, or visual images |
| Sudden tiredness or dizziness |
| Not being able to speak or understand others |

*Source:* Englander, Cifu, Diaz-Arrastia, & Model Systems Knowledge Translation Center (2014, p. 1).

seizures not attributed to other causes are referred to as posttraumatic epilepsy (PTE) (Yablon & Towne, 2012). After TBI, seizures are described as either *early* seizures (a seizure in the first week after a brain injury) or *late* seizures (a seizure more than seven days after a brain injury) (Englander et al., 2014). About 25% of individuals with early seizures will have another seizure months or years later, while 80% of those with a late seizure have another seizure (Englander et al., 2014).

In 2017, the International League Against Epilepsy (ILAE) proposed a new classification of seizures, based on: (1) the nature of the onset of the seizure (focal, generalized, unknown, or focal bilateral onset), (2) the level of awareness during the seizure (aware or not aware), and (3) the characteristics of motor and nonmotor dysfunction at the onset of a seizure. Figure 3–3 contains a summary of this classification.

The specific presentation of seizure post TBI is unique to each person, given seizure type and the area of the brain impacted. After TBI, seizures originating in the fron-

tal lobe and temporal lobes are common but can occur in any area of the brain (Hardman, 1979). Individuals with PTS and PTE have higher rates of mortality (Shavelle, Strauss, Whyte, Day, & Yu, 2001). Recurrent PTS can also have a negative impact on functional status and recovery (Ding, Gupta, & Diaz-Arrastia, 2016), particularly in individuals with open-head/penetrating TBI (Schwab, Grafman, Salazar, & Kraft, 1993; Yablon & Towne, 2013) and those with seizure characterized by status epilepticus (seizures of a prolonged nature, or two or more sequential seizures without full recovery) (Yablon & Towne, 2013). Seizure after TBI is treated with antiepileptic drugs (AEDs), but these medications can have negative side effects (Table 3–8).

## Sleep Disturbance

Sleep disturbances after TBI are common and include insomnia (inability to sleep), hypersomnia (excessive sleep), and sleep-wake cycle disturbances (Rao & Rollings, 2002). The prevalence of sleep disturbance in the general population ranges from 32% to 35% (Riggio & Wong, 2009), but in individuals with TBI this number ranges from 36% to 70% (Rao & Rollings, 2002). As with other somatic changes, persistent sleep disturbances if not properly addressed can lead to a variety of negative outcomes after TBI (Mahowald & Mahowald, 1996). For example, researchers have noted that poor sleep patterns after TBI "may exacerbate symptoms of TBI, impact the individual's ability to cope with these symptoms, increase neuropsychiatric symptoms (depression, anxiety and apathy) post-injury, and inhibit full participation in rehabilitation treatments" (Gilbert, Kark, Gehrman, & Bogdanova, 2015, p. 196). This is something to consider in the provision of treatment services for

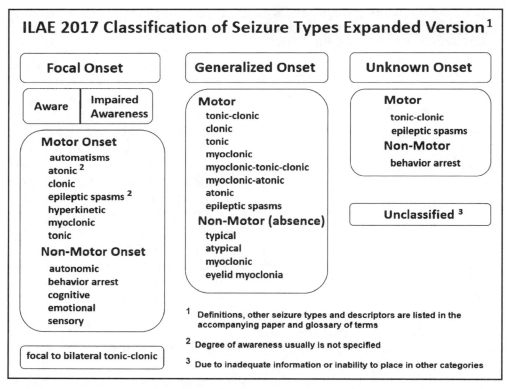

**Figure 3–3.** ILAE 2017 classification of seizure types expanded version. *Source:* International League against Epilepsy (ILAE). Permission is granted from the author (Robert Fisher, M.D., PhD). To learn more, visit: http://www.epilepsy.com/article/2016/12/2017-revised-classification-seizures

**Table 3–8.** Potential Negative Side Effects of Antiepileptic Drugs (AEDs)

Sleepiness or fatigue

Dizziness or lack of balance

Lightheadedness

Trembling

Double vision

Confusion

*Source:* Englander, Cifu, Diaz-Arrastia, & Model Systems Knowledge Translation Center (2014, p. 3).

TBI. Generally, management of sleep disturbances after TBI may include adjustments to medications, along with environmental modifications and behavioral intervention.

## Speech Concerns

TBI can impact all aspects of speech production, including respiration, phonation, and articulation (Cherney et al., 2010). After a TBI, some form of speech disorder has been reported in up to 65% of acute rehabilitation patients and 22% of outpatient rehabilitation patients (Yorkston, Honsinger, Mitsuda, & Hammen, 1989). The most commonly occurring motor speech deficit after TBI is dysarthria (Theodoros, Murdoch, & Chenery, 1994). Apraxia of speech and stuttering can also occur but are rarer after TBI (Morgan & Ward, 2009).

Dysarthria is relatively common following TBI, and particularly in closed-head injury TBI (Theodoros et al., 1994). Estimates of dysarthria in individuals after a TBI range from 8% to 100%, depending on the population studied, when the speech sample is taken after a TBI, and the degree of deficit measured (Yorkston et al., 1989, p. 2). Several researchers have noted dysarthria to be present in approximately one third of individuals with closed-head injury (Rusk, Block, & Lowmann, 1969; Sarno, 1980; Taylor Sarno, Buonaguro, & Levita, 1986). Both upper and lower motor neuron systems have been implicated in dysarthria following TBI. In severe TBI, dysarthria is one of the most persistent sequelae, often remaining beyond resolutions of concomitant language disorders (Murdoch, 2010).

As has been mentioned, individuals with TBI are unique, as is the nature of trauma associated with TBI. As such, there is wide variability in severity and presenting characteristics of dysarthria following TBI (Murdoch, 2010). This can range from speech that has mild articulation imprecision to speech that is totally unintelligible. Although spastic, hyperkinetic/hypokinetic, ataxic, flaccid, and mixed dysarthrias are noted to occur after TBI, spastic and mixed dysarthias are the most common subtypes reported after TBI (Theodoros et al., 1994; Morgan & Ward, 2010; Murdoch, 2010). Speech-language pathologists play a key role in intervention for speech concerns following TBI, including assessment and treatment targeted at function and effective communication across a variety of contexts. This is often in tandem with cognitive rehabilitation therapy.

## Swallowing Concerns

The presence of swallowing impairments (dysphagia) after TBI is common. Incidence of dysphagia following TBI range from 41% to 65% of individuals with TBI (Cherney & Halper, 1996; Halper, Cherney, Cichowski, & Zhang, 1999). The presence of dysphagia and its severity is linked to TBI severity and several risk markers. In general, the more severe the TBI, the more likely and more severe the dysphagia. For example, increased intracranial pressure and coma duration greater than 24 hours are closely associated with moderate to severe dysphagia, following closed-head TBI (Lazarus & Logemann, 1987). Similarly, lower scores on the Glasgow Coma Scale (GCS) and Rancho Los Amigos Scale (RLAS) (Mackay, Morgan, & Bernstein, 1999), as well as poor performance in outcome measures suggestive of a more severe TBI are also linked to increased risk and severity of dysphagia following TBI (Hansen, Engberg, & Larsen, 2008).

Dysphagia following TBI can be multifaceted and can impact any of the three phases of the swallow (oral preparatory phase, the oral phase, and the pharyngeal phase) (Howle, Baguley, & Brown, 2014). Table 3–9 contains a list of common oropharyngeal abnormalities following TBI. Dysphagia after TBI is caused and influenced by a number of factors unique to TBI, such as oropharyngeal neuromuscular, sensory, cognitive-communication, and behavioral impairments, as well as physical injury to the head and neck, medications, and concomitant injuries and prolonged endotracheal ventilation (Howle et al., 2014). Individuals with TBI are also at risk for acute aspiration and associated pulmonary complications due to an unprotected airway as a result of loss of consciousness, or due to acute intubation, either at the scene of the trauma or during acute hospitalization (Morgan & Mackay, 1999).

As with speech concerns, the SLP is a key team member in providing intervention services for dysphagia follow TBI. The

| **Table 3–9.** Common Oropharyngeal Abnormalities Following TBI |
| --- |
| Abnormal oral reflexes |
| Reduction in lingual range of motion or coordination of lingual movement |
| Increased muscle tone of the oral musculature |
| Reduction in labial strength |
| Delay in triggering the pharyngeal swallow |
| Reduction in velopharyngeal closure |
| Reduction in strength of the base of the tongue |
| Abnormal pharyngeal constrictor activation |
| Reduction in laryngeal elevation |

*Source:* Morgan & Mackay (1999, p. 458).

| **Table 3–10.** Common Visual Effects of TBI |
| --- |
| Double vision (diplopia) |
| Changes in visual acuity |
| Sensitivity to light |
| Problems with visual convergence and accommodation |
| Visual field deficits/visual neglect |

*Source:* ASHA (n.d., Visual Effects).

imperative nature of immediate and effective assessment and treatment in this area cannot be understated, given the critical role that adequate nutrition and hydration play in healing, but also given the risk for mortality and significant medical complications associated with aspiration pneumonia (Howle, Nott, & Baguley, 2011).

## Visual Concerns

Impairments in vision after a TBI are common. Research suggests that the incidence of visual disturbance after a TBI ranges from 30% to 85%, depending on the nature of the TBI and the type of visual deficit measured (Kapoor & Ciuffreda, 2002). Vision concerns can vary from blurred vision to double vision, or even blindness (Kelts, 2010, p. 225). Table 3–10 contains a list of some common visual effects resulting from TBI. The origins of visual deficits after TBI can result from direct trauma to the occipital cortex or from indirect trauma to the brainstem and oculomotor nerves (Kelts, 2010; Van Stavern, Biousse, Lynn, Simon, & Newman, 2001). The visual system is susceptible to injury given that it comprises a broad expanse of cortical territory, consisting of both afferent and efferent pathways (Kelts, 2010). Afferent pathways receive and process visual input, carrying impulses from the eye to the central nervous system (CNS), whereas efferent pathways carry impulses from the CNS to the eye, controlling eye movements (Kelts, 2010). In a meta-analysis of research studies in the area, Van Stavern et al. (2001) reported that abnormal neuro-ophthalmic examinations were present in 56.7% of individuals with TBI. Of those, 58% had efferent pathway deficits, while 50% had afferent pathway deficits. The most common efferent deficit reported was ocular motor cranial nerve palsy. The most common afferent deficits reported were visual field defects.

Any deficits in vision after TBI are particularly relevant to the treatment offered by an SLP, due to the integral role of written language (both expression and comprehension) in functional recovery following a

TBI, but also given the routine use of visual modes of stimulus presentation in the types of treatment provided by an SLP. Individuals with vision concerns after a TBI should be assessed by an optometrist or ophthalmologist with experience evaluating and treating visual dysfunction after TBI (Kelts, 2010).

Treatment options may include surgery, vision rehabilitation therapy, and/or compensatory strategies and devices (Powell, Weintraub, Deer, & Novack, 2015). Common compensatory strategies and devices used to address vision deficits after TBI are listed in Table 3–11.

**Table 3–11.** Examples of Compensatory Strategies and Devices for Visual Deficits after TBI

Corrective glasses or bifocals

Specialized glasses, such as prism glasses to address double vision

Patching for double vision

Frequent breaks when reading, watching television, or using a computer or other electronic devices

Increased contrast on visual surfaces

Avoiding certain light sources, such as fluorescent lights

Reducing glare by wearing tinted sunglasses and covering shiny surfaces that reflect light

Avoiding visual distraction by minimizing clutter in home and work environments

Devices such as talking timers, alarm clocks, screen-reading software for computers, and various mobile phone apps to aid in loss of vision

*Source:* Powell, Weintraub, & Deer (2015, pp. 1933–1934). Used with permission.

## References

American Psychiatric Association. (2013). *Diagnostic and statistical manual of mental disorders* (5th ed.). Washington, DC: Author.

American Speech-Language-Hearing Association. (n.d.). *Traumatic brain injury in adults* (Practice Portal). Retrieved from http://www.asha.org/Practice-Portal/Clinical-Topics/Traumatic-Brain-Injury-in-Adults/

Andersson, S., & Bergedalen, A. M. (2002). Cognitive correlates of apathy in traumatic brain injury. *Neuropsychiatry, Neuropsychology, and Behavioral Neurology, 15*(3), 184–191.

Andersson, S., Krogstad, J. M., & Finset, A. (1999). Apathy and depressed mood in acquired brain damage: Relationship to lesion localization and psychophysiological reactivity. *Psychological Medicine, 29*(2), 447–456.

Arnould, A., Dromer, E., Rochat, L., Van der Linden, M., & Azouvi, P. (2016). Neurobehavioral and self-awareness changes after traumatic brain injury: Towards new multidimensional approaches. *Annals of Physical and Rehabilitation Medicine, 59*(1), 18–22.

Arnould, A., Rochat, L., Azouvi, P., & Linden, M. (2013). A multidimensional approach to apathy after traumatic brain injury. *Neuropsychology Review, 23*(3), 210–233.

Baandrup, L., & Jensen, R. (2005). Chronic posttraumatic headache—a clinical analysis in relation to the International Headache Classification, 2nd edition. *Cephalalgia, 25*(2), 132–138.

Bergemalm, P. O. (2003). Progressive hearing loss after closed head injury: A predictable outcome? *Acta Otolaryngologia, 123*(7), 836–845.

Bombardier, C. H., Fann, J. R., Temkin, N. R., Esselman, P. C. Barber, J., & Dikmen, S. S. (2010). Rates of major depressive disorder and clinical outcomes following traumatic brain injury. *Journal of the American Medical Association, 303*, 1938–1945.

Bushnik, T., Englander, J., & Wright, J. (2008). The experience of fatigue in the first 2 years after moderate-to-severe traumatic brain injury: A preliminary report. *Journal of Head Trauma Rehabilitation, 23*(1), 17–24.

Cantor, J., Ashman, T., Gordon, W., Ginsberg, A., Engmann, C., Egan, M., . . . Flanagan, S. (2008). Fatigue after traumatic brain injury and its impact on participation and quality of life. *Journal of Head Trauma Rehabilitation, 23*(1), 41–51.

Carlson, K. F., Kehle, S. M., Meis, L. A., Greer, N., MacDonald, R., Rutks, I., . . . Wilt, T. J. (2011). Prevalence, assessment, and treatment of mild traumatic brain injury and posttraumatic stress disorder: A systematic review of the evidence. *Journal of Head Trauma Rehabilitation, 26*(2), 103–115.

Chamelian, L., & Feinstein, A. (2006). The effect of major depression on subjective and objective cognitive deficits in mild to moderate traumatic brain injury. *Journal of Neuropsychiatry and Clinical Neurosciences, 18*, 33–38.

Cherney, L. R., Gardner, P., Logemann, J. A., Newman, L. A., O'Neil-Pirozzi, T., Roth, C. R., & Solomon, N. P. (2010). The role of speech-language pathology and audiology in the optimal management of the service member returning from Iraq or Afghanistan with a blast-related head injury: Position of the communication sciences and disorders clinical trials research group. *Journal of Head Trauma Rehabilitation, 25*(3), 219–224.

Cherney, L. R., & Halper, A. S. (1996). Swallowing problems in adults with traumatic brain injury. *Seminars in Neurology, 16*(4), 349–353.

Choi, C. (2012). Mechanisms and treatment of blast induced hearing loss. *Korean Journal of Audiology, 16*(3), 103.

Coelho, D. H., & Hoffer, M. (2013). Audiologic impairment. In N. Zasler, D. I. Katz, R. D. Zafonte, D. B. Arciniegas, M. B. Bullock, & J. S. Kreutzer (Eds.), *Brain injury medicine: Principles and practice* (2nd ed.). New York, NY: Demos Medical.

Defrin, R. (2014). Chronic post-traumatic headache: Clinical findings and possible mechanisms. *Journal of Manual & Manipulative Therapy, 22*(1), 36–43.

Diaz, A. P., Schwarzbold, M. L., Thais, M. E., Hohl, A., Bertotti, M. M., Schmoeller, R., . . . Walz, R. (2012). Psychiatric disorders and health-related quality of life after severe traumatic brain injury: A prospective study. *Journal of Neurotrauma, 29,* 1029–1037.

Ding, K., Gupta, P. K., & Diaz-Arrastia, R. (2016). Epilepsy after traumatic brain injury. In D. Laskowitz & G. Grant (Eds.), *Translational research in traumatic brain injury* (pp. 299–314). Boca Raton, FL: CRC Press/Taylor and Francis Group. Retrieved from: https://www.ncbi.nlm.nih.gov/books/NBK326716/

Englander, J., Cifu, D. X., Diaz-Arrastia, R., & Model Systems Knowledge Translation Center. (2014). Seizures after traumatic brain injury. *Archives of Physical Medicine and Rehabilitation, 95*(6), 1223–1224. https://doi.org/10.1016/j.apmr.2013.06.002

Fausti, S. A., Wilmington, D. J., Gallun, F. J., Myers, P. J., & Henry, J. A. (2009). Auditory and vestibular dysfunction associated with blast-related traumatic brain injury. *Journal of Rehabilitation Research & Development, 46*(6), 797–809.

Garcia, J. (1994). Behavior after a traumatic brain injury: Toward a classification based on three outcome categories. *Rehabilitation Education, 8*(3), 259–274.

Gilbert, K., Kark, S., Gehrman, P., & Bogdanova, Y. (2015). Sleep disturbances, TBI and PTSD: Implications for treatment and recovery. *Clinical Psychology Review, 40,* 195–212.

Glaesser, J., Neuner, F., Lütgehetmann, R., Schmidt, R., & Elbert, T. (2004). Posttraumatic stress disorder in patients with traumatic brain injury. *BMC Psychiatry, 4,* 5.

Glenn, M. B., Burke, D. T., O'Neil-Pirozzi, T., Goldstein, R., Jacob, L., & Kettell, J. (2002). Cutoff score on the apathy evaluation scale in subjects with traumatic brain injury. *Brain Injury, 16*(6), 509–516.

Goverover, Y., & Chiaravalloti, N. (2014). The impact of self-awareness and depression on subjective reports of memory, quality-of-life and satisfaction with life following TBI. *Brain Injury, 28*(2), 174–180.

Gray, J. M., Shepherd, M., & McKinley, W. W. (1994). Negative symptoms in the traumatically brain injured during the first year post-discharge, and their effect on rehabilitation status, work status and family burden. *Clinical Rehabilitation, 8*(3), 188–197.

Greenspan, A. I., Stringer A. Y., Phillips, V. L., Hammond, F. M., & Goldstein, F. C. (2006). Symptoms of post-traumatic stress: Intrusion and avoidance 6 and 12 months after TBI. *Brain Injury, 20,* 733–742.

Griffen, J., & Hanks, R. (2014). Cognitive and behavioral outcomes from traumatic brain injury. In M. Sherer & A. Sander (Eds.), *Handbook on the neuropsychology of traumatic brain injury.* New York, NY: Springer.

Halper, A. S., Cherney, L. R., Cichowski, K., & Zhang, M. (1999). Dysphagia after head trauma: The effect of cognitive-communicative impairments on functional outcomes. *Journal of Head Trauma Rehabilitation, 14*(5), 486–496.

Hammon, F. M., & Masel, T. (2013). Cranial Nerve Disorders. In N. Zasler, D. I. Katz, R. D. Zafonte, D. B. Arciniegas, M. B. Bullock, & J. S. Kreutzer (Eds.), *Brain injury medicine: Principles and practice* (2nd ed.). New York, NY: Demos Medical.

Hansen, T. S., Engberg, A. W., & Larsen, K. (2008). Functional oral intake time to reach unrestricted dieting for patients with traumatic brain injury. *Archives of Physical Medicine Rehabilitation, 89,* 1556–1562.

Hardman, J. M. (1979). The pathology of traumatic brain injuries. *Advances in Neurology, 22,* 15–50.

Hart, T., Hoffman, J., Pretz, C., Kennedy, R., Clark, A., & Brenner, L. A. (2012). A longitudinal study of major and minor depression following traumatic brain injury. *Archives of Physical Medicine and Rehabilitation, 93*(8), 1343–1349.

Harvey, A. G., & Bryant, R. A. (2000). Two-year prospective evaluation of the relationship between acute stress disorder and posttraumatic stress disorder following mild traumatic brain injury. *American Journal of Psychiatry, 15,* 626–628.

Henrie, M., & Elovic, E. (2013). Fatigue: Assessment and treatment. In N. Zasler, D. I. Katz, R. D. Zafonte, D. B. Arciniegas, M. B. Bullock, & J. S. Kreutzer (Eds.), *Brain injury medicine: Principles and practice* (2nd ed.). New York, NY: Demos Medical.

Hoge, C., & Castro, C. (2014). Treatment of generalized war-related health concerns: Placing

TBI and PTSD in context. *Journal of American Medical Association, 312*(16), 1685.

Horn, L. J., Siebert, B., Patel, N., & Zasler, N. D. (2013). Post traumatic headache. In N. Zasler, D. I. Katz, R. D. Zafonte, D. B. Arciniegas, M. B. Bullock, & J. S. Kreutzer (Eds.), *Brain injury medicine: Principles and practice* (2nd ed.). New York, NY: Demos Medical.

Howle, A. A., Baguley, I. J., & Brown, L. (2014). Management of dysphagia following traumatic brain injury. *Current Physical Medicine and Rehabilitation Reports, 2*(4), 219–230.

Howle, A., Nott, M., & Baguley, I. (2011). Aspiration pneumonia following severe traumatic brain injury: Prevalence and risk factors for long-term mortality. *Brain Impairment, 12*(3), 179–186.

Howlett, J. R., & Stein, M. B. (2016). Post-traumatic stress disorder: Relationship to traumatic brain injury and approach to treatment. In D. Laskowitz & G. Grant (Eds.), *Translational research in traumatic brain injury*. Boca Raton, FL: CRC Press/Taylor and Francis Group. Retrieved from https://www.ncbi.nlm.nih.gov/books/NBK326723/

Jorge, R., & Robinson, R. G. (2003). Mood disorders following traumatic brain injury. *International Review of Psychiatry, 15*(4), 317–327.

Kapoor, N., & Ciuffreda, K. (2002). Vision disturbances following traumatic brain injury. *Current Treatment Options in Neurology, 4*(4), 271–280.

Kelts, E. (2010). Traumatic brain injury and visual dysfunction: A limited overview. *NeuroRehabilitation, 27*(3), 223–229.

Kennedy, J. E., Leal, F. O., Lewis, J. D., Cullen, M. A., & Amador, R. R. (2010). Posttraumatic stress symptoms in OIF/OEF service members with blast-related and non-blast-related mild TBI. *NeuroRehabilitation, 26*(3), 223–231.

Kennedy, R. E., Livingston, L., Riddick, A., Marwitz, J. H., Kreutzer, J. H., & Zasler N. D. (2005). Evaluation of the Neurobehavioral Functioning Inventory as a depression screening tool after traumatic brain injury. *Journal of Head Trauma Rehabilitation, 20*, 512–526.

Kessler R. C., Berglund, P., Demler, O., Jin, R., Merikangas, K. R., & Walters, E. E. (2005). Lifetime prevalence and age-of-onset distributions of DSM-IV disorders in the National Comorbidity Survey Replication. *Archives of General Psychiatry, 62*(6), 593–602.

Kocka, A., & Gagnon, J. (2014). Definition of impulsivity and related terms following traumatic brain injury: A review of the different concepts and measures used to assess impulsivity, disinhibition and other related concepts. *Behavioral Sciences, 4*(4), 352–370.

Lane-Brown, A., & Tate, R. (2011). Apathy after traumatic brain injury: An overview of the current state of play. *Brain Impairment, 12*(1), 43–53.

Lazarus, C., & Logemann, J. A. (1987). Swallowing disorders in closed head trauma patients. *Archives of Physical Medicine Rehabilitation, 68*, 79–84.

Lengenfelder, J., Goverover, Y., Cagna, C., Smith, A., & Chiaravalloti, N. (2016). The relationship between apathy and health-related quality of life in individuals with traumatic brain injury (TBI). *Archives of Physical Medicine and Rehabilitation, 97*(10), e78.

Lucas, S., Hoffman, J., Bell, K., Walker, W., & Dikmen, S. (2012). Characterization of headache after traumatic brain injury. *Cephalalgia, 32*(8), 600–606.

Mackay, L. E., Morgan, A. S., & Bernstein, B. A. (1999). Swallowing disorders in severe brain injury: Risk factors affecting return to oral intake. *Archives of Physical Medicine and Rehabilitation, 80*(4), 365–371.

Mahowald, M. W., & Mahowald, M. L. (1996). Sleep disorders. In M. Rizzo & D. Tranel (Eds.), *Head injury and postconcussive syndrome* (pp. 285–304). New York, NY: Churchill Livingstone.

Malec, J. F., Testa J. A., Rush B. K., Brown A. W., & Moessner A. M. (2007). Self assessment of impairment, impaired self-awareness, and depression after traumatic brain injury. *Journal of Head Trauma Rehabilitation, 22*, 156–166.

McAllister, T. (2011). Neurobiological consequences of traumatic brain injury. *Dialogues in Clinical Neuroscience, 13*(3), 287–300.

McMillan, T. M. (1991). Post-traumatic stress disorder and severe head injury. *British Journal of Psychiatry, 159*, 431–433.

McMillan, T. M. (1996). Posttraumatic stress disorder following minor and severe closed head injury: 10 single cases. *Brain Injury,10*, 749–758.

Morgan, A. S., & Mackay, L. E. (1999). Causes and complications associated with swallowing disorders in traumatic brain injury. *Journal of Head Trauma Rehabilitation, 14*(5), 454–461.

Morgan, A. T., & Ward, E. C. (2009). Traumatic brain injury. In E. C. Ward & A. T. Morgan (Eds.), *Dysphagia post trauma* (pp. 31–65). San Diego, CA: Plural.

Mulin, E., Leone, E., Dujardin, K., Delliaux, M., Leentjens, A., Nobili, F., . . . Robert, P. H. (2011). Diagnostic criteria for apathy in clinical practice. *International Journal of Geriatric Psychiatry, 26*(2), 158–165.

Murdoch, B. E. (2010). Speech-language disorders associated with traumatic brain injury. In B. E. Murdoch (Ed.), *Acquired speech and language disorders: A neuroanatomical and functional neurological approach* (2nd ed., pp. 118–152). Oxford, UK: Wiley-Blackwell.

Murdoch, B. E., Theodoros, D. G., Stokes, P. D., and Cherney, H. J. (1993). Abnormal patterns of speech breathing in dysarthria following severe closed head injury. *Brain Injury, 7*, 295–308.

National Institute of Mental Health. (2016). *Depression.* Retrieved from https://www.nimh.nih.gov/health/topics/depression/index.shtml

Ouellet, M. C., Beaulieu-Bonneau, S., & Morin, C. M. (2013). Sleep-wake disturbances. In N. Zasler, D. I. Katz, R. D. Zafonte, D. B. Arciniegas, M. B. Bullock, & J. S. Kreutzer (Eds.), *Brain injury medicine: Principles and practice* (2nd ed.). New York, NY: Demos Medical.

Padula, W. V., Singman, E., Vicci, V., Munitz, R., & Magrun, W. M. (2013). Evaluating and treating visual dysfunction. In N. Zasler, D. I. Katz, R. D. Zafonte, D. B. Arciniegas, M. B. Bullock, & J. S. Kreutzer (Eds.), *Brain injury medicine: Principles and practice* (2nd ed.). New York, NY: Demos Medical.

Paniak, C., Reynolds, S., Phillips, K., Toller-Lobe, G., Melnyk, A., & Nagy, J. (2002). Patient complaints within 1 month of mild traumatic brain injury: A controlled study. *Archives of Clinical Neuropsychology, 17*(4), 319–334.

Powell, J., Weintraub, A., Dreer, L., & Novack, T. (2015). Vision problems after traumatic brain injury. *Archives of Physical Medicine and Rehabilitation, 96*(10), 1933.

Ramchand, R., Schell, T. L., Karney, B. R., Osilla, K. C., Burns, R. M., & Caldarone, L. B. (2010). Disparate prevalence estimates of PTSD among service members who served in Iraq and Afghanistan: Possible explanations. *Journal of Trauma Stress, 23*(1), 59–68.

Rao, V., & Rollings, P. (2002). Sleep disturbances following traumatic brain injury. *Current Treatment Options in Neurology, 4*(1), 77–87.

Riggio, S. (2010). Traumatic brain injury and its neurobehavioral sequelae. *Psychiatric Clinics of North America, 33*(4), 807–819.

Riggio, S., & Wong, M. (2009). Neurobehavioral sequelae of traumatic brain injury. *Mount Sinai Journal of Medicine: A Journal of Translational and Personalized Medicine, 76*(2), 163–172.

Rochat, L., Beni, C., Annoni, J., Vuadens, P., & Van der Linden, M. (2013). How inhibition relates to impulsivity after moderate to severe traumatic brain injury. *Journal of the International Neuropsychological Society: JINS, 19*(8), 890–898.

Rochat, L., Beni, C., Billieux, J., Azouvi, P., Annoni, J., & Van der Linden, M. (2010). Assessment of impulsivity after moderate to severe traumatic brain injury. *Neuropsychological Rehabilitation, 20*(5), 778–797.

Rogers, J. M., & Read, C. A. (2007). Psychiatric comorbidity following traumatic brain injury. *Brain Injury, 2*, 1321–1333.

Rusk, H., Block, J., & Lowmann, E. (1969). Rehabiliation of the brain injured patient: A report of 157 cases with long-term follow-up of 118. In E. Walker, W. Caveness, & M. Critchley (Eds.), *The late effects of head injury* (pp. 327–332). Springfield, IL: Charles C. Thomas.

Sarno, M. T. (1980). The nature of verbal impairment after closed head injury. *Journal of Nervous and Mental Disorders, 168*, 685–692.

Schneiderman A. I., Braver E. R., & Kang H. K. (2008). Understanding sequelae of injury mechanisms and mild traumatic brain injury incurred during the conflicts in Iraq and Afghanistan: Persistent postconcussive symptoms and posttraumatic stress disorder. *American Journal of Epidemiology, 167*(12), 1446–1452.

Schwarzbold, M., Diaz, A., Martins, E. T., Rufino, A., Amante, L., Thais, M. E., . . . Walz, R. (2008). Psychiatric disorders and traumatic brain injury. *Neuropsychiatric Disease and Treatment*, Issue 4, 797–816.

Shavelle, R. M., Strauss, D., Whyte, J., Day, S. M., & Yu, Y. L. (2001). Long-term causes of death after traumatic brain injury. *American Journal of Physical Medicine and Rehabilitation, 80*(7), 510–516.

Sohlberg, M. M., & Mateer, C. M. (2001). *Cognitive rehabilitation: An integrative neuropsychological approach*. New York, NY: Guilford Press.

Taylor Sarno, M., Buonaguro, A., & Levita, E. (1986). Characteristics of verbal impairments in closed head injured patients. *Archives of Physical Medicine and Rehabilitation, 67*, 400–403.

Theodoros, D. G., & Murdoch, B. E. (1994). Laryngeal dysfunction in dysarthric speakers following severe closed head injury. *Brain Injury, 8*, 667–684.

Theodoros, D. G., Murdoch, B. E., & Chenery, H. J. (1994). Perceptual speech characteristics of dysarthric speakers following severe closed head injury. *Brain Injury, 8*(2), 101–124.

Theodoros, D. G., Murdoch, B. E., & Stokes, P. D. (1995). A physiological analysis of articulatory dysfunction in dysarthric speakings following severe closed head injury. *Brain Injury, 9*, 237–254.

Theodoros, D. G., Murdoch, B. E., Stokes, P. D., & Cherney, H. J. (1993). Hypernasality in dysarthric speakers following severe closed head injury: A perceptual and instrumental analysis. *Brain Injury, 7*, 59–69.

Vander Werff, K. R. (2012). Auditory dysfunction among long-term consequences of mild traumatic brain injury (mTBI). *SIG 6 Perspectives on Hearing and Hearing Disorders: Research and Diagnostics, 16*, 3–17.

van Reekum, R., Cohen, T., & Wong, J. (2000). Can traumatic brain injury cause psychiatric disorders? *Journal of Neuropsychiatry Clinical Neuroscience, 12*, 316–327.

Van Stavern, G., Biousse, V., Lynn, M., Simon, D. J., & Newman, M. J. (2001). Neuro-ophthalmic manifestations of head trauma. *Journal of Neuro-ophthalmology 21*(2), 112–117.

Whiteside, S. P., & Lynam, D. R. (2001). The five factor model and impulsivity: Using a structural model of personality to understand impulsivity. *Personality and Individual Differences, 30*(4), 669–689.

Yablon, S. A., & Towne, A. R. (2013). Post-traumatic seizures and epilepsy. In N. Zasler, D. I. Katz, R. D. Zafonte, D. B. Arciniegas, M. B. Bullock, & J. S. Kreutzer (Eds.), *Brain injury medicine: Principles and practice* (2nd ed.). New York, NY: Demos Medical.

Yorkston, K. M., Honsinger, M. J., Mitsuda, P. M., & Hammen, V. (1989). The relationship between speech and swallowing disorders in head-injured patients. *Journal of Head Trauma Rehabilitation, 4*(4), 1–16.

Zimmerman, W. D., Ganzel, T. M., Windmill, I. M., Nazar, G. B., & Phillips, M. (1993). Peripheral hearing loss following head trauma in children. *Laryngoscope, 101*, 1, 87–91.

# 4 Cognition and Communication

*The brain is more than an assemblage of autonomous modules, each crucial for a specific mental function. Every one of these functionally specialized areas must interact with dozens or hundreds of others, their total integration creating something like a vastly complicated orchestra with thousands of instruments, an orchestra that conducts itself, with an ever-changing score and repertoire.*

—Oliver Sacks

This chapter will review the scope of cognitive and communication deficits common to TBI, including defining aspects of "cognitive-communicative" disorders. Cognitive impairments described in this chapter are parsed into the categories of attention, memory, executive function, and social cognition, patterned after the categorical nature of the research literature on this topic. However, as the quote at the start of this chapter suggests, the brain and human beings are non-categorical. Communication and cognition are inescapably interconnected, as are the domains of cognition to one another. Communication and cognition are also both at the heart of all the domains of daily function (Figure 4–1).

## Communication

Many decades of research have consistently shown communication impairments after TBI to be both common and enduring in nature (Coelho, Liles, & Duffy, 1995; Ghayoumi et al., 2015; McDonald, 1993; O'Flaherty & Douglas, 1997; Rousseaux, Verigneaux, & Kozlowski, 2010; Snow, Douglas, & Ponsford, 1999; Togher, Hand, & Code, 1997). Table 4–1 contains an example of common communication deficits associated with TBI (ASHA, n.d.-a). These are defined as cognitive-communication disorders. According to the American Speech-Language-Hearing Association (ASHA), cognitive-communication disorders "encompass difficulty with any aspect of communication that is affected by disruption of cognition" (ASHA, 2005, para. 1). Cognitive-communication disorders are further defined as:

A set of communication features that result from underlying deficits in cognition. Communication difficulties can include issues with hearing, listening, understanding, speaking, reading, writing, conversational interaction and social communication. These disorders may occur as a result of underlying deficits with cognition, that is: attention, orientation, memory, organization, information processing, reasoning,

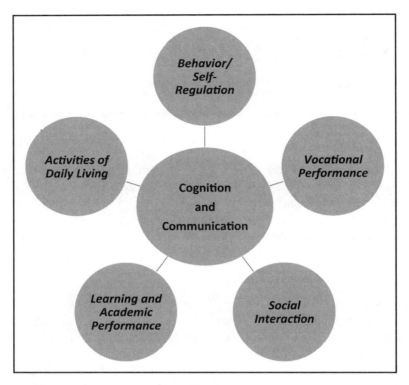

**Figure 4–1.** Foundational aspects of the intersections of cognition, communication, and important life functions.

problem solving, executive functions, or self-regulation. (College of Audiologists and Speech-Language Pathologists of Ontario, CASLPO, 2015, p. 2)

One aspect to consider further in defining cognitive-communication disorders is the relationship to cognition and language. As highlighted by ASHA, "cognition and language are intrinsically and reciprocally related. . . . An impairment of language may disrupt one or more cognitive processes, and, similarly, an impairment of one or more cognitive processes may disrupt language." (ASHA, n.d.-a, Signs and Symptoms) Although the two can co-occur, the presence of aphasia in individuals with TBI (and in particular those with closed-head injury) is rare. In one of the largest stud-

ies on this topic, aphasia due to TBI was noted to be diagnosed in only 2% of those individuals with closed-head injury (Heilman, Safran, & Geschwind, 1971). When standardized tests of aphasia are utilized, presenting features most closely resemble anomic aphasia after closed-head injury (Heilman et al., 1971). However, overall performance on these types of measures is not usually impaired enough in individuals with TBI to meet the criteria of aphasia (Levin, Grossman, & Kelly, 1976; Levin, Grossman, & Rose, 1979). Delayed word retrieval and self-cueing of correct responses using semantic association and circumlocution are generally noted in individuals with TBI on tests of this nature, with error patterns more similar to those of controls than individuals with aphasia.

| **Table 4–1.** Common Cognitive-Communication Deficits Following TBI |
| :--- |

*Comprehension deficits including:*

- Deficits in processing abstract language/concepts (e.g., figurative speech)
- Difficulty in interpreting the subtleties of conversation (e.g., humor, sarcasm)
- Impaired interpretation of nonverbal communication, such as tone of voice, facial expression, and body language
- Increased auditory processing time

*Verbal expression deficits including:*

- Anomia or word retrieval deficits
- Difficulty with discourse, including
  - coherence, confabulatory speech
  - content
  - story grammar
- Increased response latencies
- Perseveration of verbal responses
- Reduced word fluency

*Difficulty with pragmatics/social communication, including:*

- Conversational topic selection and maintenance marked by verbosity
- Initiating conversation
- Producing/interpreting nonverbal communication, such as facial expressions and body language
- Turn-taking
- Using an appropriate tone of voice

*Reading deficits, including difficulty in reading comprehension, especially with complex syntax and figurative language (e.g., idioms, metaphors, similes)*

*Writing deficits that may mirror deficits in verbal communication—writing difficulty may also be a result of motor deficits in the dominant hand and/or visuospatial deficits*

*Source:* ASHA (n.d.-a, Signs and Symptoms).

Contemporary views on language impairments in individuals with TBI, and specifically those with closed-head injury, hold that the communication difficulty following TBI occurs either secondary to cognitive disruptions common to TBI (e.g., due to attention, memory, executive function impairments) or interdependently of these disrupted processes (McDonald, Togher, & Code, 2014; Murdoch, 2010). This is reflected in Figure 4–2 with communication at the center of the process of cognition: attention, memory, executive function, and social cognition (Strutchen, n.d.). Regardless of the origin of difficulty, if one reflects more deeply on the nature of cognitive-communication deficits listed in Table 4–1, it is easy to see why any combination thereof could pose a substantial barrier to individuals with TBI across a variety of contexts.

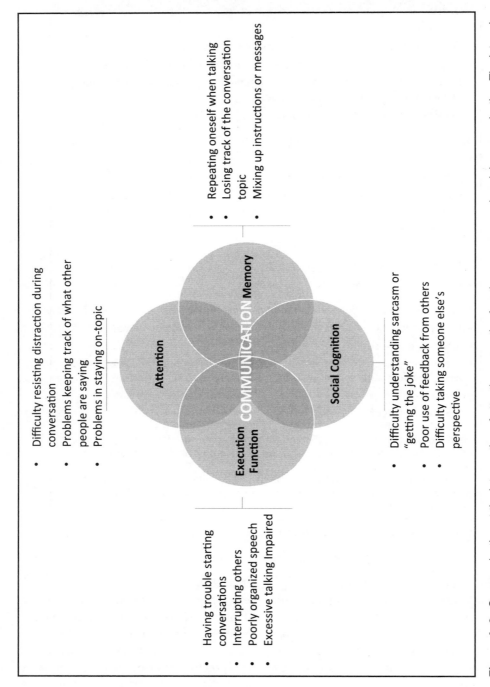

**Figure 4–2.** Communication at the intersection of attention, executive function, memory, and social communication. The interrelationship between all cognition and communication.

## Cognition

Cognition is commonly impaired in individuals with TBI (Dikmen, Machamer, Winn, & Temkin, 1995; Draper & Ponsford, 2008; Spitz, Ponsford, Rudzki, Maller, & Rao, 2012). Table 4–2 lists several common cognitive impairments following TBI. Attention, memory, executive function, and social cognition will be discussed in the sections that follow, including additional examples of the "Key to Communication" in relation to deficits in these areas.

## Attention

Table 4–3 contains examples of the potential impact on communication due to impairments in attention (Key to Communication). There are varying definitions and conceptual frames to describe attention. Despite differing perspectives, these definitions are consistent in identifying attention as multifaceted and requiring a vast array of diffuse and interconnected neural systems. Table 4–4 describes three broad systems that subserve attention, their general purpose, and areas in the brain thought to mediate that function.

Attention can be thought of in two broad categories: (1) intensity and (2) selectivity (Van Zomeren & Brouwer, 1994; Ponsford et al., 2014). Intensity involves the *level of attention* required, such as arousal, alertness, and vigilance, while selectivity involves the *level of filtering* required, such as inhibiting irrelevant sensory information (auditory, visual, tactile, or cognitive). More recent models of attention also include the concept of a central or strategic control mechanism that allows for direction of these attentional processes as needed, such as maintaining attention over time, inhibiting distracting influences, shifting attention to changing goals and priorities, and dividing attention between tasks (Ponsford et al., 2014, p. 322).

| **Table 4–2.** Common Cognitive Impairments Following TBI |
|---|
| Impaired attention |
| Decreased concentration |
| Easy distractibility |
| Impaired visual spatial conceptualization |
| Slow verbal/visual information processing |
| Impaired memory |
| Communication disorders |
| Poor judgment |
| Poor executive function |

*Source:* Barman, Chatterjee, & Bhide (2016).

| **Table 4–3.** Key to Communication: Attention |
|---|
| Difficulty responding appropriately to incoming information |
| Difficulty learning new information |
| Difficulty filtering out irrelevant stimuli |
| Difficulty conversing in situations with distractions, background noise, and multiple participants |
| Difficulty managing the demands of high-level activity |
| Difficulty sustaining attention when reading complex and/or lengthy material |
| Difficulty shifting attention as needed |
| Difficulty maintaining or changing topics in conversation |
| Tangential discourse |
| Social avoidance to compensate for sense of overstimulation |

*Source:* Cornis-Pop et al. (2012, Traumatic Brain Injury).

**Table 4–4.** Attention Systems: Purpose and Mediation

| System | Purpose | Mediation |
|---|---|---|
| Sensory Selective Attention System | Responsible for orienting, engaging, and disengaging attention and object recognition | Mediated by the parieto-temporo-occipital area |
| Arousal, Sustain Attention, and Vigilance System | Responsible for controlling arousal, sustained attention, vigilance, mood, motivation, salience (prominence), and readiness to respond | Mediated by the midbrain reticular activating system and limbic structures |
| Selection and Control System | Responsible for selection and control of responses, involving intentional and strategic control, switching, and inhibition | Mediated by the frontal lobes, anterior cingulate gyrus, and basal ganglia, with the thalamus relaying incoming information and outgoing responses |

*Source:* Ponsford, Bayley, Wiseman-Hakes, Togher, Velikonja, et al. (2014, p. 322).

From a clinical perspective, a widely referenced framework discussing and describing attention is by Sohlberg and Mateer (1987, 2001, 2010), which includes the division of attention into the following five categories:

### Focused Attention

Focused attention encompasses the ability to recognize and acknowledge sensory information (visual, auditory, tactile, or cognitive). This is the most basic level of attention in response to external or internal stimuli (Sohlberg & Mateer, 2001), such as looking toward a source of noise.

### Sustained Attention

Sustained attention is the ability to maintain attention over time. An example of sustained attention is performing a simple typing task in a distraction-free environment. Sohlberg and Mateer (2001) described sustained attention as comprising vigilance (continual response over time) and working memory (mental control necessary to hold and manipulate information). Other authors have differentiated vigilance from sustained attention, with vigilance used to describe attention over a longer period of time and given performance of a task that requires attention to a target that occurs randomly or infrequently (O'Donnell, 2002), such as a lifeguard monitoring a pool for distressed swimmers.

### Selective Attention

Selective attention is the ability to maintain attention in the presence of distraction, thereby selectively attending to important information and inhibiting irrelevant information or distractions, such as external distractions (e.g., noise, light) or internal distractions (e.g., worry, excitement). An example of selective attention is a listener focused on the conversation of her dinner partner in the middle of a noisy restaurant.

## Alternating Attention

Alternating attention is the ability to shift attention between two or more tasks that have different cognitive demands. An example of alternating attention is a receptionist shifting between typing and answering the phone.

## Divided Attention

Divided attention is the ability to respond to two or more events simultaneously, such as talking on the phone while cooking dinner. Newer models of attention suggest that this level of attention may actually be rapid alternating attention versus true divided attention.

Regardless of severity of injury (mild, moderate, or severe), impairments in attention are a common symptom following TBI (Stierwalt & Murray, 2002). These deficits can be long-standing in nature, persisting years after the initial injury (Draper & Ponsford, 2008) and negatively impact important life roles and social interaction (Ponsford et al., 2014).

Numerous studies have shown that individuals with TBI have a variety of attentional impairments. During the period of posttraumatic amnesia (PTA), all levels of attention may be impaired, but once PTA resolves, impairments in arousal and basic orienting responses commonly resolve, but impairments in higher-level attention tend to persist (Stierwalt & Murray, 2002, p. 130). These include impaired levels of vigilance and sustained attention (Ziino & Ponsford, 2006), difficulty dividing attention (Asloun et al., 2008; Azouvi, Vallat-Azouvi, & Belmont, 2009; Willmott, Ponsford, Hocking, & Schönberger, 2009), difficulty with working memory (Vallat-Azouvi, Weber, Legrand, & Azouvi, 2007), and problems with goal-directed attention for multi-step tasks and tasks with changing demands (Ponsford et al., 2014). These difficulties tend to be more impaired in completion of tasks that require high cognitive demand, and less impaired in completion of routine activities that can be performed automatically (Stierwalt & Murray, 2002).

## Information Processing Speed

Information processing speed is also a topic sometimes included in discussion in relation to attention (Mathias, Wheaton, & Becker, 2007; Ponsford et al., 2014). This is in part due to debate as to how to describe the component processes of attention, with some definitions that include aspects of processing speed and others that do not (Ponsford et al., 2014). The research in this area is consistent, however, in noting a general reduction in speed of information processing following TBI (Ponsford & Kinsella, 1992). This is particularly true for individuals with severe TBI (Mathias et al., 2007; Sarno, Erasmus, Lipp, & Schlaegel, 2003) but has also been noted across the spectrum of severity, including in those with more mild TBI (MacFlynn, Montgomery, Fenton, & Rutherford, 1984). Deficits in information processing speed have been noted in both simple and complex tasks (Mathias et al., 2007), but slowed reaction time is particularly evident in individuals with TBI for tasks of increasing difficulty, in circumstances with greater informational load, and when fatigue is present (Stuss et al., 1989). Madigan and colleagues also reported differential slowing based on modality, with disproportionately slower performance on auditory tasks, compared with visual tasks (Madigan, Deluca, Diamond, Tramontano, & Averill, 2000). Table 4–5 contains examples of the potential impact on communication due to impairments in processing speed (Key to Communication).

| **Table 4–5.** Key to Communication: Processing Speed |
| --- |
| Delayed responses |
| Difficulty making decisions |
| Difficulty comprehending rapid rate of speech |
| Difficulty staying on topic |
| Long pauses within discourse |

*Source:* Cornis-Pop et al. (2012, Traumatic Brain Injury).

| **Table 4–6.** Key to Communication: Memory |
| --- |
| Difficulty recalling instructions or messages |
| Difficulty learning new information |
| Difficulty remembering names of individuals, appointments, directions, and/or location of personal effects |
| Difficulty recalling details when reading complex and/or lengthy material |
| Difficulty maintaining topic or remembering purpose of conversation |
| Repetition of ideas, statements, questions, conversations, or stories |
| Failure to use compensatory strategies to improve performance on everyday tasks |

*Source:* Cornis-Pop et al. (2012, Traumatic Brain Injury).

## Memory

Table 4–6 contains examples of the potential impact on communication due to impairments in memory (Key to Communication). Generally speaking, memory is an act of encoding, storing, and retrieving information from short- and long-term memory systems (Figure 4–3; Velikonja et al., 2014; Wilson, 2009). Memory is a complex composite of skills, subserved by perception, attention, and executive function (Wilson, 2009). This is represented in the complex and diffuse neural pathways and interconnecting brain regions involved in memory, including areas susceptible to TBI (Table 4–7).

Encoding involves the processes of initial analysis of information, such as encoding of phonological characteristics for verbal information or graphic representations for visual information (Sohlberg & Mateer, 2001). Wilson (2009, p. 9) recommends the following guidelines for improving the encoding process:

1. Simplify information to be coded.
2. Ask individuals to remember one thing at a time (e.g., single words versus multiple words).
3. Confirm that the person understands the information to be learned. This is commonly done by asking the client to

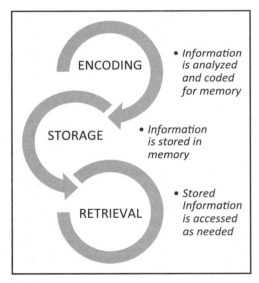

**Figure 4–3.** Stages of memory: encoding, storage, and retrieval.

repeat back the information in his her own words.
4. Ask the individual to link the information with something already known

**Table 4–7.** Stages of Memory and Associated Brain Regions

| Stages of Memory | Associated Brain Regions |
|---|---|
| Encoding | Encoding is thought to be mediated by subcortical-cortical sensory-perceptual systems and prefrontal resources (Eslinger, Zappala, Chakara, & Barrett, 2013). |
| | Memory problems secondary to encoding issues have been reported in individuals with lateralized damage involving language and visual systems (Sohlberg & Mateer, 2001). |
| | Impairments associated with encoding have also been noted with damage in diencephalic structures, such as the dorsomedial thalamus and frontal lobe systems. |
| Storage | Storage involves interactive processing between cortical sensory areas and limbic system structures (particularly the hippocampus) (Zola-Morgan & Squire, 1993). |
| | Difficulty with storage has been noted in individuals with damage in the hippocampus and bilateral medial temporal lobes (Sohlberg & Mateer, 2001). |
| Retrieval | The neural basis of retrieval is less clear than those of encoding and storage but is thought to be mediated by prefrontal structures to leverage large-scale coordination among cortical, subcortical, and limbic system structures (Eslinger, Zappala, Chakara, & Barrett, 2013). |
| | Difficulty with retrieval has been noted in individuals with damage in the frontal lobe, including errors of distortion and confabulation and those of poor source memory and retrieval of facts not in the context which they were acquired (Sohlberg & Mateer, 2001, p. 165). |

(e.g., remembering a name by linking it to another person with that same name).

5. Space out opportunities to learn information in small pieces over time. Wilson refers to this as the "little and often rule."

6. Avoid trial and error learning. Instead create opportunities to learn information in an errorless fashion.

7. Ask individuals to be active in the encoding and memory process.

Storage involves the transfer of information to a more permanent form. This process is also referred to as consolidation (Eslinger, Zappala, Chakara, & Barrett, 2013). Consolidation is more efficient after effective encoding (Eslinger et al., 2013; Wilson, 2009). It is susceptible to retroactive interference (interference due to presentation of information *after* new learning) and proactive interference (interference due to information presented *prior* to new learning) (Sohlberg & Mateer, 2001). Retrieval refers to the process of searching for and activating stored memory (Sohlberg & Mateer, 2001), through either recall or recognition (Eslinger et al., 2013).

Memory is also classically discussed given the length of time and amount of information retained, including the concepts of short-term memory, working memory, and long-term memory. Short-term memory provides for retention of a small amount of information (five to seven items) for a brief period of time (generally a few seconds) (Radomski et al., n.d.). It is susceptible to distraction but can also be extended temporarily with repetition of information, such as repeating a telephone number until you are able to write it down. Working memory is conceptually linked to short-term memory. Working memory has limited capacity and decays within a few seconds but is thought to be dynamic in nature, providing for conscious manipulation of information to be stored or retrieved (e.g., planning, organizing, sequencing) (Radomski et al., n.d.). Working memory is conceived of as the "mental workspace" for memory, where strategies for more complex cognitive processes can be applied. For example, working memory is utilized in a task like adding mentally $(12 + 14) − (8 + 7)$ (Brookshire, 2015 p. 87). In this example, working memory aids in storing the intermediate calculations of 26 and 15 so that subtraction of these two numbers can occur. Long-term memory is a more permanent repository for information over minutes to years. It has a rather large capacity for storage and is thought to decay slowly, if at all (Brookshire, 2015, p. 87).

From a temporal (time) perspective, memory is also described in terms of memory loss (retrograde and anterograde) and given the type and timing of information to be recalled (retrospective versus prospective). As was discussed in Chapter 2 (Classification and Recovery), memory loss for events immediately *before* a brain injury are referred to as retrograde memory loss (or retrograde amnesia), whereas difficulty forming new memories *after* the injury is referred to as anterograde memory loss (or anterograde amnesia) (Cantu, 2001; Sohlberg & Mateer, 2001). Retrospective memory refers to retention and recall of information about past experiences and events. Prospective memory refers to memory for carrying out intentions, or "remembering to remember" (Brookshire, 2015; Sohlberg & Mateer, 2001).

Lastly, memory is also conceptualized by the type of information to be recalled: declarative/(explicit) and non-declarative/(implicit) (Vakil, 2005). Table 4–8 offers an overview of each of these memory types.

Impairments in memory following TBI are a very common cognitive deficit (Vakil,

| Table 4–8. Memory Types (Declarative and Non-Declarative) |
|---|
| **Declarative Memory (Explicit) Memory**<br>Memory for "what we know about things" (Brookshire, 2015, p. 89) |

| Semantic Memory | Episodic Memory |
|---|---|
| Memory for world knowledge, such as word meanings, classes of information, facts, and ideas. This includes knowledge gained from educational context (e.g., book learning). | Memory for autobiographical information learned based on personal experiences (associated with events), such as the birth of a child, wedding, and so forth. This is memory specific to time and place. |

| **Non-Declarative (Implicit) Memory**<br>Memory for the "how to" (applied) portions of a skill that is learned through practice |
|---|

| Procedural Memory | Primed Memory |
|---|---|
| Memory for motor skills or action patterns, such as brushing teeth, tying shoelaces | Memory that occurs due to a paired connection with a past experience or previous exposure |

2005) and are among the most frequent complaints from individuals with TBI and their significant others. Memory deficits have been reported using a variety of measures, including neuropsychological and subjective assessment, quality of life measures, and both short-term and long-term outcome measures (Hoofien, Gilboa, Vakil, & Donovick, 2001; Kaitaro, Koskinen, & Kaipio, 1995; Ponsford, Olver, & Curren, 1995; Van Zomeren & Van Den Berg, 1985). Memory impairments after a TBI can be long-standing in nature (Zec et al., 2001) as well as recover more slowly than cognitive functions (Lezak, 1979; Zec et al., 2001). They are also associated with many debilitating functional consequences across all daily tasks (Ponsford et al., 2014).

Memory impairments after a TBI cross the span of memory categories. Generally, they manifest as problems in learning new information, including difficulty with encoding, storage, and retrieval (Sander & van Veldhoven, 2014; Velikonja et al., 2014). Severe retrograde impairments are not common (Sander & van Veldhoven, 2014). Individuals may experience memory failure during the entire day of injury or several days before, but information learned prior to the injury (e.g., autobiographical information, life events, procedures) is generally retained (Sohlberg & Mateer, 2001). One of the most common memory difficulties following TBI is impaired prospective memory (Mateer, Sohlberg, & Crinean, 1987; Roche, Fleming, & Shum, 2002). Declarative memory is also often impacted more greatly than procedural memory after a TBI (Bhatnagar, Iaccarino, & Zafonte, 2016).

Memory impairments after TBI are often closely related to impairments in attention, organization, and/or processing speed (Sanders & van Veldhoven, 2014). Memory impairments following TBI (particularly relative to encoding and storage) also generally encompass visual/spatial and verbal information. Although they can occur, modality-specific memory impairments (e.g., intact verbal recall but impaired visual recall) are rare in closed-head injury TBI, due to the diffuse nature of neural networks impacted (Vanderploeg , Curtiss, Schinka, & Lanham, 2001).

## Executive Function

Table 4–9 contains examples of the potential impact on communication due to impairments in executive function (Key to Communication). As with the other areas of cognition discussed thus far, there are varying ways to describe/define executive function. Cicerone and colleagues describe it as:

> those integrative cognitive processes that determine goal-directed behavior and are superordinate in the orderly execution of daily life functions . . . the ability to formulate goals; to initiate behaviour; to anticipate the consequences of action; to plan and organize behavior according to spatial, temporal, topical or logical sequences; and to monitor and adapt behavior to fit a particular task or context (Cicerone et al., 2000, p. 1605).

Executive function is the cornerstone of all life tasks. Researchers have noted a strong correlation between executive function deficits and negative functional and psychosocial outcomes (Hanks, Rapport, Millis, & Deshpande, 1999; Spitz, Ponsford, Rudski, & Maller, 2012). Spitz et al. (2012) noted that this was true for several aspects of cognition (attention, memory, process-

**Table 4–9.** Key to Communication: Executive Function

Lack of coherence in discourse

Lack of organization in planning daily activities

Difficulty implementing plans and actions

Difficulty initiating conversations

Problems recognizing and repairing conversational breakdowns

Inability to determine the needs of communication partners

Difficulty making inferences or drawing conclusions

Difficulty assuming another person's perspective

Difficulty interpreting the behavior of others

Difficulty evaluating validity of information

Verbose; lack of conciseness in verbal expression

Decreased comprehension of abstract language, humor, and/or indirect requests

Difficulty meeting timelines

Difficulty formulating realistic goals

Difficulty recognizing complexity of tasks and need for simplification

Difficulty anticipating consequences of actions

Inappropriate comments

*Source:* Cornis-Pop et al. (2012).

ing speed), but even more so for deficits in executive function. Sohlberg and Mateer (2001), based on the work of Mateer (1999), offer an illustrative description of the core aspects of executive function and their relevance to task completion. These are represented visually in Figure 4–4 and described below (Sohlberg & Mateer, 2001, pp. 235–236).

### Initiation and Drive

Initiation and drive are responsible for starting or "activating" behavior in response to information or internal intentions. Without this first initial act of directing executive function systems to respond, no task can be completed.

### Response Inhibition

Response inhibition serves to stop (inhibit) non–task-related behaviors, such as preventing non-relevant automatic or "prepotent" response tendencies (p. 235). Without response inhibition, behaviors would be impulsive, in either overresponding to non-relevant environmental information or acting reflexively. Preservation or getting stuck on a specific task without moving to the next important step can also occur without response inhibition (response stopping).

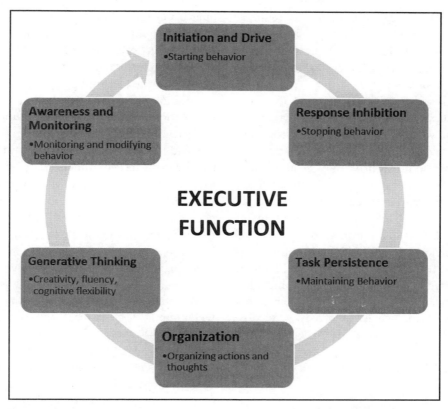

**Figure 4–4.** Domains of executive function. The core domains of executive function described by Sohlberg and Mateer (2001).

### Task Persistence

Task persistence is closely related to response inhibition and provides for maintenance of attention and persistence on the task through to completion. Without it, tasks would be discontinued prior to final completion.

### Organization

Organization involves organizing and sequencing actions and thoughts toward relevant task completion. It allows for clarity in avoiding nonessential responses and includes goal management, planning, time sense, and sequencing.

### Generative Thinking

Generative thinking allows for "creativity, fluency, and cognitive flexibility" (p. 235). This results in the generation of novel ideas and solutions during task execution.

### Awareness and Monitoring

Awareness is involved in "monitoring and modifying one's own behavior" (p. 236). Awareness includes the integrated aspects of: (1) self-knowledge (awareness of one's own abilities and beliefs), (2) self-monitoring (ongoing evaluation of one's performance and capacity to identify errors), and (3) self-regulation (capacity to adjust performance in response to task demands) (Ownsworth, Fleming, Desbois, Strong, & Kuipers, 2006). Each is critical in successful task completion.

Given the broad scope of executive function, it is no surprise that a large neural network of interconnected cortical and subcortical systems is needed for it. It is likely also no surprise that executive function is heavily integrated with attention, memory, and information processing (Tate et al., 2014). Deficits in executive function are referred to as "frontal lobe syndrome" in acknowledgment of the predominant role of the frontal lobe in executive function. In particular the prefrontal cortex, including orbital, medial, and dorsolateral prefrontal networks, is heavily involved in executive function (Eslinger et al., 2013). These are each areas vulnerable to injury due to TBI (Bigler & Maxwell, 2011; Courville, 1945).

## Social Cognition

Deficits in social interaction are common following TBI (Dahlberg et al., 2006; Finch, Copley, Cornwell, & Kelly, 2016; Finset, Dyrness, & Krogstad, 1995, Ylvisaker, Turkstra, & Coelho, 2005). Social interactions after a TBI have a strong correlation to negative psychological consequences of TBI, such as depression, loneliness, social withdrawal, and negative concepts of self (Finch et al., 2016; Morton & Wehman, 1995; Ylvisaker et al., 2005). Impairments of this nature are also often "judged by family members, teachers, employers, friends, and others to be the most problematic consequences of the injury" (Ylvisaker et al., 2005, p. 275). Relatives have reported changes in social behavior and personality of individuals with TBI that include "childishness, self-centeredness, disinterest or dislike of others,

quarrelsomeness, unreasonable or socially inappropriate behavior, unhappiness, and excitation" (McDonald, 2013, p. 233).

As the discussion above suggests, any number of the presenting aspects of communication difficulties as a result of deficits in attention, memory, or executive function could lead to breakdowns in social interaction and communication, particularly those listed under executive function (e.g., inability to determine the needs of communication partners, difficulty assuming another person's perspective, difficulty interpreting the behavior of others). Research has also begun to explore in more depth contributions specific to deficits in *social cognition* in this area (Bibby & McDonald, 2005; Byom & Turkstra, 2013; Turkstra, McDonald, & DePompei, 2001). For example, Ubukata et al. (2014) studied the relationship between tests specifically designed to measure aspects of social cognition (emotional perception and theory of the mind) and outcomes of individuals with TBI. These researchers found a significant correlation between social cognition and functional outcome, noting that measures in the area of social cognition may be a good predictor of functional outcomes after TBI. Admittedly, studies of this nature are challenging given that most tasks designed to assess social cognition also require perceptual, language, memory, and executive abilities. Further compounding study in this area is the fact that neuropsychological studies on topics related to social cognition have identified specific brain regions that tend to be activated when perceiving and interpreting social messages. Notably, these areas include regions also vulnerable to TBI and those also implicated in deficits associated with attention, memory, or executive function, such as the "medial prefrontal cortex, both ventral (bottom) and dorsal (top) (including the anterior cingulate gyrus), the amygdala, the temporal lobe poles, and the junction between the temporal and parietal lobe in the right hemisphere" (Ylvisaker, Hibbard, & Feeney, 2006, Development of Theory of Mind).

Social communication is defined as an "amalgamation of verbal and nonverbal skills that enable individuals to express themselves and understand the meanings intended by others in a diverse array of environments and with varying communication partners" (Finch et al., 2016, p. 1353). Social *cognition* is "the capacity to attend to, recognize, and interpret interpersonal cues that enable us to understand and predict the behaviors of others, to share experiences, and communicate effectively" (McDonald et al., 2014, p. 119).

As Figure 4–5 illustrates, social cognition consists of the interplay between perception/representation of social information (e.g., perception of face, speech, movement), the evaluation and interpretation of hot and cold social cognition, and the regulation of social behavior (e.g., self-awareness/reflection, cognitive control, monitoring) (McDonald, 2013). Many of the aspects of regulation in social cognition overlap with those discussed in the area of executive function. The concepts of hot

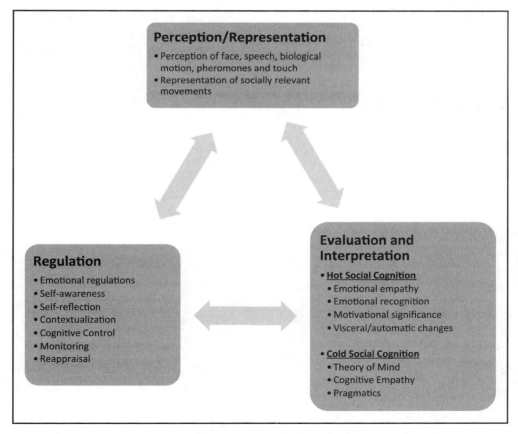

**Figure 4–5.** Processes of social cognition: perception/representation, evaluation and interpretation, and regulation. *Source:* Adapted from McDonald (2013). Copyright © Cambridge University Press. Used with permission.

and cold social cognition (interpretation and evaluation) relative to TBI will be discussed below.

## Hot Social Cognition

Individuals with TBI have been noted to present with impairments in the area of hot social cognition (McDonald, 2013). This includes differences on self-report measures of emotional empathy compared with neurotypical controls (Williams & Wood, 2010; Wood & Williams, 2008). Deficits in recognition of photographs of facial expressions and recognition of emotional expression in voice have also been reported in individuals with TBI (McDonald & Saunders, 2005; Milders, Fuchs, & Crawford, 2003; Milders, Ietswaart, Crawford, & Currie, 2008; Spell & Frank, 2000).

## Cold Social Cognition

Cold social cognition includes cognitive empathy, pragmatics, and theory of mind (ToM).

### Cognitive Empathy

Cognitive empathy is related to the concept of ToM (below) and is defined as "an individual's capacity to consider another person's perspective (as opposed to emotional empathy, which refers to engaging with their feelings)" (McDonald et al., p. 124). Studies that have purported to measure cognitive empathy following brain injury note lower self-reported cognitive empathy in individuals with TBI compared with matched controls (de Sousa et al., 2010; Wells, Dywan, & Dumas, 2005). These lower levels of cognitive empathy have also been found to be associated with high distress in caregivers (Wells et al., 2005).

### Pragmatics

Pragmatics is an area familiar to speech-language pathologists. Although definitions vary, it is broadly defined as "rules associated with the use of language in conversation and broader social situations" (ASHA, n.d., Language). Studies in the area of pragmatics have shown a wide range of deficits following TBI (Bosco, Parola, Sacco, Zettin, & Angeleri, 2017). These have been described *in general* as difficulty in managing social interactions in everyday tasks (Struchen, Pappadis, Sander, Burrows, & Myszka, 2011) and disorders of narrative discourse (Marini et al., 2011; Marini, Zettin, & Galetto, 2014).

Examples of specific impairments in this area include deficits in comprehending linguistic information affiliated with pragmatic interpretation, such as difficulty in understanding sentences with sarcasm (Channon et al., 2007; McDonald, 1992; McDonald & Pearce, 1996) and humor (Braun, Lissier, Baribeau, & Ethier, 1989; Docking, Murdoch, & Jordan, 2000). Difficulties in linguistic aspects of pragmatic production following TBI have also been noted, including:

1. Poor ability negotiating requests (McDonald & Van Sommers, 1993)
2. Difficulty giving the right amount of information to an interlocutor (McDonald, 1993)
3. Difficulties in managing turn taking during conversation (Murphy, Huang, Montgomery, & Turkstra, 2015).

Deficits in extralinguistic aspects of pragmatics following TBI have also been reported, including difficulty effectively communicating pragmatic information through gestures, facial expressions, and body posture (Bara, Cutica, & Tirassa, 2001; Rousseaux et al., 2010).

### Theory of Mind (ToM)

ToM includes the processes used to reason about beliefs, emotions, and mental states (Byom & Turkstra, 2013). ToM allows individuals not only to perceive social cues, but also to predict the behavior of others (Premack & Woodruff, 1978). According to Ylvisaker et al. (2006), to "say a person has a fully developed theory of mind is to say at least the following:

1. She knows that she and other people have minds, that is, they have thoughts, beliefs, feelings, desires, intentions, and the like.
2. She is able to understand her own thoughts and feelings, and infer other people's thoughts, beliefs, feelings, desires, and intentions from their behavior (including what they say) with reasonable accuracy.
3. She is disposed to use this information about other people's thoughts, beliefs, feelings, desires, and intentions in making decisions about how to act in social contexts. In particular, she is able to see the world from the perspective of other people" (What are Egocentrism and Theory of the Mind?).

A growing number of studies have demonstrated impairments in ToM in individuals with TBI (Martin-Rodriguez & Leon-Carrion, 2010). Examples of results in this area include:

1. Poorer performance than controls on tasks designed to infer mental states from photographs (Havet-Thomassin et al., 2006; Turkstra, 2008)
2. Lower scores than controls on tasks requiring individuals to predict the conclusion of a comic-strip story based on a character's intentions (Havet-

Thomassin, Allain, Etcharry-Bouyx, & LeGall, 2006)
3. Poorer performance than controls on tasks measuring "faux-pas" recognition and false belief (e.g., understanding that an individual's belief or representation about the world may contrast with reality) (Milders, Ietswaart, & Crawford, 2006)
4. Deficits given video-based scenarios in interpreting second-order false beliefs (e.g., attributing false belief to another person, based on interpreting that person's thoughts about another person) (McDonald & Flanagan, 2004; Turkstra, Dixon, & Baker, 2004; Turkstra, 2008)
5. Fewer thought-related and feeling-related words in conversation and use of words in inappropriate contexts (Byom & Turkstra, 2013)

### References

American Speech-Language-Hearing Association. (n.d.-a). *Traumatic brain injury in adults.* Retrieved from http://www.asha.org/PRP SpecificTopic.aspx?folderid=8589935337& section=Signs_and_Symptoms

American Speech-Language-Hearing Association. (2005). *Roles of speech-language pathologists in the identification, diagnosis, and treatment of individuals with cognitive-communication disorders: Position statement.* Retrieved from http://www.asha.org/policy

Asloun, S., Soury, S., Couillet, J., Giroire, J. M., Joseph, P. A., Mazauk, J. M., & Azouvi, P. (2008). Interactions between divided attention and working-memory load in patients with severe traumatic brain injury. *Journal of Clinical Experimental Neuropsychology, 30*(4), 481–490.

Azouvi, P., Vallat-Azouvi, C., & Belmont, A. (2009). Cognitive deficits after traumatic coma. *Progress in Brain Research, 177,* 89–110.

Bara, B. G., Cutica, I., & Tirassa, M. (2001). Neuropragmatics: Extralinguistic communication after closed head injury. *Brain and Language, 77,* 72–94.

Barman, A., Chatterjee, A., & Bhide, R. (2016). Cognitive impairment and rehabilitation strategies after traumatic brain injury. *Indian Journal of Psychological Medicine, 38*(3), 172–181.

Bhatnagar, S., Iaccarino, M., & Zafonte, R. (2016). Pharmacotherapy in rehabilitation of post-acute traumatic brain injury. *Brain Research, 1640,* 164–179.

Bibby, H., & McDonald, S. (2005). Theory of mind after traumatic brain injury. *Neuropsychologia, 21*(5), 515–531.

Bigler, E. D., & Maxwell, W. L. (2011). Neuroimaging and neuropathology of TBI. *Neuro-Rehabilitation, 28,* 1–12.

Bosco, F., Parola, A., Sacco, K., Zettin, M., & Angeleri, R. (2017). Communicative-pragmatic disorders in traumatic brain injury: The role of theory of mind and executive functions. *Brain and Language, 168,* 73–83.

Braun, C. M. J., Lissier, F., Baribeau, J. M. C., & Ethier, M. (1989). Does severe traumatic closed head injury impair sense of humor? *Brain Injury, 3,* 345–354.

Brookshire, R. (2015). *Introduction to neurogenic communication disorders.* St. Louis, MO: Mosby.

Byom, L., & Turkstra, L. (2013). Effects of social cognitive demand on theory of mind in conversations of adults with traumatic brain injury. *International Journal of Language & Communication Disorders, 47*(3), 310–321.

Cantu, R. C. (2001). Posttraumatic retrograde and anterograde amnesia: Pathophysiology and implications in grading and safe return to play. *Journal of Athletic Training, 36*(3), 244–248.

Channon, S., Rule, A., Maudgil, D., Martinos, M., Pellijeff, A., Frankl, J., . . . Shieff, C. (2007). Interpretation of mentalistic actions and sarcastic remarks: Effects of frontal and posterior lesions on mentalising. *Neuropsychologia, 45,* 1725–1734.

Cicerone, K., Dahlberg, C., Kalmar, K., Langenbahn, D., Malec, J., Bergquist, T. F., . . . Morse, P. A. (2000). Evidence-based cognitive rehabilitation: Recommendations for clinical practice. *Archives of Physical Medicine and Rehabilitation, 81*(12), 1596–1615.

Coelho, C., Liles, B., & Duffy, R. (1995). Impairments of discourse abilities and executive functions in traumatically brain injured adults. *Brain Injury, 9,* 471–477.

College of Audiologists and Speech-Language Pathologists of Ontario. (2015). *Practice standards and guidelines for acquired cognitive communication disorders.* Ontario, Canada: College of Audiologists and Speech-Language Pathologists of Ontario. Retrieved from http://www.caslpo.com/sites/default/uploads/files/PSG_EN_Acquired_Cognitive_Communication_Disorders.pdf

Cornis-Pop, M., Mashima, P. A., Roth, C. A., MacLennan, D. L., Picon, L. M., Smith Hammond, C., . . . Frank, E. M. (2012). Cognitive-communication rehabilitation for combat-related mild traumatic brain injury. *Journal of Rehabilitation Research and Development, 49*(7), xi–xxxi.

Courville, C. B. (1945). *Pathology of the nervous system* (2nd ed.). Mountain View, CA: California Pacific Press.

Dahlberg, C., Hawley, L., Morey, C., Newman, J., Cusick, C. P., & Harrison-Felix, C. (2006). Social communication skills in persons with post-acute traumatic brain injury: Three perspectives. *Brain Injury, 20*(4), 425–435.

de Sousa, A., McDonald, S., Rushby, J., Li, S., Dimoska, A., & James, C. (2010). Why don't you feel how I feel? Insight into the absence of empathy after severe traumatic brain injury. *Neuropsychologia, 48,* 3585–3595.

Dikmen, S. S., Machamer, J. E., Winn, H. R., & Temkin, N. R. (1995). Neuropsychological outcome at 1-year post head injury. *Neuropsychology, 9,* 80–90.

Docking, K., Murdoch, B. E., & Jordan, F. M. (2000). Interpretation and comprehension of linguistic humor by adolescents with head injury: A group analysis. *Brain Injury, 14,* 89–108.

Draper, K., & Ponsford, J. (2008). Cognitive functioning ten years following traumatic brain injury and rehabilitation. *Neuropsychology*, *22*, 618–625.

Eslinger, P. J., Zappala, G., Chakara, F., & Barrett, A. M. (2013). Cognitive Impairments. In N. Zasler, D. I. Katz, R. D. Zafonte, D. B. Arciniegas, M. B. Bullock, & J. S. Kreutzer (Eds.), *Brain injury medicine: Principles and practice* (2nd ed.). New York, NY: Demos Medical.

Finch, E., Copley, A., Cornwell, P., & Kelly, C. (2016). Systematic review of behavioral interventions targeting social communication difficulties after traumatic brain injury. *Archives of Physical Medicine and Rehabilitation*, *97*(8), 1352–1365.

Finset, A., Dyrness, S., & Krogstad, J. M. (1995). Self-reported social networks and interpersonal support 2 years after severe traumatic brain injury. *Brain Injury*, *9*(2), 141–150.

Ghayoumi, Z., Yadegari, F., Mahmoodi-Bakhtiari, B., Fakharian, E., Rahgozar, M., & Rasouli, M. (2015). Persuasive discourse impairments in traumatic brain injury. *Archives of Trauma Research*, *4*(1), 1–7.

Hanks, R. A., Rapport, L. J., Millis, S. R., & Deshpande, S. A. (1999). Measures of executive functioning as predictors of functional ability and social integration in a rehabilitation sample. *Archives of Physical Medicine Rehabilitation*, *80*(9), 1030–1037.

Havet-Thomassin, V., Allain, P., Etcharry-Bouyx, F., & LeGall, D. (2006). What about Theory of Mind after severe brain injury? *Brain Injury*, *20*(1), 83–91.

Heilman, K. M., Safran, A., & Geschwind, N. (1971). Closed head trauma and aphasia. *Journal of Neurology, Neurosurgery, and Psychiatry*, *34*(3), 265–269.

Hoofien, D., Gilboa, A., Vakil, E., & Donovick, P. J. (2001). Traumatic brain injury (TBI) 10 to 20 years later: A comprehensive outcome study of psychiatric symptomatology, cognitive abilities and psychosocial functioning. *Brain Injury*, *15*, 189–209.

Levin, H. S., Grossman, R. G., & Kelly, P. J. (1976). Aphasia disorder in patients with closed head injury. *Journal of Neurology, Neurosurgery, and Psychiatry*, *39*, 1062–1070.

Levin, H. S., Grossman, R. G., & Rose, S. E. (1979). Long term neuropsychological outcome of closed head injury. *Journal of Neurosurgery*, *50*, 412–422.

Lezak, M. D. (1979). Recovery of memory and learning functions following traumatic brain injury. *Cortex*, *15*, 63–72.

Kaitaro, T., Koskinen, S., & Kaipio, M. L. (1995). Neuropsychological problems in everyday life: A 5-year follow-up study of young severely closed head injured patients. *Brain Injury*, *9*, 713–727.

MacFlynn, G., Montgomery, E. A., Fenton, G. W., & Rutherford, W. (1984). Measurement of reaction time following minor head injury. *Journal of Neurology, Neurosurgery, and Psychiatry*, *47*, 1326–1331.

Madigan, N., Deluca, J., Diamond, B., Tramontano, G., & Averill, A. (2000). Speed of information processing in traumatic brain injury: Modality-specific factors. *Journal of Head Trauma Rehabilitation*, *15*(3), 943–956.

Marini, A., Galetto, V., Zampieri, E., Vorano, L., Zettin, M., & Carlomagno, S. (2011). Narrative language in traumatic brain injury. *Neuropsychologia*, *49*, 2904–2910.

Marini, A., Zettin, M., & Galetto, V. (2014). Cognitive correlates of narrative impairment in moderate traumatic brain injury. *Neuropsychologia*, *64*, 282–288.

Martin-Rodriguez, J. F., & Leon-Carrion, J. (2010). Theory of Mind deficits in patients with acquired brain injury: A quantitative review. *Neuropsychologia*, *48*(5), 1181–1191.

Mateer, C. A., Sohlberg, M. M., & Crinean, J. (1987). Perceptions of memory function in individuals with closed-head injury. *Journal of Head Trauma Rehabilitation*, *2*, 74–84.

Mathias, J., Wheaton, P., & Becker, J. (2007). Changes in attention and information-processing speed following severe traumatic brain injury: A meta-analytic review. *Neuropsychology*, *21*(2), 212–223.

McDonald, S. (1992). Differential pragmatic language loss after closed head injury: Ability to comprehend conversational implicature. *Applied Psycholinguistics*, *13*, 295–312.

McDonald, S. (1993). Pragmatic language skills after closed head injury: Ability to meet the informational needs of the listener. *Brain and Language, 44*, 28–46.

McDonald, S. (2013). Impairments in social cognition following severe traumatic brain injury. *Journal of the International Neuropsychological Society, 19*(3), 231–246.

McDonald, S., & Flanagan, S. (2004). Social perception deficits after traumatic brain injury: Interaction between emotion recognition, mentalizing ability, and social communication. *Neuropsychology, 18*(3), 572–579.

McDonald, S., & Pearce, S. (1996). Clinical insight into pragmatic theory: Frontal lobe deficits and sarcasm. *Brain and Language, 61*, 88–104.

McDonald, S., & Saunders, J. C. (2005). Differential impairment in recognition of emotion across different media in people with severe traumatic brain injury. *Journal of the International Neuropsychological Society, 11*(4), 392–399.

McDonald, S., Togher, L., & Code, C. (2014). *Social and communication disorders following traumatic brain injury.* New York, NY: Psychology Press.

McDonald, S., & Van Sommers, P. (1993). Pragmatic language skills after closed head injury: Ability to negotiate requests. *Cognitive Neuropsychology, 10*, 297–315.

Milders, M., Fuchs, S., & Crawford, J. R. (2003). Neuropsychological impairments and changes in emotional and social behavior following severe traumatic brain injury. *Journal of Clinical and Experimental Neuropsychology, 25*(2), 157–172.

Milders, M., Ietswaart, M., & Crawford, J. R. (2006). Impairments in Theory of Mind shortly after traumatic brain injury and at 1-year follow-up. *Neuropsychology, 20*(4), 400–408.

Milders, M., Ietswaart, M., Crawford, J. R., & Currie, D. (2008). Social behavior following traumatic brain injury and its association with emotion recognition, understanding of intentions, and cognitive flexibility. *Journal of the International Neuropsychological Society, 14*(2), 318–326.

Morton, M. V., & Wehman, P. (1995). Psychosocial and emotional sequelae of individuals with traumatic brain injury: A literature review and recommendations. *Brain Injury, 9*, 81–92.

Murdoch, B. E. (2010). Speech-language disorders associated with traumatic brain injury. In B. E. Murdoch (Ed.), *Acquired speech and language disorders: A neuroanatomical and functional neurological approach* (2nd ed., pp. 118–152). Oxford, UK: Wiley-Blackwell.

Murphy, A., Huang, H., Montgomery, E. B., & Turkstra, L. S. (2015). Conversational turn-taking in adults with acquired brain injury. *Aphasiology, 29*, 151–168.

O'Donnell, B. (2002). Forms of attention and attentional disorders. *Seminars in Speech and Language, 23*(2), 99–106.

O'Flaherty, C., & Douglas, J. (1997). Living with cognitive communicative difficulties following traumatic brain injury: Using a model of interpersonal communication to characterize the subjective experience. *Aphasiology, 11*, 889–911.

Ownsworth, T., Fleming, J., Desbois, J., Strong, J., & Kuipers, P. A. (2006). Metacognitive contextual intervention to enhance error awareness and functional outcome following traumatic brain injury: A single-case experimental design. *Journal of the International Neuropsychological Society, 12*(1), 54–63.

Ponsford, J., Bayley, M., Wiseman-Hakes, C., Togher, L., Velikonja, D., & McIntyre, A. (2014). INCOG recommendations for management of cognition following traumatic brain injury, Part ii: Attention and information processing speed. *Journal of Head Trauma Rehabilitation, 29*(4), 321.

Ponsford. J. L., Downing, M., Olver. J., Ponsford, M., Archer, R., Carty, M., & Spitz, G. (2014). Longitudinal follow-up of patients with traumatic brain injury: Outcome at 2, 5, and 10 years postinjury. *Journal of Neurotrauma, 31*(1), 64–77.

Ponsford, J. L., & Kinsella, G. (1992). Attentional deficits following closed-head injury. *Journal of Clinical Experimental Neuropsychology, 14*(5), 822–838.

Ponsford, J. L., Olver, J. H., & Curran, C. (1995). A profile of outcome: 2 years after traumatic brain injury. *Brain Injury, 9,* 1–10.

Premack, D., & Woodruff, G. (1978). Does the chimpanzee have a theory of mind? *Behavioral Brain Science, 1,* 515–526.

Radomski, M. V., Goo-Yoshino, S., Smith Hammond, C., Isaki, E., Maclennan, D., Manning, K., . . . Zola, J. (n.d.). Cognitive assessment and intervention. In M. Weightman, M. Vining Radomski, P. Mashima, and C. R. Roth, *Mild traumatic brain injury rehabilitation toolkit.* Fort Sam Houston, TX: Borden Institute.

Roche, N. L., Fleming, J., & Shum, D. H. (2002). Self-awareness of prospective memory failure in adults with traumatic brain injury. *Brain Injury, 16,* 931–945.

Rousseaux, M., Verigneaux, C., & Kozlowski, O. (2010). An analysis of communication in conversation after severe traumatic brain injury. *European Journal of Neurology, 17*(7), 922–929.

Sander, A. M., & van Veldhoven, L. M. (2014). Rehabilitation of memory problems associated with traumatic brain injury. In M. Sherer & A. M. Sander (Eds.), *Handbook on the neuropsychology of traumatic brain injury.* New York, NY: Springer.

Sarno, S., Erasmus, L. P., Lipp, B., & Schlaegel, W. (2003). Multisensory integration after traumatic brain injury: A reaction time study between pairings of vision, touch, and audition. *Brain Injury, 17*(5), 413–426.

Snow, P., Douglas, J., & Ponsford, J. (1999). Narrative discourse following severe traumatic brain injury: A longitudinal follow up. *Aphasiology, 13,* 529–551.

Sohlberg, M. M., & Mateer, C. A. (1987). Effectiveness of an attention-training program. *Journal of Clinical and Experimental Neuropsychology, 9*(2), 117–130.

Sohlberg, M. M., & Mateer, C. A. (2001). *Cognitive rehabilitation: An integrative neuropsychological approach.* New York, NY: Guilford.

Sohlberg, M. M., & Mateer, C. A. (2010). *APT-III: Attention process training: A direct attention training program for persons with acquired brain injury.* Youngsville, NC: Lash & Associates.

Spell, L. A., & Frank, E. (2000). Recognition of nonverbal communication of affect following traumatic brain injury. *Journal of Nonverbal Behavior, 24*(4), 285–300.

Spitz, G., Ponsford, J., Rudzki, D., Maller, J., & Rao, S. (2012). Association between cognitive performance and functional outcome following traumatic brain injury: A longitudinal multilevel examination. *Neuropsychology, 26*(5), 604–612.

Stierwalt, J., & Murray, L. (2002). Attention impairment following traumatic brain injury. *Seminars in Speech and Language, 23*(2), 129.

Strutchen, M. A. (n.d.). *Social communication and traumatic brain injury (TBI): A guide for professionals.* Houston, TX: Traumatic Brain Injury Model System at TIRR Memorial Hermann Brain Injury Research Center. Retrieved from http://www.tbicommunity .org/resources/publications/professional_ education_social_comm.pdf

Struchen, M., Pappadis, M., Sander, A. M., Burrows, C., & Myszka, K. A. (2011). Examining the contribution of social communication abilities and affective/behavioral functioning to social integration outcomes for adults with traumatic brain injury. *Journal of Head Trauma Rehabilitation, 26,* 30–42.

Stuss, D. T., Stethern, L. L., Hugenholtz, H., Picto, T., Pivik, J., & Richard, M. J. (1989). Reaction time after head injury: Fatigue, divided and focussed attention and consistency of performance. *Journal of Neurology, Neurosurgery, and Psychiatry, 52*(6), 742–748.

Tate, R., Kennedy, M., Ponsford, J., Douglas, J., Velikonja, D., Bayley, M., & Stergiou-Kita, M. (2014). INCOG recommendations for management of cognition following traumatic brain injury, Part iii: Executive function and self-awareness. *Journal of Head Trauma Rehabilitation, 29*(4), 338–352.

Togher, L., Hand, L., & Code, C. (1997). Analysing discourse in the traumatic brain injury population: Telephone interactions with different communication partners. *Brain Injury, 11,* 169–190.

Turkstra, L. S. (2008). Conversation-based assessment of social cognition in adults with traumatic brain injury. *Brain Injury, 22*(5), 397–409.

Turkstra, L. S., Dixon, T. M., & Baker, K. K. (2004). Theory of Mind and social beliefs in adolescents with traumatic brain injury. *NeuroRehabilitation*, 19(3), 245–256.

Turkstra, L. S., McDonald, S., & DePompei, R. (2001). Social information processing in adolescents: Data from normally developing adolescents and preliminary data from their peers with traumatic brain injury. *Journal of Head Trauma Rehabilitation*, 16(5), 469–483.

Ubukata, S., Tanemura, R., Yoshizumi, M., Sugihara, G., Murai, T., & Ueda, K. (2014). Social cognition and its relationship to functional outcomes in patients with sustained acquired brain injury. *Neuropsychiatric Disease and Treatment*, 10, 2061–2068.

Vakil, E. (2005). The effect of moderate to severe traumatic brain injury (TBI) on different aspects of memory: A selective review. *Journal of Clinical and Experimental Neuropsychology*, 27(8), 977–1021.

Vallat-Azouvi, C., Weber, T., Legrand, L., & Azouvi, P. (2007). Working memory after severe traumatic brain injury. *Journal of the International Neuropsychological Society*, 13(5), 770–780.

Vanderploeg, R. D., Curtiss, G., Schinka, J. A., & Lanham, R. A. Jr. (2001). Material-specific memory in traumatic brain injury: Differential effects during acquisition, recall, and retention. *Neuropsychology*, 15 (2), 174–184.

Van Zomeren, A. H., & Brouwer, W. H. (1994). *Clinical neuropsychology of attention*. New York, NY: Oxford University Press.

Van Zomeren, A. H., & Van Den Berg, W. (1985). Residual complaints of patients two years after severe head injury. *Journal of Neurology, Neurosurgery, and Psychiatry*, 48, 21–28.

Velikonja, D., Tate, R., Ponsford, J., Mcintyre, A., Janzen, S., Bayley, M., & INCOG Expert Panel. (2014). INCOG recommendations for management of cognition following traumatic brain injury, Part v: Memory. *Journal of Head Trauma Rehabilitation*, 29(4), 369–386.

Wells, R., Dywan, J., & Dumas, J. (2005). Life satisfaction and distress in family caregivers as related to specific behavioural changes after traumatic brain injury. *Brain Injury*, 19(13), 1105–1115.

Williams, C., & Wood, R. L. (2010). Alexithymia and emotional empathy following traumatic brain injury. *Journal of Clinical and Experimental Neuropsychology*, 32(3), 259–267.

Willmott, C., Ponsford, J., Hocking, C., & Schönberger, M. (2009). Factors contributing to attentional impairments following traumatic brain injury. *Neuropsychology*, 23(4), 424–432.

Wilson, B. A. (2009). *Memory rehabilitation: Integrating theory and practice*. New York, NY: Guilford Press.

Wood, R. L., & Williams, C. (2008). Inability to empathize following traumatic brain injury. *Journal of the International Neuropsychological Society*, 14, 289–296.

Ylvisaker, M., Hibbard, M., & Feeney, T. (2006). *What are egocentrism and Theory of Mind?* Albany, NY: Brain Injury Association of New York. Retrieved from http://www.projectlearnet.org/tutorials/cognitive_egocentrism_theory_of_mind.html

Ylvisaker, M., Turkstra, L., & Coelho, C. (2005). Behavioral and social interventions for individuals with traumatic brain injury: A summary of the research with clinical implications. *Seminars in Speech and Language*, 26(4), 256–267.

Zec, R. F., Zellers, D., Belman, J., Miller, J., Matthews, J., Ferneau-Belman, D., & Robbs, R. (2001). Long-term consequences of severe closed head injury on episodic memory. *Journal of Clinical and Experimental Neuropsychology*, 23, 671–691.

Ziino, C., & Ponsford, J. (2006). Vigilance and fatigue following traumatic brain injury. *Journal of the International Neuropsychological Society*, 12, 100–110.

Zola-Morgan, S., & Squire, L. (1993). Neuroanatomy of memory. *Annual Review of Neuroscience*, 16, 547.

# 5 Coordinated Care

*One day Alice came to a fork in the road and saw a Cheshire cat in a tree.*
*"Which road do I take?" she asked. "Where do you want to go?" was his response.*
*"I don't know," Alice answered. "Then," said the cat, "it doesn't matter."*

—Lewis Carroll, *Alice in Wonderland*

One of the challenges that exists for most individuals with TBI is that they may not have experienced a TBI before. The same may be true for their family and loved ones. They are thrust into an unfamiliar landscape, filled with its own complex jargon, hierarchies of services, and professionals whose roles and responsibilities may as yet not be known to them. This is a disorienting process for anyone and compounded by the fact that individuals with TBI and their family members are experiencing significant stress surrounding an uncertain future (Marsh, Kersel, Havill, & Sleigh, 1998; Winstanley, Simpson, Tate, & Myles, 2006). As the quote at the start of this chapter suggests, individuals with TBI and their families are entering a strange new land, much like Alice in Lewis Carroll's *Alice in Wonderland*. Unlike the Cheshire cat's response to Alice, the critical job of any professional interested in being of assistance to individuals with TBI is to make this new landscape understandable and easily navigated. This will require coordinated care. This chapter describes rehabilitation in the broader context, including the tenants of patient/client-centered services, common continuum of care after TBI, interdisciplinary team structure, common medical interventions for TBI, patient and family education, and special needs for individuals with TBI and their families relative to stress and coping.

## Patient/Client-Centered Care

The first step in being of service to those with a TBI and their families is to place them at the center of all aspects of health and rehabilitation services. This has not always been the case in medical-based intervention for TBI but is currently its gold standard of care (Cott, 2004). When individuals are given an opportunity to participate in treatment decisions, including setting goals, response to intervention increases (Young, Manmathan, & Ward, 2008) and overall patient satisfaction with outcomes of intervention improves (Trombly, Radomksi, Trexel, & Burnet-Smith, 2002). Within the seminal work *Through the Patient's Eyes*, the Picker Institute (Gerteis, Edgman-Levitan, Daley, & Delbanco, 1993) identified several key principles of patient-centered care still applicable in today's service delivery models. These include:

- Respect for patients' values, preferences, and expressed needs
- Coordination and integration of care
- Information, communication, and education
- Physical comfort
- Emotional support and alleviation of fear and anxiety
- Involvement of family and friends
- Continuity and transition
- Access to care (Picker Institute, n.d., para. 1)

Each of these principles serves as a cornerstone to TBI rehabilitation and should be communicated to individuals with TBI and their families. Cott (2004) further refined these principles by asking adults receiving rehabilitation (including those with acquired brain injury) about client-centered approaches and those aspects of rehabilitation which made the process easier or more challenging. These are listed in Table 5–1. Importantly, Cott also argued that implementation of these core elements of client-centered rehabilitation requires both individual team member (micro-level) implementation and organizational processes and structures (macro-level) that ensure continuity and consistency.

**Table 5–1.** Client-Centered Rehabilitation Principles from the Client Perspective

Individualization of programs to the needs of each client in order to prepare him/her for life in the real world

Mutual participation with health professionals in decision making and goal setting

Outcomes that are meaningful to the client

Sharing of information and education that is appropriate, timely, and according to the clients' wishes

Emotional support

Family and peer involvement throughout the rehabilitation process

Coordination and continuity across multiple service sectors

*Source:* Cott (2004, pp. 1418–1419).

eral guide of potential next steps can offer a helpful framework in considering potential trajectories from the point of injury forward. Figure 5–1 illustrates this continuum. Table 5–2 contains a description of several key aspects along this continuum. This is helpful information for both individuals with TBI and their familiars; however, as above, it is critical that individuals with TBI realize that their journey after a TBI is unique to them.

## Continuum of Care

Once team members have placed the client at the center of all that we do in health and rehabilitation service provision, an understanding of the continuum of care is also a helpful starting point in offering a roadmap of the path ahead for individuals with TBI and their families. Not all individuals with TBI will follow a similar path, but a gen-

## Interdisciplinary Teams

An additional facet of rehabilitation after TBI is service provision involving several disciplines within a multi- (inter-)disciplinary context (Brasure et al. 2013). As above, the most critical member of any interdisciplinary team is the individual who has experienced a TBI (and family members). The

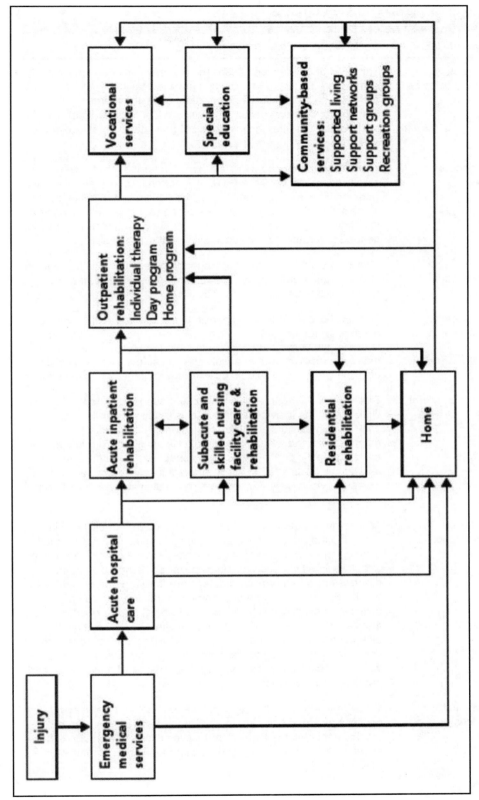

**Figure 5–1.** The flow of patients through the continuum of care. *Source:* Katz, Zasler, and Zafonte (2013). Copyright © Springer Publishing Company. Used with permission.

**Table 5–2.** Description of Continuum of Care Following TBI

| Level of Care | Description of Care/Services |
| --- | --- |
| Emergency medical services | This level of care encompasses the first medical treatment administered after a TBI, including any medical intervention provided at the scene of the injury and intervention in an emergency room. The goal of this level of care is to ensure that the individual with TBI is stabilized after the injury and to prevent further neurological damage. |
| Acute care | This level of care occurs in the hospital, after the initial emergency care is complete. For severe TBI, it is generally short-term treatment within an intensive care unit (ICU). The goals of intervention at this stage are to continue to optimize a person's medical condition and to conduct any needed diagnostics, surgical, or medical intervention needed to further stabilize an individual after an injury. |
| Acute rehabilitation | This level of care includes ongoing therapies to improve functional abilities after a brain injury. Intervention commonly focuses on relearning basic skills for everyday living. |
| Subacute rehabilitation | This level of care includes rehabilitation in a hospital or by skilled nursing, for an individual with medical needs that prevent return to home and community. The goal of intervention at this level is to maximize recovery and to ensure the safest, most active lifestyle possible when the individual does return to home and community. |
| Neurobehavioral unit | This level of care consists of a hospital-based structured environment for individuals who after an injury have difficulty controlling behaviors and impulses. Intensive behavioral management and 24-hour supervision is provided. The goal at this stage in the continuum is highly specialized treatment to assist individuals after an injury to adapt to less structured and less supervised environments in order to ultimately resume living independently. |
| Outpatient rehabilitation | This stage in the continuum includes continued rehabilitation in which the individual is no longer staying full-time within a hospital setting. It may include individual therapy within a specific discipline (e.g., speech-language pathology, physical therapy, occupational therapy) or given more coordinated care from a group of services provided, sometimes with day-long programming or given group activities. Individuals with TBI may be living at home, whether that be independently, with a family, or within group settings that offer continued support and structure. The goal of this stage is to continue to maximize recovery through ongoing support from a variety of agencies and medical professionals, including as needed outpatient rehabilitation. |
| Vocational services | Vocational services offer reeducation, training, and worksite-related services aimed at assisting the individual with TBI to return to employment or some type of productive activity. The timing of these services will vary, either in tandem with or following outpatient services. |

| **Table 5–2.** *continued* | |
|---|---|
| **Level of Care** | **Description of Care/Services** |
| Community-based services | Community-based services are an important aspect of the continuum of care after a TBI. These services serve the role of continued and ongoing care and supports utilized either in tandem with or after formal rehabilitative care. These can include supportive living, support networks and support groups (for both the individual with TBI and family), and recreational groups. Transportation, respite care for families, legal services, and mental health care services are also among the many important services and supports addressed through community-based agencies. |

*Source:* Katz, Zasler, & Zafonte (2013) and Brain Injury Alliance of Utah (n.d.).

composition of additional team members will vary based on the age of the individual with TBI, the nature of impairments, the stage of recovery, and any special training of team members. Examples of potential additional team members are listed in Table 5–3. Team members work together to establish and implement integrated rehabilitation goals, identify ways to optimize environmental and personal factors, and advocate for needed services; all for the express purpose of achieving the best possible outcome after a TBI (Joint Committee on Interprofessional Relations Between the American Speech-Language-Hearing Association and Division 40 [Clinical Neuropsychology] of the American Psychological Association, 2007).

The roles of team members may vary given their individual expertise and may overlap, depending on the disciplines involved (ASHA, 2003). It is critical, regardless of their position or expertise, for team members to establish and maintain a team dynamic that is effective in meeting established goals of rehabilitation. Appendix 5–1 contains a description of the basic components and goals of effective interdisciplinary teams for persons with acquired brain injury.

**Table 5–3.** Interdisciplinary Team Members

Primary care physician

Rehabilitation nurse

Clinical neuropsychologist

Speech-language pathologist

Audiologist

Rehabilitation psychologist

Behavioral specialist

Dietitian

Educator

Occupational therapist

Physical therapist

Psychiatrist

Social worker

Case manager

Therapeutic recreation specialist

Vocational rehabilitation counselor

Paraprofessionals

*Source:* Joint Committee on Interprofessional Relations Between the American Speech-Language-Hearing Association and Division 40 (Clinical Neuropsychology) of the American Psychological Association (2007, Interdisciplinary Team Membership).

Interdisciplinary teams also benefit from a team coordinator who is responsible for team administration/facilitation and ensuring interdisciplinary team function (Joint Committee on Interprofessional Relations Between ASHA and Division 40 [Clinical Neuropsychology] of the American Psychological Association, 2007). This could be any member of the team. This is not necessarily established solely on discipline, but rather is determined by an individual's case management skills and clinical and leadership abilities. Team members should not assume that individuals with TBI and their families understand the roles of a specific team member or the nature and purpose of an interdisciplinary team. This should be discussed among team members (including the individual with TBI) early on and frequently throughout the rehabilitation process.

## Role of the Speech-Language Pathologist

According to ASHA's scope of practice in the area of cognitive-communication disorders, an SLP's roles and responsibilities include each of the elements highlighted in Table 5–4. This includes "training discrete cognitive processes, teaching specific functional skills, developing compensatory strategies and support systems, providing caregiver training, and providing counseling and behavioral support services" (ASHA, 2005, para. Roles). Appendices 5–2 and 5–3 contain the preferred practice patterns for SLPs from ASHA in the area of cognitive-communicative disorders.

## Medical Intervention

Although it is beyond the scope of this text to describe *in detail* all aspects of medical intervention following TBI, an understanding of the important categories of medical intervention across the continuum of recovery has direct relevance to the course of rehabilitation. Prognostic indicators relative to primary and secondary injury are discussed in Chapter 2 (Classification and Recovery). Two common categories of medical intervention after a TBI are neurosurgical and pharmacological. These forms of medical intervention are sometimes necessary in the acute stage (within the first week post TBI) in order to preserve life and decrease morbidity (disease). They may also be utilized within the subacute (less than 90 days post TBI) and chronic phases (more than 90 days post TBI) to improve functional outcomes.

## Neurosurgical Intervention

Common surgical intervention to the brain (neurosurgery) includes repair of hemorrhaging (bleeding blood vessel) or removal of large hematomas (blood clot) (Amenta & Jallo, 2013). Neurosurgery is also performed to relieve critically high and life-threatening intracranial pressure. In the case of penetrating head injury, surgery may also be performed to prevent infection and cerebrospinal fluid leakage, to remove foreign bodies and debris, and to repair dural and scalp damage. Neurosurgery is either performed immediately after admittance to an emergency department or after some period of monitoring. The five most common reasons for neurosurgical intervention after a TBI are acute epidural hematomas, acute subdural hematomas, traumatic intraparenchymal lesions, posterior fossa mass lesion, and skull fracture (Amenta & Jallo, 2013). Table 5–5 contains a description of neurosurgical interventions, commonly pursued in the acute stage of medical intervention.

**Table 5–4.** Roles and Responsibilities of SLPs in the Area of Cognitive-Communication Disorders

| Primary Roles | Description |
| --- | --- |
| Identification | Identifying individuals at risk for or presenting with cognitive-communication disorders. |
| Assessment | Selecting and implementing clinically, culturally, and linguistically appropriate approaches to assessment and diagnosis, using both static and dynamic procedures. |
| | Identifying contextual factors that contribute to or can be used to ameliorate cognitive-communication disorders. |
| Intervention | Selecting and implementing clinically, culturally, and linguistically appropriate and evidence-based approaches to intervention (e.g., training discrete cognitive processes, teaching specific functional skills, developing compensatory strategies and support systems, providing caregiver training, providing counseling and behavioral support services). |
| Counseling | Providing culturally and linguistically appropriate counseling for individuals and their significant others about cognitive-communication disorders and their impact. |
| Collaboration | Collaborating with the individual with a cognitive-communication disorder, family members, teachers, other professional colleagues, care providers, and others in developing and implementing assessment and intervention plans. |
| Case management | Serving as case manager, service coordinator, or team leader by coordinating, monitoring, and ensuring the appropriate and timely delivery of a comprehensive management plan. |
| Education | Developing curricula and educating, supervising, and mentoring future SLPs in assessment and treatment options and other issues related to cognitive-communication disorders. |
| | Educating families, caregivers, and other professionals regarding the needs of individuals with cognitive-communication disorders. |
| Prevention | Educating the public on the prevention of factors contributing to cognitive-communication disorders. |
| Advocacy | Advocating for services for individuals with cognitive-communication disorders. |
| | Serving as an expert witness. |
| Research | Advancing the knowledge base on cognitive-communication disorders and their treatment through research activities. |

*Source:* ASHA (2005, Roles).

**Table 5–5.** Common Forms of Acute Neurosurgical Intervention

| | |
|---|---|
| Craniotomy | Skull fractures, hemorrhage, hematomas, and complications associated with penetrating injury are addressed surgically via a craniotomy. A craniotomy involves cutting a hole in the skull and removing a bone flap to gain access the brain. The surgeon performs any needed procedures, replaces the bone flap, and secures it in place with plates and screws. |
| Decompressive craniectomy | Critically elevated intracranial pressure is addressed surgically via a decompressive craniectomy. A decompressive craniectomy involves removing a large portion of the skull to allow room for the brain to swell. After the surgery, a biologic tissue is placed on top of the exposed brain and the skin is closed. After the swelling has resolved (anywhere from 1 to 3 months after the procedure), the bone flap is replaced in another surgery, called cranioplasty. |
| Intracranial pressure monitor | Intracranial pressure (ICP) monitors may be used to assess brain function and measure pressure inside the skull. ICP monitors are placed via inserting a catheter through a small hole in the skull, positioned inside the ventricle. If pressure increases beyond a critical threshold, surgical intervention may be needed. |
| Brain oxygen monitor | Brain oxygen monitors are placed by inserting a catheter through a small hole in the skull. Brain oxygen monitors are positioned within the brain tissue to assess oxygen levels and temperature within the brain so that adjustments in the amount of oxygen provided can be made as needed. |

*Source:* Amenta & Jallo (2013).

## Pharmacological Intervention

The use of medications after TBI can include those for the treatment of sedation, pain, seizures, intracranial pressure, fluid and electrolyte homeostasis, and infection (Rivera, 2014). Pharmacotherapy is also a growing area of interest in the research literature for the treatment of psychiatric, cognitive, and behavioral sequelae of TBI (Bhatnagar, Iaccarino, & Zafonte, 2016). Increasingly, pharmacotherapy is used within the subacute and chronic phases to address a variety of concerns, including areas within

cognitive and behavioral domains, such as hyper-arousal and agitation, hypo-arousal, inattention, slow processing speed, and memory impairment. Examples of medications studied for use in these areas (and their resulting outcomes) are listed in Table 5–6. It is important to note that the use of these and other pharmacotherapy options are mainly recommended after other non-pharmacological interventions, such as environmental modification and compensatory strategies, have been shown to be ineffective (Bhatnagar, Iaccarino, & Zafonte, 2016; O'Neil-Pirozzi, Kennedy, & Sohlberg, 2016).

**Table 5–6.** Pharmacotherapy: Common Drugs and Their Corresponding Impact on Cognitive and Behavioral Domains

| | | |
|---|---|---|
| Hyper-arousal and agitation | Beta-blockers | Non-selective beta-blockers have been shown to reduce agitation in individuals with TBI compared with other drug intervention. |
| | Buspirone | Buspirone has been shown to reduce anxiety in individuals with TBI, but benefits can be delayed 2–3 weeks. |
| | Psychotropic medications | Benzodiazepines and typical antipsychotics are not recommended for TBI-related agitation, as they have the potential to impair cognition and hinder cognitive recovery. |
| | Amantadine | Amantadine has been shown to reduce the frequency and severity of irritability (but not aggression) in individuals with TBI. |
| | Lamotrigine | Lamotrigine has been shown to reduce aggressive behaviors and improve psychosocial cognitive behavior in individuals with TBI. |
| Hypo-arousal | Anti-epileptic anti-psychotic, anti-spasticity, and medications used to treat agitation or anxiety | These classes of medication may worsen hypo-arousal in individuals with TBI. |
| | Amantadine | Amantadine has been shown to improve early arousal in the acute phase of recovery and improve overall rate of recovery in individuals with TBI. |
| | Bromocriptine | Within a small study, improvements in arousal were noted in individuals with TBI who were administered bromocriptine, but sample size was too small to make a definitive conclusion on its effects. |
| | Levodopa/carbidopa | Within a small study, individuals with TBI administered levodopa/carbidopa showed improvement in consciousness within 2 weeks of treatment, but sample size was too small to make a definitive conclusion on its effects. |
| | Zolpidem | Studies have shown zolpidem to have a temporary impact on consciousness and hemispheric activity in individuals with severe TBI. |
| | Sertraline | No significant improvements in arousal (compared with placebos) have been noted in administration of sertraline to individuals with TBI. |

*continues*

**Table 5–6.** *continued*

| | Modafinil | Results are mixed in the use of modafinil to improve excessive daytime sleepiness and fatigue. Some studies note no change in either daytime sleepiness or fatigue, while others note reduction in excessive daytime sleepiness but no change in fatigue. |
|---|---|---|
| | Pramipexole | Within a small randomized study, administration of pramipexole resulted in improvement in arousal and awareness. |
| Attention and processing speed | Methylphenidate | Some studies have noted improvement in performance speed across with administration of methylphenidate, but there have been mixed results in the area of improved attention with methylphenidate. Side effects of hyperactivity and aggression have also been reported. |
| | Donepezil | In a single study in this area, administration of donepezil was noted to improve sustained attention in individuals with moderate to severe TBI. |
| | Atomoxetine | In a single study on the topic, significant improvement was shown in attention, speed of memory, or working memory with administration of atomoxetine post TBI. |
| | Lisdexamfetamine dimesylate | A single study in this area showed improvement in attention and working memory, but not processing speed with administration of lisdexamfetamine dimesylate in individuals with moderate to severe TBI. |
| | Bromocriptine | In a single study on this medication, no improvement in attention was shown with administration of bromocriptine post TBI. |
| Memory | Donepezil | Administration of donepezil has been shown to improve memory after a TBI and in particular short-term memory. |
| | Rivastigmine | Rivastigmine, used in the treatment of Alzheimer's disease, has not shown significant improvement in memory or other cognitive functions in individuals with TBI. |

*Source:* Bhatnagar, Iaccarino, & Zafonte (2016).

## Complementary/Alternative Medicine and Neurotherapy

Although not discussed in detail within this text, complementary and alternative medicine (CAM) (Table 5–7) and the use of neurotechnology (Table 5–8) are also in the research literature on TBI rehabilitation. Readers interested in additional information about CAM are referred to Hernández, Brenner, Walter, Bormann, and Johansson (2016) and the National Center for Complementary and Integrative Health, located at https://nccih.nih.gov/. For information on neurotechnology and TBI, the reader is referred to Bonato (2013).

## Patient and Family Education

The role of each team member in providing timely and relevant information/education about a wide spectrum of content cannot be underestimated. As ASHA's scope of practice highlights, a core aspect of an SLP's role in providing services is "educating families, caregivers, and other professionals regarding the needs of individuals with cognitive-communication disorders" (ASHA, 2005, para. Role). The type of information and education provided will vary greatly, given the needs of an individual with TBI (and his/her family members). It is helpful to consider core tenets of adult learning relative to education for individuals with TBI and their adult family members. These include the seminal works of Malcolm Knowles (1984a, 1984b), which state that an adult learner:

■ Has an independent self-concept and can direct his or her own learning

**Table 5–7.** Examples of Complementary and Alternative Medicine in TBI Rehabilitation

Herbal medicine

Homeopathy

Naturopathy

Aromatherapy

Energy-based therapy
- Light therapy
- Healing touch therapy
- Reflexology
- Reiki

Mind-body medicine
- Meditation
- Relaxation techniques
  - Guided imagery
  - Autogenic training
  - Humor therapy
  - Music therapy

Spiritual healing

Alternative movement therapy
- Alexander and Feldenkrais
- Tai chi or Qigong

Massage therapy

Craniosacral manipulation

Acupuncture

Electroencephalographic biofeedback

Hyperbaric oxygen therapy

Electrical and magnetic therapy
- Magnetic therapy
- Transcutaneous electrical nerve stimulation
- Cranial electrical stimulation
- Transcranial magnetic stimulation

*Source:* McElligott, Zollman, & Kothari (2013).

**Table 5–8.** Examples of Neurotechnology in TBI Rehabilitation

Brain stimulation

- Deep brain stimulation
- Cortical stimulation
- Transcranial magnetic stimulation
- Transcranial direct current stimulation

Peripheral stimulation

- Vagus nerve stimulation (VNS)
- Functional electrical stimulation (FES)
- Mechanical and electrical stimulation via stochastic

Brain–computer interface (BCI)

Robotics

- End-effector–based interfaces
- Exoskeletal-based interfaces

*Source:* Bonato (2013).

- Has accumulated a reservoir of life experiences that is a rich resource for learning
- Has learning needs closely related to changing social roles
- Is problem centered and interested in immediate application of knowledge
- Is motivated to learn by internal rather than external factors (Merriam, 2001, p. 5)

Further, Knowles's four assumptions stipulate that

- Adults need to be involved in the planning and evaluation of their instruction.
- Experience (including mistakes) provides the basis for learning activities.
- Adults are most interested in learning about subjects that have immediate relevance to their job or personal life.

- Adult learning is problem centered rather than content oriented.

Given the potential for impairments in attention, memory, and executive function, which may alter comprehension, processing, and recall of information, team members must factor the influence of these impairments on the nature and format of information provided to meet the specific needs of individuals with TBI. The ways in which education is adjusted given current cognitive status is an important topic for team discussion. As a team member with expertise in communication (receptive and expressive), SLPs can play a key role in guiding effective practice in this area.

Across the continuum of care, team members should tailor education to the unique needs of individuals with TBI and their families but also ensure that there is a structured and standardized process for providing this information. Holland and Shigaki (1998) suggested a three-phase model for offering education and information in support of families and caregivers of individuals with TBI (Table 5–9). This is a model that can also be applied to individuals with TBI.

Within this first stage (Phase I), individuals with TBI and their families are often still experiencing the shock of the initial injury. They are forced to quickly learn complex and unfamiliar medical terminology and jargon, under a situation of significant stress. Within this stage, team members can focus on providing basic information about what is immediately happening. Team members can also clarify terms and procedures associated with medical intervention and brain injury at this stage. Team members need to be mindful of the fact that individuals at this stage in the continuum of care (both individuals with TBI and their

**Table 5–9.** Phases of Family and Caregiver Education

| Phase of Education | Stage in Continuum of Care | Emphasis of Education |
|---|---|---|
| Phase I | Emergency Department<br>Critical Care<br>Acute Care | Providing new information<br>Clarifying terms and procedures about medical management and brain injury |
| Phase II | Acute Rehabilitation<br>Subacute Rehabilitation<br>Neurobehavioral Rehabilitation | Orienting individuals with TBI and their families to the nature and purpose of rehabilitation<br>Introducing the full spectrum of possible TBI outcomes<br>Emphasizing the importance of family systems and potential for alterations in family dynamics<br>Preparing family and caregivers for community and post-acute or outpatient rehabilitation |
| Phase III | Community | Emphasizing and explaining the long-term and protracted nature of recovery<br>Explaining and preparing family and caregivers for potential changes in behavior, personality, and sexuality<br>Providing descriptions and information on home health, community, and other support services<br>Describing applicable home environment adaptations<br>Explaining the process for school and vocational reentry<br>Describing TBI recovery from the patient's perspective |

*Source:* Holland & Shigaki (1998).

families) may have limited recall and learning abilities due to the stress surrounding this stage of recovery. As such, giving information in manageable amounts is critical, as is repeating that information frequently and offering written and visual supports to enhance recall.

Within Phase II there is a larger volume of information that is provided. The emphasis of education in this phase is to help individuals with TBI and their families begin to understand the complexities of this stage of intervention as well as to prepare them for the next steps in the journey ahead. As with Phase I, information that is understandable and presented with written and visual supports is important.

Like Phase II, Phase III involves additional amounts of information, adjusted to meet the specific needs of both the individual with TBI and his/her family. The primary goals of this phase are preparation for return to a community setting and outpatient rehabilitation. Emphasis is placed on understanding the need for continued rehabilitation and long-term changes. Family members and caregivers will also take on a greater role in coordination of rehabilitation efforts. For individuals with moderate to severe TBI, a return to home and community may also mean a greater burden and expansion of family member and caregiver roles and responsibilities in everyday activities of the individual with TBI.

Information that is tailored to the individual has been shown to increase satisfaction with treatment and improve the outcome of rehabilitation (Pegg et al., 2005). Team members can also help individuals with TBI and their families identify reliable sources of information for both self-study and for future inquiry, such as brain injury association websites and community accessible service providers. There is now a wealth of information about brain injury online, tailored to individuals with TBI and their families. However, a word of caution is in order about online resources. In providing any external online resources, it is important that team members consider the phases of recovery in determining that depth and format of information provided. It is also critical that if direct links or URLs are provided, they are reviewed by team members to ensure the content is accurate and represents the best and most current evidence on the topic. Alternatively, since online sites and URLs can change, it is best to refer individuals to well-developed networks that offer easily searchable sites, with established structures for continued vetting of content and specialized expertise in assisting individuals with TBI and their families. For example, the American Speech-Language-Hearing Association (ASHA) has several patient- and family-centered resources in the area. Other reliable sources of information in this area (although not exhaustive) include the Brain Injury Association, Brain Injury Information Network, Brain Injury Resource Center, and the Washington Educational Telecommunications Association (WETA) Brainline.org .

## Coping and Emotional Adjustment After TBI

It goes without saying that a TBI is a life changing event, with the potential for many complex and longstanding emotional and psychological challenges. Chapter 3 (Compounding and Concomitant Conditions) discusses some of these challenges, including personality changes and psychological concerns such as depression and anxiety.

A topic that has received attention in the research literature is coping and adjustment after a TBI. Coping is the cognitive and behavioral strategies individuals use to address the stressful circumstances of TBI (Krpan, Anderson, & Stuss, 2013). Coping strategies in individuals without TBI generally comprise problem-focused coping and emotion-focused coping (Krpan, Anderson, & Stuss, 2013). Problem-focused coping (sometimes referred to as planful coping) seeks a solution to the problem, while emotion-focused coping (also known as avoidant coping) seeks to manage the stress emotionally, sometimes through avoiding the issue. The coping strategy an individual deploys after a TBI is not necessarily related to injury factors, such as severity, impairment, lesion location, or type of injury (Anson & Ponsford, 2006). However, demographics such as personality, age, and social factors can play a role in the coping strategies deployed after a TBI. Self-awareness of injury after a TBI may also influence the copy strategy employed (Anson & Ponsford, 2006).

Research suggests that individuals who adopt more problem-focused/planful coping after a TBI have better psychosocial outcome than those with more emotional/ avoidant coping (McMillan, Williams, & Bryant, 2003; Tomberg, Toomela, Pulver, & Tikk, 2005). For example, Anson and Ponsford (2006) found that after a TBI, individuals with behaviors such as avoidance, worry, wishful thinking, self-blame, and use of drugs and alcohol (defined as non-productive coping strategies) had higher levels of anxiety, depression, and psychosocial dysfunction, as well as lower levels of self-esteem, while individuals who actively worked on problems, using humor and enjoyable activities to manage stress (defined as adaptive coping), had higher self-esteem (Anson & Ponsford, 2006, p. 256).

Several researchers have suggested that intervention targeting reframing coping strategies is key to positive outcomes and adjustment after a TBI (Anson & Ponsford, 2006; Krpan, Anderson, & Stuss, 2013; McMillan, Williams, & Bryant, 2003; Tomberg, Toomela, Pulver, & Tikk, 2005). As with all aspects of rehabilitation, these techniques must be individualized to the client and his/her unique circumstances and experience (Krpan, Anderson, & Stuss, 2013). Neuropsychologists will play a key role in providing direct intervention and counseling in these areas (ASHA, 2003). They can also recommend to team members applicable strategies for effectively fostering adaptive coping strategies after a TBI.

## Special Needs of Family and Caregivers

Family members and caregivers of individuals with TBI are also in need of special support from interdisciplinary team members. It is well established in the research literature that family members and caregivers of individuals with TBI experience emotional turmoil and a heightened sense of distress and anxiety when a loved one experiences a TBI (Allen, Linn, Gutierrez, & Willer, 1994). This has been measured in increased rates of depression and anxiety, self-reports of increased burden, and increased help-seeking behaviors among family members and caregivers of individuals with TBI. This distress varies based on the residual sequelae of injury in the individual with TBI, the relationship of the family member or caregiver to the individual with TBI (e.g., parent, spouse, child), and the level of social support available to a family member or caregiver after an injury. The most commonly identified predictor of heightened family and caregiver distress is residual behavioral, emotional, or personality changes in the individual with TBI, such as irritability, aggressiveness, angry outburst, and egocentrism (Marsh, Kersel, Havill, & Sleigh, 1998). To a lesser degree, residual cognitive impairments, such as ongoing memory problems and slowed information process have also been shown to be related to family member distress (Kreutzer, Gervasio, & Camplair, 1994). Psychological counseling and emotional support for family and caregivers of individuals with TBI are critical. This should be provided in tandem with intervention for the individual with TBI.

## References

Allen, K., Linn, R. T., Gutierrez, H., & Willer, B. (1994). Family burden following traumatic brain injury. *Rehabilitation Psychology*, 39(1), 29–48.

Amenta, P. S., & Jallo, J. I. (2013). The surgical management of traumatic brain injury. In N. Zasler, D. I. Katz, R. D. Zafonte, D. B. Arciniegas, M. B. Bullock, & J. S. Kreutzer (Eds.), *Brain injury medicine: Principles and practice* (2nd ed.). New York, NY: Demos Medical.

American Speech-Language-Hearing Association. (1990). *Interdisciplinary approaches to brain damage* [Position statement]. Retrieved from http://www.asha.org/policy

American Speech-Language-Hearing Association. (2003). *Evaluating and treating communication and cognitive disorders: Approaches to referral and collaboration for speech-language pathology and clinical neuropsychology* [Technical report]. Retrieved from http://www.asha.org/policy

American Speech-Language-Hearing Association. (2004). *Preferred practice patterns for the profession of speech-language pathology* [Preferred practice patterns]. Retrieved from http://www.asha.org/policy

American Speech-Language-Hearing Association. (2005). *Roles of speech-language pathologists in the identification, diagnosis, and treatment of individuals with cognitive-communication disorders: Position statement*. Retrieved from http://www.asha.org/policy

Anson, K., & Ponsford, J. (2006). Coping and emotional adjustment following traumatic brain injury. *Journal of Head Trauma Rehabilitation, 21*(3), 248.

Bhatnagar, S., Iaccarino, M., & Zafonte, R. (2016). Pharmacotherapy in rehabilitation of post-acute traumatic brain injury. *Brain Research, 1640*, 164–179.

Bonato, P. (2013). Neurotechnology in traumatic brain injury rehabilitation. In N. Zasler, D. I. Katz, R. D. Zafonte, D. B. Arciniegas, M. B. Bullock, & J. S. Kreutzer (Eds.), *Brain injury medicine: Principles and practice* (2nd ed.). New York, NY: Demos Medical.

Brain Injury Alliance of Utah. (n.d.). *Continuum of care*. Retrieved from: https://biau.org/about-brain-injuries/continuum-of-care/

Brasure, M., Lamberty, G., Sayer, N., Nelson, N., Macdonald, R., Ouellette, J., & Wilt, T. J. (2013). Participation after multidisciplinary rehabilitation for moderate to severe traumatic brain injury in adults: A systematic review. *Archives of Physical Medicine and Rehabilitation, 94*(7), 1398–1420.

Cott, C. A. (2004). Client-centred rehabilitation: Client perspectives. *Disability and Rehabilitation, 26*(24), 1411–1422.

Gerteis, M., Edgman-Levitan, S., Daley, L., & Delbanco, T. (Eds.). (1993). *Through the patient's eyes.* San Francisco, CA: Jossey-Bass.

Hernández, T., Brenner, L., Walter, K., Bormann, J., & Johansson, B. (2016). Complementary and alternative medicine (CAM) following traumatic brain injury (TBI): Opportunities and challenges. *Brain Research, 1640*, 139–151.

Holland, D., & Shigaki, C. (1998). Educating families and caretakers of traumatically brain injured patients in the new health care environment: A three-phase model and bibliography. *Brain Injury, 12*(12), 993–1009.

Joint Committee on Interprofessional Relations Between the American Speech-Language-Hearing Association and Division 40 (Clinical Neuropsychology) of the American Psychological Association. (2007). *Structure and function of an interdisciplinary team for persons with acquired brain injury*. Retrieved from http://www.asha.org/policy

Katz, D. I., Zasler, N. D., & Zafonte, R. D. (2013). Clinical continuum of care and natural history. In N. D. Zasler, D. I. Katz, & R. D. Zafonte (Eds.), *Brain injury medicine: Principles and practice* (2nd ed., pp. 2–12). New York, NY: Demos Medical.

Knowles, M. (1984a). *The adult learner: A neglected species* (3rd ed.). Houston, TX: Gulf.

Knowles, M. (1984b). *Andragogy in action*. San Francisco, CA: Jossey-Bass.

Kreutzer, J. S., Gervasio, A. H., & Camplair, P. S. (1994). Primary caregivers psychological status and family functioning after traumatic brain injury. *Brain Injury, 8*(3), 197–210.

Krpan, K., Anderson, N. , & Stuss, D. (2013). Obstacles to remediating coping following traumatic brain injury. *NeuroRehabilitation, 32*(4), 721–728.

Marsh, N. V., Kersel, D. A., Havill, J. H., & Sleight, J. W. (1998) Caregiver burden at 6 months following severe traumatic brain injury. *Brain injury, 12*(3), 225–238.

McElligott, J., Zollman, F., & Kothari, S. (2013). Complementary and alternative medicine. In N. Zasler, D. I. Katz, R. D. Zafonte, D. B. Arciniegas, M. B. Bullock, & J. S. Kreutzer (Eds.), *Brain injury medicine: Principles and practice* (2nd ed.). New York, NY: Demos Medical.

McMillan, T. M., Williams, W. H., & Bryant, R. A. (2003). Posttraumatic stress disorder and traumatic brain injury: A review of causal mechanisms, assessment and treatment. *Neuropsychological Rehabilitation*, *13*, 149–164.

Merriam, S. B. (2001). Andragogy and self-directed learning: Pillars of adult learning theory. *New Directions for Adult and Continuing Education*, *89*, 3–14.

Nochi, M. (2000). Reconstructing self-narratives in coping with traumatic brain injury. *Social Science & Medicine*, *51*(12), 1795–1804.

O'Neil-Pirozzi, T., Kennedy, M., & Sohlberg, M. (2016). Evidence-based practice for the use of internal strategies as a memory compensation technique after brain injury: A systematic review. *Journal of Head Trauma Rehabilitation*, *31*(4), E1.

Pegg, P. O., Auerbach, S. M., Seel, R. T., Buenaver, L. F., Kiesler, D. J., & Plybon, L. E. (2005). The impact of patient-centered information on patients' treatment satisfaction and outcomes in traumatic brain injury rehabilitation. *Rehabilitation Psychology*, *50*(4), 366–374.

Picker Institute. (n.d.). *Principle of patient-centered care*. Retrieved from: http://cgp.pick erinstitute.org/?page_id=1319

Rivera, J. O. (2014). Pharmacological management of traumatic brain injury and implica-tions for speech language pathology. *Seminars in Speech and Language*, *35*(3), 196–203.

Tomberg, T., Toomela, A., Pulver, A., & Tikk, A. (2005). Coping strategies, social support, and life orientation and health-related quality of life following traumatic brain injury. *Brain Injury*, *19*(14), 1181–1190.

Trombly, C., Radomski, M., Trexel, C., & Burnet-Smith, S. (2002). Occupational therapy and achievement of self-identified goals by adults with acquired brain injury: Phase II. *American Journal of Occupational Therapy: Official Publication of the American Occupational Therapy Association*, *56*(5), 489.

Winstanley, J., Simpson, G., Tate, R., & Myles, B. (2006). Early indicators and contributors to psychological distress in relatives during rehabilitation following severe traumatic brain injury: Findings from the brain injury outcomes study. *Journal of Head Trauma Rehabilitation*, *21*(6), 453–466.

Young, C., Manmathan, G., & Ward, J. (2008). Perceptions of goal setting in a neurological rehabilitation unit: A qualitative study of patients, carers and staff. *Journal of Rehabilitation Medicine*, *40*(3), 190.

Zatz, D. I., Zasler, N. D., & Zafonte, R. D. (2013). Clinical continuum of care and natural history. In N. Zasler, D. I. Katz, R. D. Zafonte, D. B. Arciniegas, M. B. Bullock, & J. S. Kreutzer (Eds.), *Brain injury medicine: Principles and practice* (2nd ed.). New York, NY: Demos Medical.

## APPENDIX 5–1

# Process to Facilitate Interdisciplinary Team Function

The rehabilitation process should incorporate the following basic components:

1. Integration of information known to affect behavior and outcome, such as (a) age and premorbid and current levels of functioning, (b) effects of medications on behavior, (c) potential medical complications and their effect on behavior, (d) sensitivity to linguistic and cultural needs, (e) various service delivery models, (f) length and intensity of rehabilitation, (g) social/caregiver support, and (h) environmental facilitators and barriers.

2. Establishment and integration of specific discipline assessments and plans of care. In this connection, the following are usually thought to be necessary:
   - Collection of a complete history and interview of patient/caregivers, including a complete medical history provided by an appropriate medical facility, which can serve as a basis for structuring each assessment.
   - Discipline-specific assessments conducted individually or together in order to construct a set of accurate observations. These assessments should result in appropriate diagnosis and a framework for establishing a plan of care.
   - Inclusion of the caregiver and person with acquired brain injury in the development of treatment objectives.

3. Determination of differential diagnoses after all observations are analyzed and integrated during clinical discussion. Requisites for this would include the following:
   - An initial assessment meeting to report strengths and needs in a format that focuses on the processes necessary to develop functional skills in daily living, education, leisure, personal relationships, and work. Assessments should be designed to address body structure/function, activity/participation, and barriers and facilitators to recovery.
   - Discipline-specific assessments and observations across disciplines that are communicated to help determine the overall reliability and consistency of assessment; this process illustrates the interdisciplinary nature of team decision making.
   - Meetings to integrate clinical findings into a plan of care. Meetings should be structured to facilitate an exchange of all opinions—including those of the patient and caregiver—to enhance positive treatment outcomes and avoid negative treatment outcomes.

4. Development of an evidence-based plan of care to provide well-defined, attainable goals with relevant functional outcomes. Such a plan should include the following:
   - Clearly defined goals in various functional skill areas within a specified time frame. The goals include discipline-specific goals as well as interdisciplinary goals.

- Provision for regular review and appropriate alteration of goals.
- Discharge planning and a description of functional ability and level of independence/dependence. This process is necessary to ensure that the discharge plan proposed at admission remains consistent with the patient's skill level at discharge from rehabilitation.
- The necessary structure and content to comply with the appropriate regulatory agency standards and guidelines.

5. Involvement of the patient and caregivers as integral members of the interdisciplinary team. In this connection, the following points should be emphasized:
   - Differing opinions about diagnosis and treatment planning (including those of the patient and caregivers) should be discussed when the team develops a treatment plan.
   - Open discussion with caregivers and the person with acquired brain injury reinforces their important roles as members of the interdisciplinary team and the mutual responsibility for decision making. Provisions for education, training, support, and counseling for the caregiver and for the person with acquired brain injury should be clearly identified in the plan of treatment.

6. An understanding among team members of the relationships among different levels of assessment. Important issues to consider may include, but are not limited to, the following points:
   - In addition to appropriate assessment conducted by each

discipline, the team engages in a discussion of the outcomes from discipline-specific assessments and conducts an overall assessment of functional independence at admission, at discharge, and at a predetermined period after discharge from rehabilitation. A functional assessment demonstrates the impact of the rehabilitation process on the person's body structure/function and activity/participation.
   - Discussion of observations of patient behavior among various team members to ensure integration of various assessment and intervention findings.
   - The establishment of appropriate discharge criteria and the adoption of procedures to facilitate necessary modifications of the program as progress is observed.

7. A measurement system for determining treatment outcomes. Certain settings require use of treatment designs that permit the clinician to establish a relationship between the gain experienced during rehabilitation and the treatments rendered (e.g., pre- and posttreatment designs, single-subject experimental designs).

*Source:* Joint Committee on Interprofessional Relations Between the American Speech-Language-Hearing Association and Division 40 (Clinical Neuropsychology) of the American Psychological Association. (2007). *Structure and Function of an Interdisciplinary Team for Persons with Acquired Brain Injury.* Available from http://www.asha.org/policy. Copyright © ASHA. Used with permission.

APPENDIX 5–2

# Preferred Practice Patterns: Cognitive-Communication Assessment

Cognitive-communication assessment for children and adults addresses cognitive-communication functioning (strengths and weaknesses), including identification of impairments, associated activity and participation limitations, and context barriers and facilitators.

Assessment is conducted according to the *Fundamental Components and Guiding Principles.*

## Individuals Who Provide the Service(s)

Cognitive-communication assessments are conducted by appropriately credentialed and trained speech-language pathologists. Speech-language pathologists may perform these assessments as members of collaborative teams that may include the individual, family/caregivers, and other relevant persons (e.g., educators, medical personnel).

## Expected Outcome(s)

Consistent with the World Health Organization (WHO) framework, assessment is conducted to identify and describe:

- underlying strengths and weaknesses related to cognitive, executive function/self-regulatory, and linguistic factors, including social skills that affect communication performance;
- effects of cognitive-communication impairments on the individual's

activities (capacity and performance in everyday communication contexts) and participation;
- contextual factors that serve as barriers to or facilitators of successful communication and participation for individuals with cognitive-communication impairment.

Assessments may result in the following:

- Diagnosis of a cognitive-communication disorder.
- Clinical description of the characteristics of a cognitive-communication disorder.
- Identification of a communication difference, possibly co-occurring with a cognitive-communication disorder.
- Prognosis for change (in the individual or relevant contexts).
- Recommendations for intervention and support.
- Identification of the effectiveness of intervention and supports.
- Referral for other assessments or services.

## Clinical Indications

Cognitive-communication assessment services are provided to individuals of all ages as needed, requested, or mandated or when other evidence suggests that they have cognitive-communication impairments affecting body structure/function and/or activities/participation. Assessment is prompted by referral, by the individual's educational or medical status, or by failing a language or cognitive-communication screening that is sensitive to cultural and linguistic diversity.

## Clinical Process

Comprehensive assessment is sensitive to cultural and linguistic diversity and addresses the components within the WHO framework, including body structures/functions, activities/participation, and contextual factors. Assessment may be static (i.e., using procedures designed to describe current levels of functioning within relevant domains) and/or dynamic (i.e., using hypothesis-testing procedures to identify potentially successful intervention and support procedures) and includes the following:

- Relevant case history, including medical status, education, vocation, and socioeconomic, cultural, and linguistic background.
- Review of auditory, visual, motor, cognitive, and emotional status.
- Patient/client reports of goals and preferences, as well as domains and contexts of concern.
- Standardized and/or nonstandardized methods selected with consideration for ecological validity:
    - Observe and describe the individual's processing of varied types of information under ideal conditions (i.e., capacity) and in the context of varied activities and settings (i.e., performance) (e.g., ability to attend to, perceive, organize, and remember verbal and nonverbal information, to reason and to solve problems);
    - Observe and describe the individual's executive or self-regulatory control over cognitive, language, and social skills functioning (e.g., set goals, plan, initiate and inhibit, self-monitor and self-evaluate, solve problems, think and act strategically);
    - Analyze the cognitive and communication demands of relevant social, academic, and/or vocational tasks and identify possible facilitative effects in modification of those tasks;
    - Identify the communication and support competencies of relevant everyday people in the environment and possible facilitative effects of modification of their support behaviors;
    - Identify the individual's potential for effective compensatory behaviors and associated motivational barriers and facilitators.
- Follow-up services to monitor cognitive-communication status and ensure appropriate intervention and support for individuals with identified cognitive-communication disorders.

## Setting, Equipment Specifications, and Safety and Health Precautions

### Setting

Assessment is conducted in a clinical or educational setting, and/or other natural environments conducive to eliciting a representative sample of the patient/client's cognitive-communication functioning. The goals of the assessment and the WHO framework are considered in selecting assessment settings. Identifying the influence of contextual factors on functioning (activity and participation) requires assessment data from multiple settings.

### Equipment Specifications

All equipment is used and monitored in accordance with the manufacturer's specifications.

### Safety and Health Precautions

All services ensure the safety of the patient/client and clinician and adhere to universal health precautions (e.g., prevention of bodily injury and transmission of infectious disease). Decontamination, cleaning, disinfection, and sterilization of multiple-use equipment before reuse are carried out according to facility-specific infection control policies and services and according to manufacturer's instructions.

## Documentation

Documentation includes pertinent background information, results and interpretation, prognosis, and recommendations. Recommendations may include the need for further assessment, follow-up, or referral. When treatment is recommended, infor-mation is provided concerning frequency, estimated duration, and type of service (e.g., individual, group, home program). Documentation addresses the type and severity of the cognitive-communication disorder and associated conditions (e.g., medical diagnoses). Documentation includes summaries of previous services in accordance with all relevant legal and agency guidelines. The privacy and security of documentation are maintained in compliance with the regulations of the Health Insurance Portability and Accountability Act (HIPAA), Family Educational Rights and Privacy Act (FERPA), and other state and federal laws. Results of the assessment are reported to the individual and family/caregivers, as appropriate. Reports are distributed to the referral source and other professionals when appropriate and with written consent.

*Source:* American Speech-Language-Hearing Association. (2004). Preferred Practice Patterns for the Profession of Speech-Language Pathology [Preferred Practice Patterns]. Available from http://www.asha.org/policy. Copyright © ASHA. Used with permission.

APPENDIX 5-3

# Preferred Practice Patterns:
# Cognitive-Communication Intervention

Intervention services are provided to individuals with cognitive-communication disorders, including problems in the ability to attend to, perceive, organize, and remember information; to reason and to solve problems; and to exert executive or self-regulatory control over cognitive, language, and social skills functioning. Intervention is conducted according to the *Fundamental Components and Guiding Principles*.

## Individuals Who Provide the Service(s)

Interventions for cognitive-communication disorders are conducted by appropriately credentialed and trained speech-language pathologists, possibly supported by speech-language pathology assistants under appropriate supervision. Speech-language pathologists may provide these services as members of collaborative teams that may include the individual, family/caregivers, and other relevant persons (e.g., educators, medical personnel).

## Expected Outcome(s)

Consistent with the World Health Organization (WHO) framework, intervention is designed to:

■ capitalize on strengths and address weaknesses related to underlying structures and functions that affect communication;
■ facilitate the individual's activities and participation by assisting the person to acquire new skills and strategies;

■ modify contextual factors that serve as barriers and enhance facilitators of successful communication and participation including development and use of appropriate accommodations.

Intervention is expected to result in reduced deficits and contextual barriers, improved abilities and contextual facilitators, and measurably enhanced functioning and participation. Intervention also may result in recommendations for cognitive-communication reassessment or follow-up, or in a referral for other services.

## Clinical Indications

Treatment for cognitive-communication disorders is prompted by the results of a cognitive-communication assessment. Individuals of all ages receive intervention and/or consultation services when their ability to communicate effectively is impaired because of a cognitive-communication disorder and when there is a reasonable expectation of benefit to the individual in body structure/function and/or activity/participation. Interventions that enhance activity and participation through modification of contextual factors may be warranted even if the prognosis for improved body structure/function is limited.

## Clinical Process

Intervention services include providing information and guidance to patients/clients, families/caregivers, and other significant persons about the cognitive-communication disorder, and the course of treatment and prognosis for recovery. Intervention addresses the complexities of a cognitive-communication disorder, including possible reactions, defensive behaviors, and coping strategies of the person who has the cognitive-communication disorder and the reactions of significant others in the environment in a manner that is sensitive to cultural and linguistic diversity. Depending on assessment results, intervention addresses the following:

- Processing of varied types of information under ideal conditions (i.e., capacity) and in the context of varied activities and settings (i.e., performance) (e.g., ability to attend to, perceive, organize, and remember verbal and nonverbal information, including social cues, to reason, and to solve problems).
- Executive or self-regulatory control over cognitive, language, and social skills functioning (e.g., set goals, plan, initiate and inhibit, self-monitor and self-evaluate, solve problems, think and act strategically).
- Modification of the cognitive and communication demands of relevant social, academic, and/or vocational tasks to facilitate performance of those tasks.
- Modification of the communication and support competencies of relevant everyday people in the environment.
- Development and use of effective compensatory behaviors and communication techniques and strategies.
- Development of plans, including referral, for problems other than in cognitive-communication that may

accompany the disorder, such as hearing or visual difficulties, language or speech disorders, and emotional disturbance.

Intervention is long enough to accomplish stated objectives/predicted outcomes. The intervention ends when there is no longer any expectation for further benefit. Clinicians provide an estimate of treatment duration to patients/clients and their families/caregivers.

## Setting, Equipment Specifications, and Safety and Health Precautions

### Setting

Intervention may be conducted in clinical or educational settings and/or natural environments and are selected on the basis of intervention goals and in considerations of the social, academic, and/or vocational activities that are relevant to or desired by the individual. In any setting, intervention addresses the personal and environmental factors that are barriers to or facilitators of the patient/client's cognitive-communication function. There is a plan to generalize and maintain intervention gains and to increase participation in relevant settings and activities.

### Equipment Specifications

All equipment will be used and maintained in accordance with the manufacturer's specifications.

### Safety and Health Precautions

All services ensure the safety of the patient/client and clinician and adhere to universal health precautions (e.g., prevention of bodily injury and transmission of infectious disease). Decontamination, cleaning, disinfection, and sterilization of multiple-use equipment before reuse are carried out according to facility-specific infection control policies and services and according to manufacturer's instructions.

## Documentation

Documentation includes the following:

■ Written record of the dates, length, and type of interventions that were provided.
■ Progress toward stated goals, updated prognosis, and specific recommendations.

■ Evaluation of intervention outcomes and effectiveness within the WHO framework of body structures and functions, activities and participation, and contextual factors.

The privacy and security of documentation are maintained in compliance with the regulations of the Health Insurance Portability and Accountability Act (HIPAA), Family Educational Rights to Privacy Act (FERPA), and other state and federal laws.

*Source:* American Speech-Language-Hearing Association. (2004). Preferred Practice Patterns for the Profession of Speech-Language Pathology [Preferred Practice Patterns]. Available from http://www.asha.org/policy. Copyright © ASHA. Used with permission.

# 6 Cognitive Rehabilitation Therapy Principles

Cognitive rehabilitation therapy (CRT) is not new. CRT dates back to World War I when soldiers and civilians received treatment for war-related TBIs (American Speech-Language-Hearing Association [ASHA], 2003). In the 1970s, CRT gained momentum as a result of improvements in medical services that increased survival rates for those with severe TBI. By the 1980s, CRT was a common part of rehabilitative service offered in many rehabilitation settings (ASHA, 2003). In recent years, research evidence in this area has continued to grow, due in part to military conflicts that resulted in increases in military service members with TBI, but also due to advances in understanding about mild TBI, concussion, and sports-related brain injury.

There is now overwhelming evidence to demonstrate positive efficacy (impact in controlled environments) and effectiveness (impact under real-world circumstances) of CRT for individuals with TBI (Cicerone et al., 2000, 2005, 2011; Rohling, Faust, Beverly, Demakis, & Rao, 2009).

The purpose of this chapter is to provide a framework that clinicians can use in evaluating and implementing the CRT approaches described in Section II (Treatment in Action). The sections that follow will define CRT, place it in the context of the World Health Organization (WHO) International Classification of Functioning, Disability and Health (ICF), describe common categories of approaches, and offer additional insight into other factors to consider in implementing CRT.

## Defining Cognitive Rehabilitation

Although there are many definitions of CRT, the most commonly utilized is that of the Brain Injury Interdisciplinary Special Interest Group (BI-ISIG) of the American Congress of Rehabilitation Medicine (ACRM), which states, "Cognitive rehabilitation is a systematic, functionally oriented service of therapeutic cognitive activities, based on an assessment and understanding of the person's brain-behavior deficits. Services are directed to achieve functional changes by (1) reinforcing, strengthening, or reestablishing previously learned patterns of behavior, or (2) establishing new patterns of cognitive activity or compensatory mechanisms for impaired neurological systems" (Harley et al., 1992, p. 63; Institute of Medicine [IOM], 2011). The United States Department of Veterans Affairs states that "[c]ognitive rehabilitation is one component of a comprehensive brain injury rehabilitation program. It focuses not only on the specific cognitive deficits of the individual with brain injury, but also on their impact on social, communication, behavior, and academic/vocational performance. Some of the interventions used in cognitive rehabilitation include modeling, guided practice, distributed practice, errorless learning, direct instruction with feedback, paper-and-pencil tasks, communication skills, computer-assisted retraining programs, and use of memory aids. The interventions can be provided on a one-on-one basis or in a small group setting." (Benedict et al., 2010, as cited in Institute of Medicine, 2011, p. 78)

CRT should not be confused with Cognitive Behavioral Therapy (CBT), which differs in goals and techniques (Institute of Medicine, 2011). CBT is utilized with individuals who experience emotional and psychiatric disorders, in order to modify maladaptive thoughts and emotions, including training in anxiety management and in some cases exposure to anxiety-provoking or distressing stimuli in order to establish adaptive emotional responses (Institute of Medicine, 2011, p. 76).

In 2011, the IOM conducted a comprehensive review of the research literature in the area of CRT (IOM, 2011). Figures 6–1 and 6–2 illustrate the framework suggested by the IOM in defining CRT, given either modular or comprehensive CRT. Within

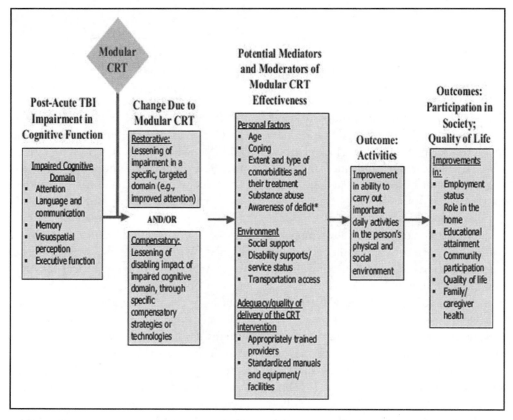

**Figure 6–1.** The IOM model of modular CRT. *For some domains, the CRT intervention may also target deficit awareness; for example, videotape of a social interaction followed by a critique will increase awareness of deficit in language and communication. Source: IOM (2011, pp. 81–82). Copyright © The National Academies Press. Used with permission.

this framework, the IOM acknowledged that a variety of professions provide CRT, using diverse methods and practices. The IOM conceptualized *modular* CRT as targeting a single cognitive domain, deployed primarily in individuals with a single or predominant cognitive impairment. *Comprehensive* CRT (also known as holistic or multi-modal CRT) targets multiple cognitive impairments/domains within a comprehensive program of services, primarily for individuals with impairments in more than one cognitive domain and/or deficits in self-awareness or psychological comorbidity.

As can be seen in Figures 6–1 and 6–2, the outcomes of either model or comprehensive CRT are framed within the WHO ICF, discussed in Chapter 2 (Classification and Recovery; WHO, 2002). The IOM envisioned Activity outcomes of CRT as improvements in ability to carry out important daily activities in the person's physical

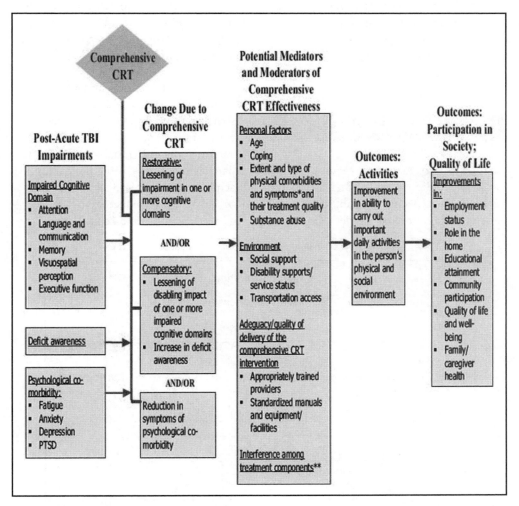

**Figure 6–2.** The IOM model of comprehensive CRT. *For example: visual impairment, headache, dizziness. **Side effect of medication for depression interferes with attention. Source: IOM (2011, pp. 81–82). Copyright © The National Academies Press. Used with permission.

and social environment, while Participation and Quality of Life outcomes of CRT are improvements in employment, role in the home, education, community participation, quality of life/well-being, and family/caregiver health. Lastly, this framework highlights the moderators and mediators of effectiveness of CRT, to include personal factors, environmental factors, and factors specific to the process of CRT, including the adequacy and quality of CRT, and in the area of comprehensive CRT, any potential interference among treatment services. This model serves as an important cornerstone in conceptualizing the treatment activities discussed in Section II (Treatment in Action).

## CRT and the WHO ICF

Chapter 2 provided an overview of the WHO ICF (Figure 6–3). CRT using the WHO ICF is expected to result in "reduced deficits and contextual barriers, improved abilities and contextual facilitators, and measurably enhanced functioning and participation" (ASHA, 2004, Expected Outcomes). Figure 6–4 illustrates the cycle for establishing applicable treatment goals of CRT within this framework, starting with comprehensive and dynamic assessment that addresses each of the three areas of the WHO ICF (Body Structure/Function, Activity, and Participation), followed by clinical reasoning and targeted questions in each of the WHO ICF categories, and concluding with the development of goals that effectively address the WHO ICF categories (ASHA, n.d.). This should lead to intervention designed to:

- Capitalize on strengths and address weaknesses related to underlying structures and functions that affect communication;
- Facilitate the individual's activities and participation by assisting the person to acquire new skills and strategies; and
- Modify contextual factors that serve as barriers and enhance facilitators

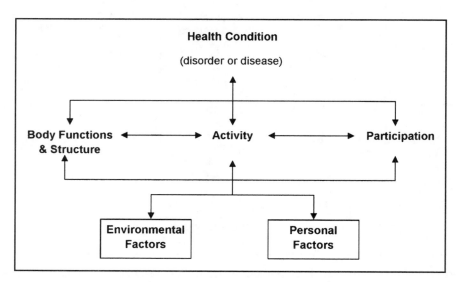

**Figure 6–3.** World Health Organizations (WHO) International Classification of Functioning, Disability and Health (ICF). Source: From "Towards a Common Language For Functioning, Disability and Health: ICF," by WHO and IFC, 2002.

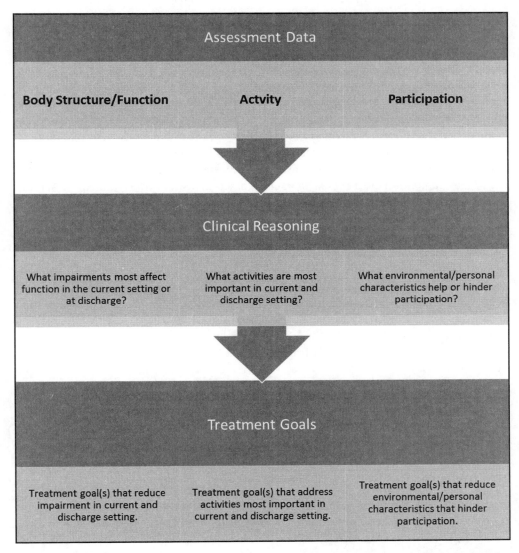

**Figure 6–4.** The process of clinical reasoning used to establish treatment goals based on the WHO ICF. Source: ASHA (n.d).

of successful communication and participation, including development and use of appropriate accommodations. (ASHA, 2004, Expected Outcomes)

Measurements of CRT effectiveness are also predicated on demonstrating clinically meaningful changes across the categories of the WHO ICF (ASHA, 2004, Documentation; Brasure et al., 2012).

## Categories of CRT Approaches

The treatment approach selected within CRT (or a combination thereof) should be guided by the established goals, the research evidence, and the theoretical foundation of a specific approach. Cognitive rehabilitation may include restorative treatments, training in compensatory strategies, caregiver training, education about cognitive consequences of TBI, and environmental manipulation (Bayley et al., p. 303). Figure 6–5 illustrates the common categories of approaches within CRT: restoration, calibration, and compensation. It is important to keep in mind that while these general categories are evident within CRT approaches, in reality the distinction between approaches is not always clear. Many approaches use a combination of theoretical frames, and several approaches may be used simultaneously. There has also been some debate of the stated outcomes of these different categories of treatment. For example, restoration approaches are said to target restoration of cognitive processes, but it is not clear whether this truly occurs or if behavioral impairments just become less visible due to restorative approaches (IOM, 2011).

The purpose of providing this framework is not to lay this argument to rest or to suggest that clinicians select one framework over the other in guiding treatment decisions. This framework is an acknowl-

edgment that the treatment approaches described in the research literature on CRT are varied and often attempt to accomplish a similar goal (improving recall, attention, problem solving, communication, and so forth in daily activities), using differing approaches (restoration, compensation, calibration, or combinations thereof). These categories should serve as an additional frame in evaluating the treatment approaches discussed in Section II (Treatment in Action).

## Restoration

Restoration approaches seek to improve, strengthen, or normalize an impaired cognitive function (IOM, 2011). Methods within restoration approaches involve repetition and drill or exercise-like activities that target a cognitive process, gradually increasing in difficulty and demand (IOM, 2011). The Society of Cognitive Rehabilitation refers to this type of treatment as process training, noting that the purpose is to "stimulate poorly functioning neurologic pathways in the brain in order to maximize their efficiency and effectiveness . . . using new undamaged pathways (redundant representation) and, sometimes, old partially damaged pathways" (Malia et al., 2004, p. 32). This frame views the act of restorative treatment as overcoming damage related to TBI.

## Compensation

Compensation approaches seek to provide alternative strategies for completing everyday activities, despite residual cognitive deficits (IOM, 2011). Compensation approaches are divided into internal and external strategy compensation (IOM, 2011; Malia et al., 2004). External strategies are

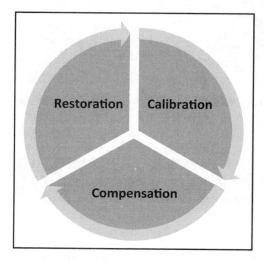

**Figure 6–5.** Different categories of cognitive rehabilitation approaches.

those that rely on items external to the individual, such as alarms, notebooks, notes, calendars, and so forth. Internal strategies are those internal processes such as mnemonics, visualization, word association, and so forth (Malia et al., 2004). The level of independence in the use of compensation will depend on several factors, including awareness and residual cognitive deficits of the individual, the task, and the environment. As such, in both internal and external, the method of compensation and treatment to train a specific strategy are tailored to the individual and the task(s) for which the compensation is meant to address.

## Calibration

As the name suggests, calibration approaches seek to refine awareness and self-measurements of cognitive performance (e.g., thinking about thinking) and use that information to shape behavior after a TBI. Calibration approaches are common within treatment that focuses on the broader construct of metacognition and executive function. Impairments in self-awareness (or the ability to recognize one's deficits) are common in individuals with TBI, particularly those with moderate to severe TBI (Sherer et al., 1998, 2003). Self-awareness is a multidimensional construct comprising both offline and online awareness (Toglia & Kirk, 2000). Offline awareness (also known as metacognitive awareness) occurs prior to task completion, while online awareness is used during and directly after a task. Online awareness includes how effectively the individual conceptualizes and evaluates the task (anticipatory awareness) and the self-monitoring skills of error recognition and adjustment of performance accordingly (self-regulation). Calibration approaches

seek to improve both online and offline awareness. After a TBI, impairments in these areas can be due to neurocognitive, psychological, and/or environmental factors. Table 6–1 contains an overview of calibration approaches that target unawareness due to neurocognitive and socio-environmental factors.

## Decontextualized/ Contextualized Approaches

An additional factor to consider in the selection of an applicable treatment approach is the presence of decontextualized and contextualized treatment frames. Historically, CRT approaches have varied in the extent to which they take place in or use materials from the patient's everyday life (IOM, 2011).

The IOM in its summary of CRT highlighted some of the distinct advantages and disadvantages of each treatment frame, as follows (IMO, 2011, paraphrase, pp. 83–84):

- Decontextualized approaches offer more control over a single cognitive dimension, in order to isolate and treat cognitive processes independently of each other and of other factors.
- Contextualized treatments that are individualized to the client likely enhance motivation, improve self-awareness, and increase the likelihood that strategies learned are generalized to the individual's personal situation.
- Individualization needed within contextualized treatment makes it more cumbersome to deliver and assess than decontextualized approaches, which can be more readily standardized for use with a wide variety of individuals.

**Table 6–1.** Awareness Intervention Approaches Due to Neurocognitive and Socio-Environmental Factors

| Basis for Unawareness | Specific Factors Contributing to Awareness Deficit | Corresponding Treatment Guidelines and Intervention Component |
|---|---|---|
| Neurocognitive factors | • Damage to the right hemisphere or parietal regions (domain-specific awareness deficits), frontal systems or diffuse brain injury (global awareness deficits and difficulty self-monitoring and assimilating experiences into self-knowledge)<br><br>• Impaired executive functioning or significant cognitive impairment contributing to the onset or maintenance of awareness deficits | • Select key task and environments in which behaviors are most important within everyday activities and roles<br><br>• Provide clear feedback and structured opportunities to help people evaluate their performance, discover errors, and compensate for deficits<br><br>• Focus on habit formation through repetition and procedural or implicit learning. Specifically train for application outside the learning environment.<br><br>• Group therapy, family education, and environmental supports to provide external compensation |
| Socio-environmental context | • Information about self is not disclosed due to concerns about how such information will be used in the referral context. Individuals have not had the relevant information or meaningful opportunities to observe post-injury changes.<br><br>• Cultural values impact individual's understanding of the assessment or rehabilitation process. | • Clarify the rationale for the assessment or rehabilitation program and help the person to identify any concerns (e.g., discuss the "pros and cons" of the individual involved in the assessment or rehabilitation program)<br><br>• Consider the timing of the intervention and need for safe and supportive opportunities to observe post-injury changes. Educate significant others to provide appropriate feedback and support. Link people to support or education groups to provide positive social context and normalize people's experiences.<br><br>• Seek advice from a cultural liaison officer and speak to family and friends of the individual to develop a shared understanding. |

Source: Fleming & Ownsworth (2006). Adapted with permission.

Table 6–2 contains additional details of the differences in these two frames of treatment. As can be seen, although there is overlap, traditional (or decontextualized) approaches align most closely with the WHO ICF of Body Structure/Function,

**Table 6–2.** Differences in Decontextualized and Contextualized Treatment Approaches

| | Decontextualized Treatment Approaches | Contextualized Treatment Approaches |
|---|---|---|
| Focus and goals | • Focus on underlying neuropsychological impairment, with the goal of restoration of cognitive functions.<br><br>• Focus on compensatory strategies if restorative intervention is unsuccessful. | • Possible focus on body structure/function, activity/participation, and/or context.<br><br>• Primary goal is to help children and adults with cognitive-communication disabilities to achieve their real-world objectives and participate in their chosen real-world activities |
| Assessment | • Standardized neuropsychological and language measures, possibly combined with customized laboratory tasks; used as diagnostic, treatment planning, and outcome measures. | Body Structure/Functions:<br>• Neuropsychological and language measures, with possible dynamic manipulation of task variables to isolate underlying processes.<br><br>Activity/Participation:<br>• Systematic behavioral observations (static assessment) and exploration of variables that affect functional performance (dynamic assessment); systematic behavioral observations of people in an individual's everyday life. |
| Treatment modalities and methods | • Cognitive exercises to restore cognitive processes or skills, possibly combined with cognitive exercises to acquire compensatory cognitive behaviors. | • Flexible combination of cognitive exercises (if indicated), task-specific training, intervention for strategic thinking and compensatory behavior in functional contexts, and environmental modifications (including changes in the support behaviors of others). |
| Organization of treatment | Exercise Hierarchies:<br>• Hierarchical ordering of targeted cognitive processes.<br><br>Sequence 1:<br>• Mastery of skills in acquisition tasks, then generalization tasks.<br><br>Sequence 2:<br>• Reduction of body/structure/function limitations first, then possibly reduction of associated activity/participation limitations; finally possibly reduction of associated limitations in varied contexts of life. | Hierarchies:<br>• Cognitive components approached nonhierarchically.<br><br>Sequence 1:<br>• Generalization promoted from outset.<br><br>Sequence 2:<br>Traditional progression possibly reversed, with context limitations first reduced by enabling functional participation with environmental supports, activity/participation limitations then reduced with compensatory behaviors and equipment, and underlying body structure/function limitations finally reduced with internalization of well-rehearsed strategies and behaviors. |

*continues*

137

| **Table 6–2.** continued | | |
|---|---|---|
| | *Decontextualized Treatment Approaches* | *Contextualized Treatment Approaches* |
| Setting, content, providers | • Clinical setting using specialized equipment, materials and tasks; cognitive retraining specialists used to deliver the service. | • Possibly clinical setting using personally relevant content (materials and tasks); possibly personally relevant settings as well as content, service delivered by specialists who also recruit the support of people in everyday life. |

Source: ASHA (2003). Copyright © ASHA. Used with permission.

while contextualized approaches align most closely with the Activities and Participation aspects of the WHO ICF. As with the theoretical foundations of restoration, compensation, and calibration, the use of a decontextualized or contextualized approach should be based on the research evidence and whether that approach is relevant to achieving an established goal.

## Treatment Format: Group Therapy

The treatment format: group and/or individual therapy is also a factor to consider when determining a CRT approach (ASHA, 2004). Group therapy (either alone or in combination with individual therapy) is a common form of CRT (Hammond et al., 2015). The recommendations of the INCOG group of researchers and clinicians in the area of CRT specific to group-based intervention state (Bayley et al., p. 302):

Group-based intervention may be considered as part of cognitive rehabilitation to address:

    a.  Social skills
    b.  Memory

    c.  Emotional self-regulation
    d.  Goal attainment
    e.  Problem solving
    f.  Communication
    g.  Attention and concentration
    h.  Sleep hygiene

In general, the purpose of group treatment varies (Roth & Worthington, 2001) but can include:

1.  Teaching participants new communication skills at an introductory level
2.  Providing participants with practice in skills established in an individual session
3.  Providing participants with socialization, self-help, and/or counseling

Table 6–3 contains several common group treatment approaches for individuals with TBI and the general goals of each. As with all treatment decisions, the use of group therapy following TBI should be predicated on the applicable research, and an assessment of the advantages and disadvantages of group format and its applicability to the goals of CRT for an individual with TBI. Table 6–4 contains a list of general advantages and disadvantages of group treatment. Specific group treatment

**Table 6–3.** Types of Group Treatment Following TBI and Sample Goals

| Type of Group | Sample Group Goals |
|---|---|
| Orientation and Recovery from Posttraumatic Amnesia (PTA) Groups | • To be oriented to person, place, and time<br>• To identify group members<br>• To distinguish staff from peers<br>• To use environmental cues/aids to facilitate orientation<br>• To recall episodic events<br>• To use a schedule card to identify next appointment |
| Attention and Information Processing Groups | • To identify auditory stimuli presented during sessions<br>• To recognize (select) target information, such as phone numbers, names, descriptions, or instructions in listening exercises<br>• To use note taking to aid in retrieval of information<br>• To shift attention from one task to another when signed<br>• To divide attention between two tasks<br>• To attend to a sequence of information to complete a task |
| Memory Book Training Groups | • To locate information in memory book<br>• To use a calendar<br>• To follow a routine schedule<br>• To use a to-do list |
| Planning and Problem Solving Groups | • To list the steps of a problem-solving model<br>• To identify each step as it is being used in a problem situation<br>• To apply the step procedure to example problems<br>• To solve problems in the rehabilitation setting using the model<br>• To solve problems in the community using the model |
| Verbal Expression Groups | • To make distinctions between clear and concise statements and wordy and/or extraneous statements<br>• To state opinions and ideas concisely<br>• To provide clear directions<br>• To use personal information and express feelings or attitudes concisely<br>• To use analogies to express opinions and ideas<br>• To respond to situations with appropriate comments and emotional tone |
| Communication Groups (Communicative Intent and Vocational) | Communicative Intent Group<br>• To list a minimum of 15 communicative intents<br>• To identify a variety of communicative intents<br>• To use a variety of communicative intents during group activities<br><br>Vocational Communication Group<br>• To obtain and provide information over the phone regarding employment opportunities<br>• To ask pertinent questions and answer questions effectively during job interview<br>• To understand job requirements and be able to discuss qualifications<br>• To identify appropriate and inappropriate types of communication to use with supervisors and coworkers<br>• To use different types of communication appropriate to workers' positions |

Source: Gillis (2007a, pp. 304–312) and Gillis (2007b, pp. 324–335).

**Table 6–4.** Advantages and Disadvantages of Group Therapy

| Advantages of Group Therapy | Disadvantages of Group Therapy |
|---|---|
| Group participants may motivate each other or offer insight and assistance that a clinician cannot readily provide. | Individual participants may receive less direct attention from the clinician. |
| More opportunities exist for natural speaking situations, socialization, and peer interactions. This may enhance carryover and generalization of a target behavior. | Some participants may be reluctant to participate fully in group interactions, particularly those that are shy or self-conscious. |
| Participants have an opportunity to observe group members and may recognize that others have problems similar to their own. | Some participants may monopolize group interactions. |
| Group interactions, especially when the clinician takes a non-directive role, may decrease dependence of the clinician and thereby increase client independence. | Generally there are fewer opportunities per participant, per increment of time, to engage in a specific behavior (compared with individual sessions). This may mean fewer opportunities to address specific weaknesses and less direct practice of a specific skill. |
| | The pace of the group (or the rate of progress) may not be exactly matched with each participant. |

Source: Roth & Worthington (2001, p. 26).

approaches with demonstrated efficacy will be discussed in Section II (Treatment in Action) as applicable.

## Assistive Technology for Cognition

An increasingly prominent element of CRT for individuals with TBI is assistive technology for cognition (ATC) (Leopold, Lourie, Petras, & Elias, 2015). There are many helpful books now available in this area, including studies by O'Neill (2015) and Scherer (2012). Although an in-depth discussion of ATC is beyond the scope of this text, what follows is a brief overview of several key topics. The reader is also referred to Chapters 8a and 8b (on Memory). Much of the work in the area of external compensation for memory and in particular recommendations in the area of training for assessment/anticipation, acquisition, application, and adaptation are applicable across ATC training and implementation in other areas of cognitive compensation (executive function, attention, and so forth).

Assistive technology is "any item, piece of equipment, or product system, whether acquired commercially, modified, or customized, that is used to increase, maintain, or improve functional capabilities of individuals with disabilities" (Assistive Technology Act of 1998; reauthorized in 2004). Specific to cognition, AT is designed to "increase, maintain, or improve functional capabilities for individuals whose cognitive changes limit their performance of daily activities" (Scherer, 2012, p. 159).

ATC has been described as low technology (low-tech), medium technology (mid-tech), or high technology (high-tech) (Sohlberg, 2011). Table 6–5 contains examples of ATC, categorized by these levels, given their function (task specific or multi-function) (see Table 6–5). Previous studies in this area have noted paper-based calendars, wall charts, and notebooks to be the most commonly used ATCs for individuals with TBI (Evans, Wilson, Needham, & Brentnall, 2003; Hart, Buchhofer, & Vaccaro, 2004). In a recent study among military service members, portable electronic ATCs,

**Table 6–5.** Sample Assistive Technology for Cognition Aids Categorized by Function and Level

| Task Specific | Multifunctional |
|---|---|
| *Low Tech* | |
| Calculator | Sticky notes |
| Pillbox reminder | Voice mail |
| Phone dialer | Watch beeps |
| Alarm clock | Checklists |
| Electronic speller, thesaurus, dictionary | Answering machines |
| Oven timer | Appointment calendars |
| Watch/clock | Car memo pads |
| Labeler | |
| Key finder | |
| Mail sorter baskets | |
| Map, posted directional signs | |
| Financial planner | |
| Posted instructions | |
| *Mid Tech* | |
| Camera | Voice recorder/digital recorder |
| | Cell phone |
| | Pager |
| | Data watches |
| *High Tech* | |
| Global positioning system (GPS) | Specialized task guidance systems (Planning and Executive Assistant and Trainer—PEAT, ISSAC, Pocket Coach) |
| Specialized software programs for facilitated writing, reading, or email | Smartphones |
| | Personal digital assistants |

Source: Sohlberg (2011, p. 15).

especially smartphones and a variety of apps, were reported to be widely used by the participants to compensate for cognitive limitations (Wang, Ding, Teodorski, Mahajan, & Cooper, 2016).

Assistive technology can significantly enhance the independence and quality of life for individuals with disabilities (Parette & Stoner, 2008; Riemer-Reiss & Wacker, 2000), including those with TBI (Sohlberg & Mateer, 2001). It can also help to reduce the demands that are often placed on the caregivers of individuals with disabilities (Lopresti, Mihailidis, & Kirsch, 2004).

The growth in ATC associated with TBI has occurred in parallel with the growth of mainstream *high* technology, such as smartphones and tablet technology for occupational and entertainment purposes. One potential advantage of this parallel growth is the use of mainstream technology for ATC lends itself to greater inclusion in mainstream society for individuals with TBI (Hart et al., 2004). In addition, new high tech AT devices, such as smartphones, tablets, and related apps, also have the potential for multi-purpose use, such as providing entertainment and social connection, in addition to cognitive support (Gillette & DePompei, 2004). Despite the growing research in this area, there are several challenges to successful implementation of ATC for individuals with TBI, including a significant paucity of research, especially on newly evolving apps and mainstream technology use for AT applications (Leopold et al., 2015; Ostergren & Montgomery, 2014).

Foundational knowledge in this area suggests that one key aspect of long-term assistive technology success is careful selection of aids to ensure that they are well matched to the user and the environment (Scherer et al., 2007). This is important considering that an average of one-third of all assistive devices are abandoned by the user (Goodman, Tiene, & Luft, 2002). Several reasons for device "abandonment" include (ASHA, 2004):

1. Poor performance of the device
2. Lack of significant changes in the individual's functional performance
3. Difficulty operating the device
4. High cost
5. Limited availability of service and repair

Feature matching is the process whereby "devices are selected based on relationships between an individual's strengths . . . capabilities and communication needs in relation to various features of a device (ASHA, 2004, p. 9). ATC selection must also be a team-based decision that includes the user's preferences and considers contextual factors likely to contribute to ultimate success (Sohlberg, 2011). It is also important to evaluate ATC at different stages in recovery from TBI, given the potential for needs and available options to change over time (Johnson & Harniss, 2016). Appropriate training in ATC use is also critical (Bartfai & Boman, 2014).

Sohlberg and Mateer (2001) offer a helpful framework to approach feature matching for ATC, given a needs assessment that includes an individual's cognitive profile, physical profile, personal factors (e.g., device preference, available resources and support), and situational factors (e.g., current or historical factors that impact use). These are displayed in Figure 6–6 and combined with common device analysis principles, such as ease of use, access, portability, environment, and modifications and costs. As this figure illustrates, at the intersection of needs and device analysis is the appropriate ATC "match." As an additional resource in this area, Appendix 6–1 contains a checklist for incorporating both these areas specific to individuals with TBI and cognitive deficits.

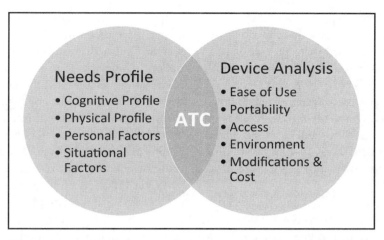

**Figure 6–6.** ATC feature match: Needs profile and device analysis. A suggested framework for identifying ATC, given the needs of the individuals (Needs Profile) and device features (Device Analysis).

## Treatment in Action

In implementing CRT, general treatment recommendations include (Bayley et al., pp. 302–303):

1. Cognitive rehabilitation should be tailored to the patient's neuropsychological profile, premorbid cognitive characteristics, and goals for life activities and participation.
2. Cognitive rehabilitation should:
   a. Focus on engaging in activities that are meaningful to the patient and relevant stakeholders;
   b. Include therapy interventions in the affected person's own environment and/or applicable to the person's own life; and
   c. Incorporate strategizes for generalization.
3. Reassessment of cognition should be undertaken on a regular basis using standardized function outcome measures to determine effectiveness of intervention.

The chapters that follow in Section II (Treatment in Action) address treatment from the perspective of: (1) attention and information processing speed, (2) memory, (3) executive function and awareness, and (4) social communication. Included are treatment approaches recommended within the research literature in each of these areas, including recommended candidacy, level of research evidence, theoretical frame, background, and suggested principles and practices in implementation. Candidacy recommendations for CRT within this text are based on individuals in the post-acute phases of recovery. The majority of studies in the area of CRT have been conducted in the post-acute phases, and in particular the chronic phase of recovery. This is not to suggest that only individuals within the chronic phase of recovery benefit from CRT. Rather, the study of mostly individuals within this stage of recovery is likely the artifact of experimental designs and a need to rule out spontaneous recovery as the source of changes in performance due to treatment.

Further, the approaches in the sections that follow are applicable to individuals who are no longer within the period of post-traumatic amnesia (PTA). As discussed in Chapter 2 (Classification and Recovery), PTA is the period of "generalized cognitive disturbance characterized by confusion, disorientation, retrograde amnesia, inability to store new memories, and sometimes agitation and delusions" (Ponsford et al., 2014, p. 307).

Cognitive (and language) assessment and therapy are *not* recommended while individuals are within PTA (Ponsford et al., 2014). Rather, intervention for individuals with TBI who are experiencing PTA includes strategies to reduce agitation and improve orientation, such as those listed in Table 6–6. Chapter 2 contains a description of applicable measures for monitoring PTA, as per these recommendations. As can be seen in Table 6–6, an additional recommendation in this area is to provide orienting information, as tolerated by the individual with TBI. Haskins and colleagues recommend that individuals within PTA be cued by staff and family to refer to an autobiographical orientation page, in order to promote orientation and reduce anxiety and agitation (Haskins et al., 2012, p. 48). An example of an autobiographical orientation page is shown in Figure 6–7. Typical person, place, time, and situational orientation information is included, such as:

- **Person:** Name, age, birthdate, and birth location
- **Place:** Current location (place and city)

---

**Table 6–6.** Recommendations for Individuals in PTA

Avoid restraint and allow person to move around freely.

Maintain a quiet environment and stay on ward.

Avoid overstimulation.

Avoid daytime sedative medication.

Evaluate the impact of visitors and limit visitors if causing agitation.

Allow frequent rest times.

Try to keep consistent staff.

Establish most reliable means of communication.

Provide frequent reassurance.

Monitor using an appropriate PTA scale.

Do not perform cognitive/language assessment and therapy, as it is generally inappropriate

Present orienting or familiarizing information only as tolerated by the person. If this causes agitation, refrain from providing such information and acknowledge their understanding in the situation.

Help family members to understand how to approach the person with information to reduce triggering agitation.

Source: Ponsford, Janzen, Mcintyre, Bayley, Velikonja, et al. (2014, p. 315).

My name is John Allen Smith

I am 25 years old

I was born May 5, 1992 in Long Beach, California

Today's date is Wednesday, April 15, 2017

Right now I am at Long Beach Memorial Hospital

I was injury in car accident on April 12, 2017

**Figure 6–7.** A sample autobiographical page that can be used to orient individuals within PTA to person, place, time, and situational information.

- **Time:** Current day and time
- **Situation:** Date of injury and type of injury

Pilot studies in the area of reality orientation (ROT) (Langhorn, Holdgaard, Worning, Sørensen, & Pedersen, 2015) recommend similar information be present at least twice a day, using various props (e.g., orientation clipboard, calendars, watches, maps). Langhorn and colleagues also recommend providing information about the person visiting or interacting with the individual with TBI (e.g., the visitor's name, relationship to the patient, reason for visit). ROT studies (De Guise, Leblanc, Feyz, Thomas, & Gosselin, 2005; Langhorn, Holdgaard, Worning, Sørensen, & Pedersen, 2015; Thomas Feyz, LeBlanc, Brosseau, Champoux, Christopher, & Lin, 2003) have assessed the impact of these practices on duration of PTA and improvements in overall outcome of individuals with TBI using ROT. To date, efficacy of ROT for the purposes of reducing the period of PTA

(or improvements on overall outcome) has yet to be established across a variety of individuals with TBI, or using large-scale, randomized controlled studies.

## References

American Speech-Language-Hearing Association. (n.d.). *Person-centered focus on function: Traumatic brain injury*. Rockville, MD: Author. Retrieved from http://www.asha.org/uploadedFiles/ICF-Traumatic-Brain-Injury.pdf

American Speech-Language-Hearing Association. (2003). *Rehabilitation of children and adults with cognitive-communication disorders after brain injury* [Technical report]. Retrieved from http://www.asha.org/policy

Bartfai, A., & Boman, I. L. (2014). A multiprofessional client-centred guide to implementing assistive technology for clients with cognitive impairments. *Technology and Disability*, *26*(1), 11–21.

Bayley, M., Tate, R., Douglas, J., Turkstra, L., Ponsford, J., Stergiou-Kita, M., Kua, A., Bragge, P.; INCOG Expert Panel. (2014). INCOG guidelines for cognitive rehabilitation following traumatic brain injury: Methods and overview. *Journal of Head Trauma Rehabilitation, 29*(4), 290–306.

Benedict, S. M., Belanger, H. G., Ceperich, S. D., Cifu, D. X., Cornis-Pop, M., Lew, H. L., & Meyer, K. (2010). *Veterans health initiative on traumatic brain injury.* U.S. Department of Veterans Affairs.

Brasure, M., Lamberty, G. J., Sayer, N. A., Nelson, N. W., MacDonald, R., Ouellette, J., . . . Wilt, T. J. (2012). *Multidisciplinary postacute rehabilitation for moderate to severe traumatic brain injury in adults* [Internet]. Rockville (MD): Agency for Healthcare Research and Quality (US) (Comparative Effectiveness Reviews, No. 72.) Executive Summary. Retrieved from https://www.ncbi.nlm.nih.gov/books/NBK98999/

Cicerone, K. D., Dahlberg, C., Kalmar. K., Langenbahn, D. M., Malec, J. F., Bergquist, T. F., . . . Morse, P. A. (2000). Evidence-based cognitive rehabilitation: recommendations for clinical practice. *Archives of Physical Medicine Rehabilitation, 81*(12), 1596–1615.

Cicerone, K. D., Dahlberg, C., Malec, J. F., Langenbahn, D. M., Felicetti, T., Kneipp, S., . . . Catanese, J. (2005). Evidence-based cognitive rehabilitation: Updated review of the literature from 1998 through 2002. *Archives of Physical Medicine Rehabilitation, 86*, l681–l692.

Cicerone, K., Langenbahn, D., Braden, C., Malec, J., Kalmar, K., Fraas, M., . . . Ashman T. (2011). Evidence-based cognitive rehabilitation: Updated review of the literature from 2003 through 2008. *Archives of Physical Medicine and Rehabilitation, 92*(4), 519–530.

Evans, J. J., Wilson, B. A., Needham, P., & Brentnall, S. (2003). Who makes good use of memory aids? Results of a survey of people with acquired brain injury. *Journal of the International Neuropsychological Society, 9*(6), 925–935.

Fleming, J., & Ownsworth, T. (2006). A review of awareness interventions in brain injury rehabilitation. *Neuropsychological Rehabilitation, 16*(4), 474–500.

Gillette, Y., & DePompei, R. (2004). The potential of electronic organizers as a tool in the cognitive rehabilitation of young people. *Neurological Rehabilitation, 19*, 233–243.

Gillis, R. (2007a). Traumatic brain injury: Early intervention. In R. J. Elman (Ed.), *Group treatment of neurogenic communication disorders: The expert clinician's approach.* San Diego, CA: Plural.

Gillis, R. (2007b). Community oriented group treatment for traumatic brain injury. In R. J. Elman (Ed.), *Group treatment of neurogenic communication disorders: The expert clinician's approach.* San Diego, CA: Plural.

Goodman, G., Tiene, D., & Luft, P. (2002). Adoption of assistive technology for computer access among college students with disabilities. *Disability and Rehabilitation, 24*, 80–92.

Hammond, F. M., Barrett, R., Dijkers, M. P., Zanca, J. M., Horn, S. D, . . . Dunning, M. R. (2015). Group therapy use and its impact on the outcomes of inpatient rehabilitation after traumatic brain injury: Data from traumatic brain injury–practice based evidence project. *Archives of Physical Medicine and Rehabilitation, 96*(8), S282–S292.e5.

Harley, J. P., Allen, C., Braciszewski, T. L., Cicerone, K. D. Dahlberg, C. Evans, S., . . . Smigelski, J. S. (1992). Guidelines for cognitive rehabilitation. *NeuroRehabilitation, 2*(3), 62–67.

Hart, T., Buchhofer, R., & Vaccaro, M. (2004). Portable electronic devices as memory and organizational aids after traumatic brain injury: A consumer survey study. *Journal of Head Trauma Rehabilitation, 19*(5), 351–365.

Institute of Medicine. 2011. *Cognitive rehabilitation therapy for traumatic brain injury: Evaluating the evidence.* Washington, DC: National Academies Press. https://doi.org/10.17226/13220

Johnson, K., & Harniss, M. (2016). Assistive technology in traumatic brain injury. In F. Zollman (Ed.), *Manual of traumatic brain injury: Assessment and management* (2nd ed.). New York, NY: Demos Medical.

Leopold, A., Lourie, A., Petras, H., & Elias, E. (2015). The use of assistive technology for cognition to support the performance of daily activities for individuals with cognitive disabilities due to traumatic brain injury: The current state of the research. *NeuroRehabilitation, 37*(3), 359.

LoPresti, E. F., Mihailidis, A., & Kirsch, N. L. (2004). Assistive technology for cognitive rehabilitation: State of the art. *Neuropsychological Rehabilitation, 14*, 5–39.

Malia, K., Law, P., Sidebottom, K., Danziger, S., Schold-Davis, E., Martin-Scull, R., . . . Vaidya, A. (2004). *Recommendations for best practice in cognitive rehabilitation therapy: Acquired brain injury.* Surrey, UK: The Society of Cognitive Rehabilitation. Retrieved from https://www.societyforcognitiverehab.org/membership-and-certification/documents/EditedRecsBestPrac.pdf

O'Neill, B. (2015). *Assistive technology for cognition: A handbook for clinicians and developers.* London, UK: Psychology Press.

Ostergren, J., & Montgomery, J. (2014). Smartphone technology use in individuals with cognitive communicative impairments: A survey of speech-language pathologists (SLPs). *Journal of Medical Speech-Language Pathology, 21*(3), 267–278.

Parette, H. P., & Stoner, J. B. (2008). Benefits of assistive technology user groups for early childhood education professionals. *Early Childhood Education Journal, 35*, 313–319.

Riemer-Reiss, M. L., & Wacker, R. R. (2000). Factors associated with assistive technology discontinuance among individuals with disabilities. *Journal of Rehabilitation, 66*(1), 44–50.

Rohling, M., Faust, M., Beverly, B., Demakis, G., & Rao, S. (2009). Effectiveness of cognitive rehabilitation following acquired brain injury: A meta-analytic re-examination of Cicerone et al.'s (2000, 2005) systematic reviews. *Neuropsychology, 23*(1), 20–39.

Roth, F. R., & Worthington, C. K. (2001). *Treatment resource manual for speech-language pathology.* Albany, NY: Delmar.

Scherer, M. J. (2012). *Assistive technologies and other supports for people with brain impairment* (p. 160). New York, NY: Springer.

Sherer, M., Bergloff, P., Levin, E., High, W., Oden, K., & Kathryn, E. (1998). Impaired awareness and employment outcome after traumatic brain injury. *Journal of Head Trauma Rehabilitation, 13*(5), 52–61.

Sherer, M., Hart, T., Nick, T. G., Whyte, J., Thompson, R. N., & Yablon, S. A. (2003). Early impaired self-awareness after traumatic brain injury. *Archives of Physical Medicine and Rehabilitation, 84*, 168–176.

Scherer, M., Jutai, J., Fuhrer, M., Demers, L., & DeRuyter, F. (2007). A framework for modeling the selection of assistive technology devices (ATDs). *Disability and Rehabilitation: Assistive Technology, 2*(1), 1–8.

Sohlberg, M. (2011). Assistive technology for cognition. *ASHA Leader, 16*(2), 14.

Sohlberg, M. M., & Mateer, C. A. (2001). *Cognitive rehabilitation: Integrative neuropsychological approach.* New York, NY: Guilford.

Toglia, J., & Kirk, U. (2000). Understanding awareness deficits following brain injury. *NeuroRehabilitation, 15*, 57–70.

Wang, J., Ding, D., Teodorski, E., Mahajan, H., & Cooper, R. (2016). Use of assistive technology for cognition among people with traumatic brain injury: A survey study. *Military Medicine, 181*(6), 560–566.

World Health Organization (WHO). (2002). *Towards a common language for functioning, disability and health: ICF.* Geneva: WHO. Retrieved from http://www.who.int/classifications/icf/training/icfbeginnersguide.pdf

# Assistive Technology for Cognition Checklist

Client Name: _____ Age: _____

Dx: _____ Date of Assessment: _____

**PART 1: COGNITIVE PROFILE** (Indicate with an X in applicable category: strength/ weakness)

| Strength | **MEMORY** | Weakness |
|---|---|---|
| | Memory for events | |
| | Memory for fact | |
| | Memory for routines | |
| | Remembers to remember | |
| | Memory for biographical information | |
| | Compensates for weaknesses *in memory* | |
| | Comments: | |

| Strength | **ATTENTION** | Weakness |
|---|---|---|
| | Attention in a quiet environment | |
| | Attention for extended periods | |
| | Attention in distracting environments | |
| | Can switch between tasks, maintaining attention | |
| | Can divide attention between simultaneous tasks | |
| | Compensates for weaknesses *in attention* | |
| | Comments: | |

| Strength | **EXECUTIVE FUNCTION** | Weakness |
|---|---|---|
| | Initiates tasks | |
| | Inhibits counterproductive behaviors | |
| | Sets realistic goals | |
| | Identifies steps to accomplish goals | |
| | Identifies barriers to task completion | |
| | Organizes steps for task completion | |

| Strength | EXECUTIVE FUNCTION | Weakness |
|---|---|---|
| | Follows through with steps for task completion | |
| | Evaluates task performance | |
| | Aware of strengths and weaknesses *in cognition* | |
| | Compensates for weaknesses *in executive function* | |
| | Comments: | |

Part 2: **PHYSICAL PROFILE** (Indicate with an X in applicable category: present/absent)

| Present | VISION | Absent |
|---|---|---|
| | Blindness | |
| | Vision for small print | |
| | Vision for items at a distance | |
| | Double vision | |
| | Difficulty visually tracking | |
| | Visual neglect (side: _____ ) | |
| | Vision field cut (side: _____ ) | |
| | Comments: | |

| Present | HEARING | Absent |
|---|---|---|
| | Deaf | |
| | Difficulty hearing voices | |
| | Difficulty hearing high pitch noises | |
| | Difficulty understanding synthesized/recorded speech | |
| | Uses hearing aids (status: _____ ) | |
| | Comments: | |

| Present | MOTOR | Absent |
|---|---|---|
| | Walks without assistance | |
| | Uses wheelchair for daily tasks | |
| | Uses walker or cane for daily tasks | |

*continues*

| Present | MOTOR | Absent |
|---------|-------|--------|
| | Able to carry items while walking (size limit: _____ ) | |
| | Hemiparesis/paralysis<br>LUE ___ RUE ___ LLE ___ RLE ___ | |
| | Tremors | |
| | Spasticity/Dystonia | |
| | Dexterity for fine motor movements with hands/fingers (Direct Select). Note any limitations in hand/finger access:<br><br>If unable to access device directly with hands/fingers (In-Direct Selection), note access recommendations: | |

**Part 3: PERSONAL PROFILE** (Indicate level with an X along continuum)

| | |
|---|---|
| Family/client reported needs | |
| Past experience with AT | |
| Motivation | Unmotivated -------------------------------------Motivated<br>Comments: |
| Comfort with technology | Uncomfortable------------------------------Comfortable<br>Comments: |
| Awareness of need for AT | Unaware ----------------------------------------------Aware<br>Comments: |
| Willingness to learn AT | Unwilling -------------------------------------------Willing<br>Comments: |

**Part 4: SITUATIONAL FACTORS** (Indicate level with an X along continuum)

| | |
|---|---|
| Independence/level of support | ___ Independent in daily tasks<br>___ Needs some level of support in daily tasks<br>Level of Support Needed:<br>Minimal Support ------------------------Maximal Support<br>Comments: |
| Number of settings | Limited --------------------------------------------Multiple<br>List typical environments: |
| Amount of funding | Minimal Support ------------------------Maximal Support<br>___ Insurance/medical coverage<br>___ Out of pocket<br>___ School<br>___ Other (List: _____ ) |

**Part 5: SYSTEM RECOMMENDATIONS**

| | Category | Notes: |
|---|---|---|
| | Reminders | |
| | Voice recorder | |
| | Pager | |
| | Timer | |
| | Watch/clock | |
| | Organizer | |
| | Calendar/planner | |
| | To-do lists | |
| | Task monitoring | |
| | Memory aids | |
| | Object locators | |
| | Goal setting | |
| | Note taking | |

*continues*

| | Category | Notes: |
|---|---|---|
| | Text-to-speech | |
| | Camera | |
| | Medication management | |
| | Other | |
| | | |
| | | |

| Indicate level with an X along the continuum<br>Client is able to use or could benefit from a device that requires: | Barriers/Notes |
|---|---|
| Minimal Cognition ----------------------------Maximal Cognition<br>(e.g., Attention, memory, and learning needed for device use/training) | |
| Minimal Fine Motor--------------------------Maximum Fine Motor<br>(e.g., Dexterity and control needed for using the device) | |
| Minimal Vision------------------------------------Maximum Vision<br>(e.g., Vision for small print, tracking,<br>frequently changing screens, etc.) | |
| Minimal Hearing------------------------------Maximum Hearing<br>(e.g., Hearing for beeps, tones, and recorded speech) | |
| Stationary Use------------------------------------------Portable Use | |
| Minimal Modification---------------------Maximum Modification<br>(e.g., Ongoing changes and updates needed for device use) | |
| Minimal Expense------------------------------Maximum Expense<br>(e.g., Subjective-dependent on the individual's funding) | |

*Source:* Ostergren, Montgomery, & Carey (2011).

# SECTION II

## Treatment in Action

# 7 Attention and Information Processing Speed

> a. Introduction
> b. Time Pressure Management (TPM)
> *Jennifer A. Ostergren and Carley B. Crandall*
> c. Attention Processing Training (APT)
> *Jennifer A. Ostergren and Carley B. Crandall*
> d. Dual-Task Training (DTT)

## a. Introduction

International Cognitive (INCOG) treatment recommendations in the area of attention and information processing speed deficits include (Ponsford et al., 2014, pp. 324–328):

1. Metacognitive strategy training using functional everyday activities should be considered, especially in patients with mild-to-moderate attention deficits.
2. Training in dual tasking should be used to improve dual-task performance on tasks similar to those trained.
3. Cognitive behavior therapy techniques should be considered to develop strategies to maximize attention in individuals with mild-to-moderate TBI in whom anxiety and depression are impacting on attentional function.
4. Screening for and treatment of comorbid sleep-wake disorders may help to optimize attentional processes.

5. Alterations to the environment and tasks may be used to reduce the impact of attentional problems on daily activities.
6. Reliance on repeated exposure and practice on decontextualized computer-based attentional tasks is NOT recommended due to lack of demonstrated impact on everyday attentional functions.
7. Training with periodic random auditory alerting tones for patients with attentional deficits should not be conducted in therapy outside of a research protocol, as current evidence is conflicting.
8. Training in mindfulness-based meditation techniques is not recommended for remediation of attention deficits outside of a research protocol due to lack of demonstrated efficacy.

Similarly, the American Congress of Rehabilitation Medicine (ACRM), given multiple meta-analyses in this area (Cicerone, Dahlberg, Kalmar, et al., 2000; Cicerone et al., 2005; Cicerone et al., 2011, p. 521) recommends:

1. Remediation of attention is recommended during post-acute rehabilitation after TBI. Remediation of attention deficits after TBI should include direct attention training and metacognitive training to promote development of compensatory strategies and foster generalization to real-world tasks. Insufficient evidence exists to distinguish the effects of specific attention training during acute recovery and rehabilitation from spontaneous recovery or from more general cognitive interventions (Practice Standard).

2. Computer-based interventions may be considered as an adjunct to clinician-guided treatment for the remediation of attention deficits after TBI or stroke. Sole reliance on repeated exposure and practice on computer-based tasks without some involvement and intervention by a therapist is not recommended (Practice Option).

Attention and information processing speed treatment approaches are addressed within this chapter using the hierarchical diagram in Figure 7–1, to include sections on:

1. Time Pressure Management (TPM)
2. Dual-Task Training (DTT)
3. Attention Processing Training (APT)

Table 7–1 contains a list of several possible environmental modifications and strategies, stratified by attention level. At present, there has not been extensive and systematic research conducted on the use of environmental support approaches and their efficacy specific solely for attention deficits (Ponsford et al., 2014). Specific to assistive technology for cognition (ATC), this body

of evidence continues to grow. The general principles outlined in Chapter 6 (Cognitive Rehabilitation Therapy Principles) can be used to guide decisions in the area of ATC relative to attention deficits.

## Assessment

Table 7–2 contains examples of common assessment measures in the area of attention, including direct measures and rating scales. These are helpful measures in identifying particular strengths and weaknesses, and in the case of standardized assessment, comparison to a normative data set. The rehabilitative process also benefits from ongoing structured evaluation of performance in real-world tasks (Sohlberg & Mateer, 2001). Table 7–3 contains examples of real-world tasks, stratified by level of attention. These can be individualized to the client's home, recreational, vocational, and educational experiences. Important factors applicable to each client, such as duration, accuracy, complexity of task, type of attention, and nature and awareness of errors, can be assessed using these structured activities before, during, and after intervention, regardless of the approach utilized. Appendix 7–1 contains an example of a data recording sheet that can be modified for this purpose.

Engaging the client in an ongoing self-assessment can be a valuable exercise in the rehabilitation process. Several authors have noted awareness after a brain injury to be an important factor across a variety of rehabilitation approaches (Bergquist & Jacket, 1993; Ezrachi et al., 1991; Prigatano, Altman, & O'Brien, 1990). A helpful first step in this process is self-observation. This can be done by asking the client to keep a structured attention journal or log about attention performance during daily tasks.

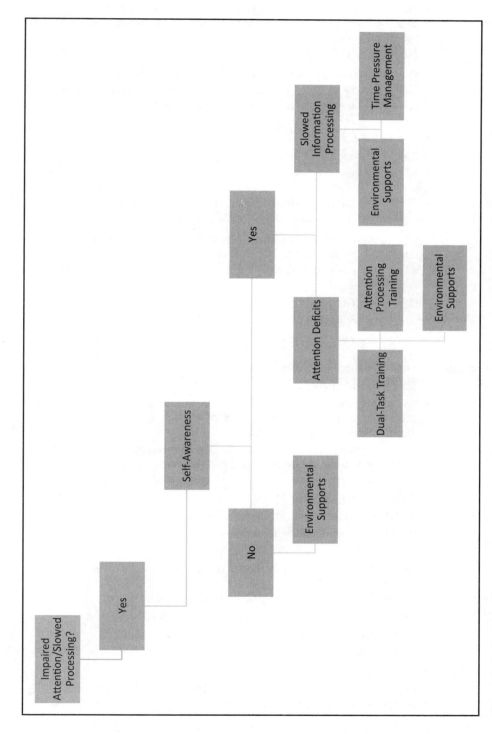

**Figure 7–1.** Suggested treatment approaches in the area of attention and information processing speed, given level of awareness and nature of difficulty.

**Table 7–1.** Possible Modifications/Strategies Associated with Levels of Attention

| | |
|---|---|
| **Focused attention** | • Check with physician or psychologist on current medications; avoid sedating medications; consider stimulants such as coffee, colas, or tea, if not contraindicated.<br>• Take frequent breaks.<br>• Schedule higher consequence tasks when most alert.<br>• Use external cues to stay on task, such as alarms on cell phones or other devices to initiate a task, and timers set for certain durations to stay on task.<br>• Use pause cues.<br>• Sustain attention.<br>• Allow extra time for tasks. |
| **Selective attention** | • Control environmental distractions when able; for example:<br>    ○ Run errands or tend to social activities at non-peak hours<br>    ○ Choose to sit in an area with the least number of distractions (corner booth by the wall, etc.).<br>    ○ Use a personal music player to cancel out background noises, when appropriate.<br>• Rest prior to demanding situations.<br>• Take frequent breaks.<br>• Politely ask others not to visit with you while you are working. |
| **Alternating attention** | • Control environmental distractions.<br>• Take frequent breaks.<br>• Use stop notes, including cues in your environment that show you where you left off, and notes that indicate what you did last and what your next thought or action was or would be.<br>• Alternate attention between tasks that are high-consequence or difficult and those that are not. Allow phone calls to go to voicemail and address them later.<br>• Do not answer people until you have reached a stop point in your work.<br>• Politely ask others not to visit with you while you are working.<br>• Rest prior to demanding situations.<br>• Take frequent breaks.<br>• Use alarms to decrease the need to watch the clock. |
| **Divided attention** | • Do not divide attention on high-consequence and difficult tasks.<br>• Limit divided attention on high-consequence tasks that are easy.<br>• Do not talk on a cell phone while driving.<br>• Limit conversation while driving.<br>• Take frequent breaks.<br>• Rest prior to situations that require divided attention. Use alarms to decrease the need to watch the clock. |

*Source:* Radomski, Goo-Yoshino, Smith Hammond, Isaki, Maclennan, Manning, Mashima, Picon, Roth, & Zola (n.d., p. 232).

**Table 7–2.** Common Attention Measures: Direct Measures and Questionnaires/Rating Scales

**DIRECT ATTENTION MEASURES**

*Comprehensive Attention Batteries*
- Test of Everyday Attention (TEA)
- Attention Processing Training Test

*Component Assessment*

**Processing Speed**
- Oral Symbol Digit Test  (NIH Toolbox)
- Pattern Comparison Processing Speed Test (NIH Toolbox)
- Speed and Capacity of Language Processing Test
- Trail Making Test, Part A

**Sustained Attention (Continuous Performance Tests)**
- Conners Continuous Performance Test
- Test of Variables of Attention
- Visual and Auditory Continuous Performance Test

**Selective Attention**
- Ruff 2 & 7 Selective Attention Test
- Stroop Color and Word Test
- Symbol Digit Modality
- Test of Sustained Selective Attention

**Divided Attention**
- Brief Test of Attention (Auditory Divided Attention)
- Paced Auditory Serial Addition Test (PASAT)
- Trail Making Test, Part B
- Test for Divided Attention

**QUESTIONNAIRES/RATING SCALES**
- Attention Rating Scale (Ponsford & Kinsella, 1991)
- Brock Adaptive Functioning Questionnaire (Attention Domain)
- Moss Attention Rating Scale

The SLP can collaborate with the client to identify good times for this observation (e.g., during specific periods of the day, while performing specific tasks). Based on the psychosocial composition of the client, Sohlberg and colleagues recommend logs that capture successes and/or challenges. This could be done by alternating observation periods (one day of tracking success in attention/one day of tracking lapses in attention) or by requesting that the client record attention successes and lapses in a given time period of observation (Sohlberg, Johnson, Paule, Raskin, & Mateer, 2005). Appendix 7–2 contains a sample data collection sheet that can be modified for this purpose. As with all aspects of self-reflection, this would begin with and include ongoing

**Table 7–3.** Examples of Functional Attention Tasks

Sustain Attention

*Have the client engage in a familiar task, in a quiet environment, such as:*

- Sorting familiar home or vocational items based on a specific rule (e.g. personal mail versus bills, sorting laundry based on colors, placing recipes into piles based on dessert, main meal, appetizer)
- Listening to a list of numbers for a winning ticket number

Selective Attention

*Have the client engage in any of the tasks above, while in a visually or auditorily distracting environment, such as:*

- Sorting a jar of coins by type, while sitting in distracting environment, such as the busy kitchen while meals are being prepare, a coffee shop, and so forth
- Performing an "I Spy," "Where is Waldo," or similar hidden visual object task
- Placing pills into a weekly medicine container while the radio is playing

Alternating Attention

*Have the client engage in any of the above tasks, but switching between them at regular intervals, such as:*

- Alternating between preparing a meal and doing the laundry
- Alternating between filling out a job application and searching for information on a map

Divided Attention

*Have the client perform 2 tasks at a time, such as:*

- Balancing a checkbook or pay bills while engaging in a conversation
- Searching for information in a directory while listening to the radio for for next week's weather forecast
- Preparing a meal while listing items in categories (favorite movies by genre, types of animals by type)
- Completing a word search while describing the recent events of the day

conversations with the client about types of attention (sustained, selective, alternating, divided) and what they mean specifically to the client's daily tasks and his/her unique needs/skills.

Overall self-assessment after self-observation is also valuable. Using a framework based on levels of awareness (Flashman et al., 1998), this self-assessment could include reflection on: (1) the nature of a specific deficit (knowledge); (2) the source of the deficit/difficulty (attributes); (3) how the individual feels about that deficit/difficulty (emotion); and (4) how that deficit/difficulty affects daily tasks (impact). Appendix 7–3 contains a sample worksheet for overall reflection and discussion between the SLP and the client in the area of attention. This should be tailored to meet each individual's needs and abilities and pursued after an effective and trusting therapeutic relationship has been established between the client and the SLP (Flashman & McAllister, 2002). Individuals with ongoing strong negative emotions in this area should be referred to a psychologist or neuropsychologist team member for additional support (American Speech-Language-Hearing Association, 2003).

## b. Time Pressure Management (TPM)

## Candidacy Recommendations

Based on a composite of research in this area (Fasotti, Kovacs, Eling, & Brouwer, 2000; Winkens, Van Heugten, Fasotti, & Wade, 2009; Winkens, Van Heugten, Wade, & Fasotti, 2009), time pressure management (TPM) is recommended in the post-acute stages after TBI for:

1. **Individuals who experience slowed mental processing.** Examples of recommended measures in this area are listed in Table 7–4. In addition, because the relationship between formalized attention tests and actual performance in daily activities is not consistently matched in individuals with brain injury (Ylvisaker, Hanks, & Johnson-Greene, 2002), measures assessing the perceptions of those with TBI are also recommended. The *Mental Slowness*

*Questionnaire* can be used for this purpose (Appendix 7–4).

2. **Individuals who experience time pressure failures in everyday activities.** The *Mental Slowness Observation Test* (or similar online performance evaluation tools) can be used to assess both speed and errors on familiar daily tasks (Appendix 7–5). This is also a measure that can be utilized throughout TPM training to reflect on changes in performance over time.

3. **Individuals who have sufficient awareness to benefit from and generalize TPM strategies to daily activities.** Although not specific to TPM, Ylvisaker and Holland (1985) recommend that successful compensatory training comprise certain characteristics of the patient and the strategy itself (Table 7–5). These can also be applied to TPM in establishing sufficient levels of awareness for implementation of TPM. It should also be noted that Step 1 of TPM is *Identifying the Problem* (Winkens, Van Heugten, Fasotti, & Wade, 2009). As such, candidacy for this approach may be contingent on implementation of this first TPM step in order to determine if awareness is sufficient to proceed to the remaining two steps of TPM: *Teaching the Strategy* and *Generalization*.

## Treatment Evidence

Multiple meta-analyses and systematic reviews have recommended the use of "metacognitive strategy training" during functional activities in individuals with attention deficits following TBI (Ponsford et al., 2014, p. 324). Specific to TPM, there is Level A evidence to support its use in developing strategies to prevent or manage time pressures in individuals with slowed

**Table 7–4.** TPM Related Measures of Mental Slowness and Attention

Paced Auditory Serial Addition Task (PASAT)[1,2]

Auditory Concentration Task (ACT)[1]

Choice Reaction Time Task[1]

Symbol Digit Modalities Test[2]

Trail Making Test[2]

*Note.* [1]Recommended by Fasotti, Kovacs, Eling, & Brouwer, 2000. [2]Recommended by Winkens, Van Heugten, Fasotti, & Wade, 2009.

**Table 7–5.** Requisite Patient and Strategy Variable for Successful Compensatory Training

| Patient | Strategy |
|---|---|
| The patient must recognize the existence of impairments that cannot be alleviated by restitution of underlying problems | The strategy must be fitted to the patient's needs, personality, and abilities |
| The patient must be capable of recognizing problems as they occur or, better yet, anticipate problems before they occur | The strategy must fulfill an obvious and apparent need that personally is felt by the patient |
| The patient must be capable of invoking a strategy based on recognition of a present or potential problem situation | The strategy must fit the personal inclination and the attitudes of patient |
| | The strategy must be easy enough that the patient can invoke it automatically and effortlessly |

*Source:* Ylvisaker & Holland (1985).

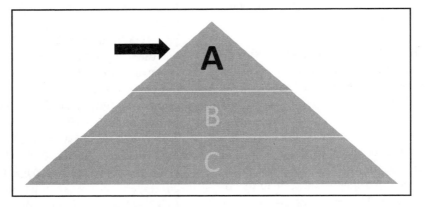

**Figure 7–2.** Level A evidence for the use of TPM following TBI. Level A consists of "recommendation supported by at least one meta-analysis, systematic review or randomized controlled trial study of appropriate size and relevant control group" (Bayley et al., 2014, p. 295).

processing following TBI (Figure 7–2; Ponsford et al., 2014).

## Theoretical Frame

TPM combines compensation and calibration treatment techniques (Figure 7–3). TPM targets compensation by providing training in the use of specific strategies to prevent or reduce time pressures due to slowed mental processing speed (Fasotti et al., 2000; Winkens, Van Heugten, Fasotti, & Wade, 2009). TPM also uses calibration (and metacognitive techniques) to: (1) bring awareness to slowed mental processes after a TBI, (2) highlight the relationship of slowed mental processing to time pressures in daily activities, and (3) foster an understanding of the relationship between compensation and persisting deficits of this nature (Ponsford et al., 2014, pp. 324–325).

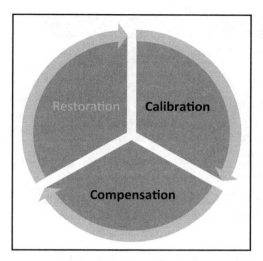

**Figure 7–3.** Theoretical framework of time pressure management. The predominant treatment approaches present in TPM.

## Background Introduction

After a TBI, slowed mental processing is common (Mathias, Wheaton, & Becker, 2007). This can be observed in standardized testing, but also experienced by individuals with TBI as a sense of "information overload," due to a lack of sufficient time to act and think, especially during complex tasks with time constraints (Fasotti et al., 2000, p. 47). Slowed information processing can be disruptive to any real-world task where increased time pressure is created due to slowed information processing, such as difficulty driving in traffic, holding a conversation, preparing a meal, performing time-based work or school tasks, and so forth.

The goals of TPM are to bring awareness to how mental slowness impacts daily activities and to assist individuals with TBI in developing strategies to prevent or manage time pressures created by slowed mental processing (Fasotti et al., 2000; Winkens, Van Heugten, Fasotti, & Wade, 2009; Winkens, Van Heugten, Wade, & Fasotti,

2009). Essentially, TPM seeks to reorganize the execution of tasks so that individuals with TBI "learn to give themselves enough time to deal with the task at hand" (Fasotti et al., 2000, p. 48). Depending on the task, some examples of TPM strategies include additional planning prior to task completion, reorganizing of task steps, rehearsing a task in advance of performance, and modifying the environment prior to or during task completion. TPM addresses both preventative and management strategies (Winkens, Van Heugten, Wade, Habets, & Fasotti, 2009). Preventive strategies are those strategies that anticipate decisions to be made and seek to reduce time pressure during task execution, while management strategies are those that seek to prevent increases in time pressure and deal with existing time pressures while the task is occurring.

Decision making in TPM is stratified into three different levels, based on their impact on time pressure in task execution (Fasotti et al., 2000; Winkens, Van Heugten, Wade, & Fasotti, 2009). Namely, decisions and resulting actions are either strategic, tactical, or operational (Table 7–6). A strategic level of decision making occurs when there are no time pressures. At this level, there is usually sufficient time to plan, as time pressure is not present. Michons (1979, as cited in Fasotti et al., 2000, p. 49) illustrated this level of decision making as analogous to the stage before driving a car, when the driver can plan that route and time for departure to minimize time pressure while driving. At the tactical level, an individual is engaged in a task and time pressure is present, but it has not increased to the point where it is unmanageable. At this level of decision making, there is still the potential to adjust decisions to minimize time pressure, such as when a driver allows for greater distance from the car in front and

**Table 7–6.** Levels of Decision Making: Task Analysis on Information Intake

| | |
|---|---|
| Strategic level:<br>Before task execution<br>No time pressure | Decisions of high anticipatory nature to prevent time pressure: *preventive steps*<br><br>1. Make a plan including:<br> &bull; Questions about the assignment<br> &bull; The rehearsal of the most important instructions<br> &bull; The optimalisation of the conditions under which information intake takes place<br><br>2. Make an emergency plan |
| Tactic level:<br>During task execution<br>Slight time pressure | Decisions of medium anticipatory nature to prevent and/or deal with time pressure: *preventive and managing steps*<br><br>1. Look regularly at the plan<br>2. Interrupt the video as soon as something is not clear, and:<br>3. Ask for a clarification or pause<br>4. Repeat the information for yourself |
| Operational level:<br>During task execution<br>Much time pressure | Decisions of low anticipatory nature to deal efficiently with time pressure: *managing steps*<br><br>1. Interrupt the video as soon as possible and look at your emergency plan |

*Source:* Michon (1979, as cited in Fasotti, Kovacs, Eling, & Brouwer, 2000, p. 50). Copyright © Taylor and Francis. Used with permission.

drives at a slower speed to allow for less time pressure demands, should the need arise to react quickly. At the last level of decision making, the operational level, time pressure is present and the individual must react quickly to avoid failure, such as needing to turn quickly or slam on the brakes to avoid a collision.

As Figure 7–4 illustrates, time demands are relatively low at the strategic level, increasingly present at the tactical level, and relatively high at the operational level. Given these variations in time constraints, execution of decisions at the strategic and tactical levels are thought to be less impaired by slowed mental processing, while those at the operational level are thought to be highly impacted by deficits in this area (Wilkins, Van Heugten, Fasotti, & Wade, 2009). The

potential for decision at each level to reduce time pressure also varies. Decisions at the strategic level are thought to have a high potential to reduce time pressure, while those at the tactical level have slightly less potential to reduce time pressure. Those at the operational level have relatively little impact on reducing time pressure (Wilkins, Van Heugten, Fasotti, & Wade, 2009).

## Treatment in Action

Training in TPM is implemented in three distinct stages: (1) identifying the problem, (2) teaching the strategy, and (3) generalization (Fasotti et al., 2000; Haskins, Shapiro-Rosenbaum, Dams-O'Connor, Eberle, Cicerone, & Langenbahn, 2012; Ponsford

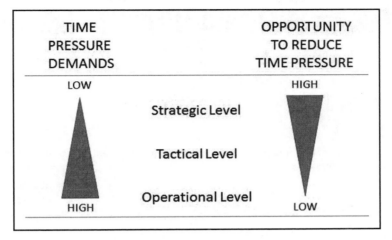

**Figure 7–4.** The relationship of decision-making levels to the time pressure demands and opportunities to reduce time pressure.

et al., 2014; Winkens, Van Heugten, Wade, & Fasotti, 2009; Winkens, Van Heugten, Wade, Habets, & Fasotti, 2009). These stages are illustrated in Table 7–7.

### Stage 1: Identifying the Problem

In stage 1 of TPM training, the main objective is to foster awareness of deficits and of the potential effects of those deficits on task completion. Specifically, it is vital for both the SLP and the individual with TBI to acknowledge the presence of mental slowness, identify activities that are adversely affected, and develop a shared understanding of secondary consequences (e.g., emotional changes, fatigue, or forgetfulness) encountered by the client in the face of increasing time pressures (Winkens, Van Heugten, Wade, Habets, et al., 2009, p. 1673).

In solidifying awareness, a diagnosis of mental slowness needs to be confirmed. As was mentioned above, there may be discrepancies between objectively measured slowness and what a client experiences as slowness. Hence, it is important to incorporate both the client's impressions of the problem and his/her objective performance in daily activities into this discussion of awareness (Winkens, Van Heugten, Wade, & Fasotti, 2009, p. 82). This can be achieved through administration of a battery of neuropsychological tests (see Table 7–4), psychosocial questionnaires (e.g., *Mental Slowness Questionnaire*), and behavioral observations (e.g., *Mental Slowness Observation Test*).

It is important to note that mental slowness "may be present even if the patient does not complain about it directly"; in fact, unawareness or denial is not uncommon after TBI and may occur for a number of reasons (e.g., lack of information or prior performance feedback, psychological denial, organic and/or neurological reasons [damage to areas of the brain leading to inaccurate self-reflection]; Winkens, Van Heugten, Wade, & Fasotti, et al., 2009, pp. 82–83). Nevertheless, an awareness of mental slowness and its connection to time pressure is an important aspect of TPM. An individual with TBI needs to understand that some aspects of daily activities can be impaired by an inability to react quickly or

**Table 7–7.** TPM Treatment Stages: Components, Prerequisites, and Assessment Tools

| Stages | Components | Stage Specific Prerequisites | Can Be Achieved By |
|---|---|---|---|
| **Stage 1: Identifying the problem** | Diagnosis of mental slowness | Awareness of clinician | Neuropsychological tests<br><br>Mental Slowness Questionnaire |
| | Patient accepting the problem | Awareness of patient | Mental Slowness Observation Test<br><br>Feedback and demonstration<br><br>Practice, explanation and feedback |
| **Stage 2: Teaching the strategy** | Patient learning the strategy<br>  Analyze the task for time pressure<br>  Make a plan of decisions and actions to undertake before the task starts<br>  Make an emergency plan<br>  Execute the task and monitor | Anticipatory awareness and emergent awareness<br><br>Sufficient learning ability<br><br>Adequate cognitive skills<br><br>Enough rest<br><br>Sufficient motivation | Distributed practice<br><br>Meaningful and personalized information and examples |
| | Apply the strategy | Patient should agree that it works<br><br>Awareness that the strategy is a general strategy that can be applied to other situations as well | Practice, feedback and demonstration |
| **Stage 3: Generalization** | Apply the strategy in new and more difficult situations | Sufficient cognitive skills | Practice, feedback and demonstration |

*Source:* Winkens, Van Heugten, Wade, Habets, & Fasotti (2009, p. 81). Used with permission.

with sufficient speed (Winkens, Van Heugten, Wade, & Fasotti, 2009; Winkens, Van Heugten, Wade, Habets, et al., 2009). Education, demonstration, and feedback may be beneficial at this stage of training (Winkens, Van Heugten, Wade, & Fasotti, 2009).

Fundamentally, this stage in TPM promotes the understanding that "slowness is a common thread in activities that are impaired" and that this has negative implications on daily operations (Winkens, Van Heugten, Wade, & Fasotti, 2009, p. 83).

Choosing information, examples, and activities that are personalized and meaningful will expedite attainment of this level of awareness. It is also helpful to review test results, or alternatively, to ask the client to predict his or her own performance, juxtaposing predictions and actual performance (Winkens, Van Heugten, Wade, & Fasotti, 2009). With this additional education and discussion, clients should exhibit a *general* recognition of deficits in everyday functioning due to slowed mental processing, as success in stage 2 of TPM is contingent upon it.

### Stage 2: Teaching the Strategy

The second stage in TPM training is composed of strategy acceptance, acquisition, and application. The strategy *Let Me Give Myself Enough Time* is introduced (Fasotti et al., 2000, p. 52). Patients are made aware that although speed of processing may not improve, there is a strategy that will allow them to better deal with slowness, which may in turn result in improved task performance. The aim of this strategy is to ameliorate consequences brought about by time pressure, allowing patients ample time to better prepare for or deal with the task at hand (Fasotti et al., 2000).

*Let Me Give Myself Enough Time* is broken into four parts: analyze, prevent, emergency plan, and implement and monitor. These are described briefly in Table 7–8 and displayed visually in Figure 7–5. A short variant of the self-instruction method by Meichenbaum (1977, 1980) is also helpful as a theoretical framework in deploying *Let Me Give Myself Time* (Fasotti et al., 2000; Winkens, Van Heugten, Wade, & Fasotti, 2009; Winkens, Van Heugten, Wade, Habets, et al., 2009). This self-instructional method is displayed in Table 7–9 and will be referenced throughout the following section in

order to describe how the speech-language pathologist (SLP) guides the individual in strategy learning and implementation processes. Appendix 7–6 contains a sample data collection sheet, stratified by the stages within *Let Me Give Myself Enough Time* for use during TPM implementation.

The first aspect of *Let Me Give Myself Enough Time* strategy learning, according to Meichenbaum's self-instructional method is for the SLP to introduce and demonstrate the strategy using cognitive modeling (see Table 7–9). It is recommended that the SLP choose a fairly easy task (e.g., cooking a meal, watching TV) to demonstrate, explaining aloud how the activity should be performed while using the strategy (Haskins et al., 2012; Winkens, Van Heugten, Wade, & Fasotti, 2009). Demonstrating the first step of *Let Me Give Myself Enough Time* (i.e., analyze), the SLP promotes the understanding that the client's first and primary concern should be on-task analysis and establishing any time pressure present (Winkens, Van Heugten, Wade, & Fasotti, 2009, p. 84). Prior to beginning a task, the client should be taught to "analyze a task for time pressures and to identify where preventing or handling strategies might help" (Winkens, Van Heugten, Wade, & Fasotti, 2009, p. 84). For example, when cooking a meal, there are several things that need to be done at once, such as gathering, washing, and mixing ingredients on the stove ("Are there two or more things to be done at the same time?"), which may lead to situations of information overload. The clinician should make all such pressures explicitly clear through modeling the *Questions to Ask* in *Let Me Give Myself Enough Time* (i.e., "Are there two or more things to be done at the same time?"; "Could I be overwhelmed or distracted?," see Table 7–8) and assist the individual with recognition of such instances.

**Table 7–8.** TPM *Let Me Give Myself Enough Time* Questions and Goals

| Questions to Ask | Goals |
|---|---|
| | *Analyze* |
| Are there two or more things to be done at the same time? Could I be overwhelmed or distracted? If yes, go to step 2 (Prevent) | To recognize and analyze the time pressure in the task at hand |
| | *Prevent* |
| Which things can be done before the task begins? Make a short plan of things to be done before the actual task begins. | To prevent as much time pressure as possible |
| | *Emergency Plan* |
| What to do in case of unexpected, overwhelming time pressure? Make an emergency plan. | To make an emergency plan to deal with time pressure as quickly as possible |
| | *Implement and Monitor* |
| Are plans and emergency plans ready? If plan and emergency plan are ready, use them to perform the task | To implement the task and monitor performance for successes and challenges |

*Source:* Modified from Fasotti, Kovacs, Eling & Brouwer (2000, p. 53). Copyright © Taylor and Francis. Used with permission.

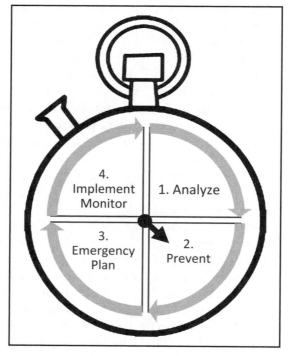

**Figure 7–5.** Stages of *Let Me Give Myself Enough Time* visual representation.

| **Table 7–9.** Implementation of TPM Using Self-Instruction | |
|---|---|
| *Phase* | *Procedure* |
| Strategy Learning | |
|     Cognitive modeling | The instructor demonstrates the task, verbalizing each action as it is performed |
|     Overt, external guidance | The client instructs himself/herself aloud and writes down the four steps of TPM |
| Strategy Practice/Implementation | |
|     Overt self-guidance | The client performs that task, while instructing himself/herself aloud. |
|     Covert self-instruction | The client performs that task, while guiding his or her performance via private speech. |

*Source:* Miechenbaum (1977, 1980).

The next step in *Let Me Give Myself Enough Time* is to address pressure situations (e.g., precooking predictions) using strategic and tactical planning. Here the client learns to "identify which decisions can be taken and which actions can be performed before actually starting the activity, and to make a plan to undertake these preparatory tasks" (Winkens, Van Heugten, Wade, & Fasotti, 2009, p. 84). For example, before starting to cook, the plan might involve reading the recipe in its entirety, opening cans and wrappings, and scanning the task environment to eliminate distractions (e.g., turning off the television). The clinician should model plan development based on answers to questions asked in Step 1 (i.e., *Questions to Ask*) and execute these preparatory tasks.

It is not possible to anticipate all possible pressures that may arise during an activity. For this reason, the next aspect of *Let Me Give Myself Enough Time* is to develop an emergency plan. Emergency plans should describe what to do in instances of overwhelming or unexpected time pressure (Haskins, 2012; Winkens, Van Heugten,

Wade, & Fasotti, 2009). For example, what if the doorbell was to ring while cooking? The SLP should assist the client in considering how he or she should react, whether it be turning off the cooker before answering the door or choosing to simply ignore it. The final aspect of *Let Me Give Myself Enough Time* is to carry out the plan and monitor the success in dealing with the time pressure, acknowledging what worked and what did not work. The SLP should implement plans and describe performance with the client postdemonstration.

Once the overall strategy has been taught through cognitive modeling procedures, the SLP assists the client in memorizing the four steps in *Let Me Give Myself Enough Time* (analyze, prevent, emergency plans, implement and monitor) (Haskins, 2012; Winkens, Van Heugten, Wade, & Fasotti, 2009). To do so, the client should instruct himself or herself aloud and write down the four steps on a memory card, which can be referenced in instances when memory fails (overt, external guidance). In some cases, visuals as opposed to written information may be more helpful—in such cases the SLP may choose to utilize Figure 7–5 as a training supplement. The SLP should regularly reinforce use of these external strategies and gradually withdraw prompts for recall (Fasotti et al., 2000; Winkens, Van Heugten, Wade, & Fasotti, 2009). Only when the client demonstrates that he or she can remember steps of *Let Me Give Myself Enough Time* should actual practice of implementation begin (Winkens, Van Heugten, Wade, & Fasotti, 2009, p. 84).

During implementation of tasks, initially the client is asked to instruct himself or herself aloud using these newly learned strategies (overt self-guidance; Winkens, Van Heugten, Wade, & Fasotti, 2009). This self-talk strategy allows the SLP to monitor strategy acquisition and to better assist the client in application (e.g., providing cues, asking questions; Winkens, Van Heugten, Wade, & Fasotti, 2009). The client should be allowed sufficient practice in more than one task and be provided with feedback upon completion of each task. In providing feedback, discussion of task performance and "analysis of how success or failure is linked to the use of (or failure to use) the strategy" should be a priority (Winkens, Van Heugten, Wade, & Fasotti, 2009, p. 86). Clients need to agree that the strategy works and understand that quality performance (e.g., success) is related to use of strategies. Eventually, through practice, feedback, and demonstration in a range of tasks, the client should become aware that the strategy is applicable to other situations and conditions.

At this stage in TPM training, an additional goal is to support independent use of the strategy (Fasotti et al., 2000; Haskins et al., 2012; Ponsford et al., 2014 Winkens, Van Heugten, Wade, & Fasotti, 2009). Clients need to learn to recognize problems associated with time pressure when they occur and initiate compensation without

the support of prompts or overt guidance. However, some patients may lack the "anticipatory" or "emergent awareness" required to prevent and/or manage problems on their own. When this is the case, the SLP should focus on training the client to look for internal and external warning signs as a cue to initiate strategic behavior (Haskins et al., 2012; Winkens, Van Heugten, Wade, & Fasotti, 2009). Internal warning signs could be emotional indicators, such as feelings of heightened anxiety, confusion, or fatigue. External warning signs, often based on the actions of others, "may suggest the patient is having difficulty understanding or following conversation," and might involve others speaking at a slower rate or asking the individual "if he or she understands" (Haskins et al., 2012, p. 83).

These cues should be taught as signals to implement the TPM strategy (Haskins et al., 2012; Winkens, Van Heugten, Wade, & Fasotti, 2009). Not all patients will demonstrate an ability to implement strategies independently—some individuals may not be able to accurately "read" a situation and others may "see the need" but be unable to remember planned solutions, or successfully implement them (Haskins et al., 2012, p. 83). For these individuals, the SLP may need to encourage habitual use of a strategy in certain situations or when performing certain tasks (i.e., situational compensations; Brookshire, 2015; Haskins et al., 2012; Winkens, Van Heugten, Wade, & Fasotti, 2009).

### Stage 3: Generalization

Training efforts in the last stage of TPM are directed toward strategy maintenance and transfer. In this stage, training should take place in more distracting and difficult conditions and/or in novel settings and activities. The goal is to support strategy use in different circumstances to foster maximum independence (Fasotti et al., 2000; Haskins et al., 2012; Winkens, Van Heugten, Wade, & Fasotti, 2009).

## c. Attention Processing Training (APT)

APT was developed in 1987 by Sohlberg and Mateer. It is now commercially marketed, with three versions available: APT I, APT II (specifically for mild cognitive impairment), and APT III (computerized version) Sohlberg, Johnson, Paule, Raskin, & Mateer, 2005; Sohlberg & Mateer, 2001a, 2010). Speech-language pathologists interested in purchasing these versions can do so at https://www.lapublishing.com/

### Candidacy Recommendations

APT is recommended in the post-acute stages after TBI (Sohlberg & Mateer, 2010) for:

1. **Individuals who have intact basic vigilance, sufficient to participate in treatment activities.** Individuals with deficits in vigilance will have difficulty focusing on a task for more than a few seconds to minutes, or have attention that fluctuates dramatically within brief periods of time (Sohlberg & Mateer, 2001a, p. 128).

2. **Individuals who exhibit mild-to-moderate attention deficits in any of the following areas: sustained, selective, alternating, and divided attention.** Both direct measures and those used to assess attention from the perspective of the individual with TBI are recommended (Sohlberg & Mateer, 2010). Several common measures in this area are listed at the start of this chapter (Table 7–10). Tasks within APT are also stratified by specific attentional difficulties. Candidacy recommendations of this nature from APT III (Sohlberg & Mateer, 2010) are listed in Table 7–13.

### Treatment Evidence

Although "reliance on repeated exposure and practice on decontextualized computer

**Table 7–10.** APT-III Levels Candidacy Recommendations

| Level of Training | Recommended Candidate |
|---|---|
| Basic Sustained Attention | Individuals who have a short attention space and lose concentration over time |
| Executive Control: Working Memory | Individuals who have difficulty holding onto information during task completion |
| Executive Control: Selective Attention | Individuals who are easily distracted by internal or external stimuli |
| Executive Control: Suppression | Individuals who tend to be impulsive or distracted |
| Executive Control: Alternating Attention | Individuals who tend to perseverate, lack mental flexibility, demonstrate slowed processing, or have difficulty with working memory |

*Source:* Sohlberg & Mateer (2010, p. 8).

based attentional tasks is NOT recommended due to lack of demonstrated impact on everyday attentional functions" (Ponsford et al., 2014, p. 327), there is Level B evidence to support the use of APT for individuals with TBI (Figure 7–6). Cicerone et al. (2011) recommend that APT (and other similar approaches using direct attention training) be combined with metacognitive training and the development of compensatory strategies that generalize outside of treatment settings (p. 521). Ponsford and colleagues also recommend incorporating compensatory training with this approach and note that recent iteration of APT (discussed below) have incorporated "increased emphasis on the development of compensatory strategies as part of the training" (Ponsford et al., 2014, p. 327).

## Theoretical Frame

Traditionally, APT has been described as a restorative approach, given a framework that targets repeated practice of specific attentional systems, "hypothesized to facilitate cognitive change" (Sohlberg & Mateer, 2001a, p. 134). Recent iterations have also incorporated compensatory strategy and metacognitive training (Ponsford et al., 2014, APT III manual). As such, Figure 7–7

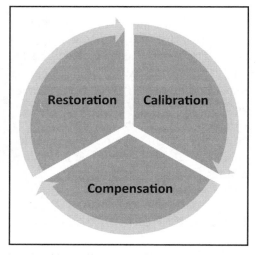

**Figure 7–7.** Theoretical framework of APT. The treatment approaches evident in contemporary versions of APT.

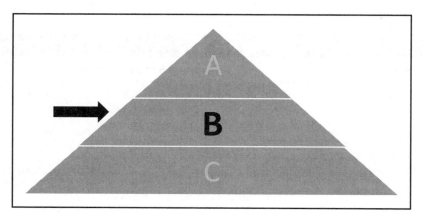

**Figure 7–6.** Level B evidence for the use of APT. Level B consists of "recommendation supported by cohort studies that at minimum have a comparison group, or supported by well-designed single subject experimental design studies or small sample size randomized controlled trial studies" (Bayley, Tate, & Douglas et al., 2014, p. 295).

is reflective of these three approaches (restoration, compensation, and calibration), with restoration being the primary historical perspective within APT.

## Background Introduction

Conceptually, APT is guided by the principles listed in Table 7–11. As can be seen, these have changed slightly with each additional version of APT but include the core tenets of:

■ Grounding treatment in hierarchical organization and theoretical models of attention

■ Providing opportunity for practice and repetition

■ Using client data to drive treatment decisions

■ Individualizing treatment and promoting generalization to relevant real-world tasks

APT is based on the hypothesis that repeated activation and stimulation of attentional systems facilitates change in cognitive capacity (Sohlberg & Mateer, 2001a). It assumes that abilities in the area of attention can be improved by providing opportunities to stimulate particular aspects of attention (Sohlberg & Mateer,

**Table 7–11.** APT Guiding Principles

| APT I[1] | APT II[2] | APT III[3] |
|---|---|---|
| *Ground Treatment in Hierarchical Organization and Theoretical Models of Attention* | | |
| Principle 1. Use a treatment model that is grounded in attention theory | Principle 1. The importance of working from a theoretical model | Principle 1. Organize therapy materials using a theoretically grounded model |
| Principle 2. Use therapy activities that are hierarchically organized | Principle 2. Use therapy programs that are hierarchically organized | |
| *Provide Opportunity for Practice and Repetition* | | |
| Principle 3. Provide sufficient repetition | Principle 3. The Importance of Repetition | Principle 2. Provide sufficient repetition |
| *Use Client Data to Drive Treatment Decisions* | | |
| Principle 4. Treatment decisions should be based upon client performance data | Principle 4. Using Data-Based Treatment | Principle 3. Use patient performance data to direct therapy |
| *Individualize Treatment and Promote Generalization to Real-World Tasks* | | |
| Principle 5. Actively facilitate generalization from the start of treatment | Principle 5. The ultimate measures of success are changes in community functioning | Principle 4. Include metacognitive training |
| Principle 6. Be flexible in adapting the therapy format | | Principle 5. Identify and practice functional goals related to attention |

*Note.* [1]Sohlberg & Mateer (2001a); [2]Sohlberg, Johnson, Paule, Raskin, & Mateer (2005); [3]Sohlberg & Mateer (2010).

2010). According to APT authors, most real-world tasks require multiple cognitive systems (e.g., several levels of attention, memory, executive function) (Sohlberg & Mateer, 2010). For this reason, APT utilizes repeated practice on specially designed discrete (non real-world) tasks, which allow practice in targeted aspects of cognitive (attentional) processes. Samples of tasks of this nature, within APT II, are located in Table 7–12. These APT exercises are hierarchically organized to systematically increase in complexity and demand with each additional step progression within APT.

APT emphasizes generalization training (early on and throughout APT tasks) so that "cognitive improvements generalize to performance of relevant everyday activities" (p. 11). Recent versions of APT also stress metacognitive and compensatory strategy development and training (Sohlberg & Mateer, 2010).

Based on changes in the foundational knowledge in the area of attention systems, the newest version of APT (APT III) addresses "executive control" of attentional processes (Sohlberg & Mateer, 2010). This newest version also targets working memory

as distinct from basic sustained attention processes. Lastly, the concept of multitasking (or rapidly shifting alternating attention) is targeted within APT III as the process of executive control of alternating attention, rather than the distinct attentional process of divided attention. Table 7–13 reflects these changes across theoretical foundations and treatment targets in APT I, II, and III.

## Treatment in Action

The APT treatment protocols described in this chapter are organized around Sohlberg and Mateer's (1987) theoretical model of attention and treatment principles. In accord, methodologies discussed will reference the updated attention framework implemented in APT III (see Table 7–14), as well as draw from prior studies implementing a direct attention training approach.

Sohlberg and colleagues acknowledge that prescription of "an exact [treatment] regimen" for individuals with TBI is not possible (Sohlberg et al., 2005, p. 12). This is readily understood, especially when considering the heterogeneity of the TBI popu-

**Table 7–12.** Sample Treatment Activities by Attention Level (APT II)

| Attention Level | Sample Tasks |
| --- | --- |
| Sustain Attention | Paragraph Listening Exercise<br>Alphabetized Sentence Exercise<br>Mental Math Activity |
| Alternating Attention | Alternating Alphabet Exercise<br>Serial Numbers Activity |
| Alternating Attention | Sustained Attention Activities with Distracter Noise<br>Sustained Attention Activities with Distracter Movement |
| Divided Attention | Read and Scan Task<br>Time Monitoring Task |

*Source:* Sohlberg, Johnson, Paule, Raskin, & Mateer (2005).

lation and resulting attentional deficits, and given the importance of individualized programming and data-based treatment articulated in APT principles. In addition, Sohlberg and Mateer (2010) highlight that by its very nature, direct attention training will rarely be implemented in isolation. This further confounds the development and application of one uniform treatment protocol. Therefore, a *general* construct to treatment implementation, based on treatment principles and trends in research literature, will be explained in the following sections.

In general, APT begins with an evaluation (baseline) stage, followed by a training stage, finally ending with a generalization stage (Figure 7–8). The aforementioned treatment principles guide the administration throughout these informal stages, making the process dynamic and not delineated into rigid stages. For example, although an "evaluation" stage is evident, a continued

| **Table 7–13.** APT Attention Targets | |
|---|---|
| ***APT I and APT II***[1] | ***APT III***[2] |
| • Focused | • Basic Sustained Attention |
| • Sustained | • Executive Control: |
| • Selective | ○ Working Memory |
| • Alternating | ○ Selective Attention |
| • Divided | ○ Suppression |
| | ○ Alternating Attention |

*Note.* [1]Sohlberg & Mateer (2001a) and Sohlberg, Johnson, Paule, Raskin, & Mateer (2005); [2]Sohlberg & Mateer (2010).

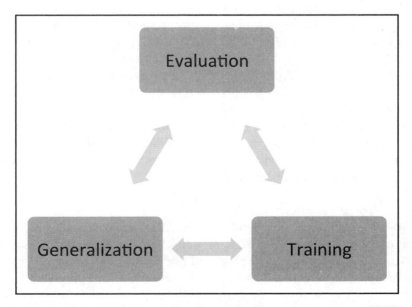

**Figure 7–8.** APT processes. The general and interrelated stages of APT.

process of data collection and monitoring of performance is prevalent throughout all stages. Likewise, despite the presence of a "generalization stage," the principles associated with obtaining functional outcomes to dictate generalization are addressed from the very beginning (at initial evaluation) and reinforced throughout the training and generalization stages.

### Evaluation

Attention, as well as a broad range of cognitive, psychological, and behavioral factors, are typically assessed in the initial stages of APT (Sohlberg et al., 2005). Table 7–2 (*Common Attention Measures: Direct Measures and Rating Scales*) at the start of this chapter contains several common measures for this purpose. The authors of the APT program also provide examples of standardized measures, "thought to capture the types of attention demands targeted" within the APT manual (Sohlberg et al., 2005; Sohlberg & Mateer, 2010). The goals of evaluation are to gain an overall impression of cognitive, psychosocial, and everyday functioning, and to develop an individualized client attentional profile (Sohlberg & Mateer, 2001a).

Sohlberg and colleague recommended that, "an assessment of attentional processing needs to include more than standardized attention measures," but also a battery of self-reported measures (e.g., psychosocial questionnaires), structured interviews, and behavioral observations (Sohlberg et al., 2005, p. 8). These measures lend themselves to an evaluation of adaptive functioning and an understanding of the impact of attention deficits in everyday contexts. This allows the clinician to design a program that will lead to improvements in real-world activities in the client's environment (Sohlberg et al., 2005).

APT authors stress the importance of facilitating and measuring generalization and transfer to naturalistic contexts (Sohlberg et al., 2005, p. 10). As was highlighted in the background summary (above), APT utilizes discrete tasks that more closely resemble laboratory tasks (Sohlberg et al., 2005, p. 79). Simply measuring performance on these treatment tasks does not necessarily translate to measurements of success in real-world functioning. This means that the clinician must plan for the "generalization" stage even before therapy begins, by using the evaluation stage to identify which tasks at home, work, or in the community will be targeted for generalization and measured to establish functional outcomes from APT training.

The APT II program provides an *Attention Questionnaire* that can be used to identify where, when, and how frequently breakdowns in attention occur (Sohlberg et al., 2005). Through interview and questioning, this questionnaire allows the client and clinician to document "the most frequent and frustrating breakdowns in attention," which aids in the creation of "an individualized attention problem list" (Sohlberg et al., p. 81). Additionally, APT contains an *Attention Lapse Log* and *Attention Success Log*, which can also be used by the client to record success and challenges in attention performance, both initially and throughout the course of treatment (Haskins et al., 2012, p. 76). Appendices 7–2 and 7–3 at the start of this chapter can also be used for this purpose.

### Training

The APT training stage involves task selection (i.e., discrete attention tasks and generalization tasks), task pacing, documentation of performance, and program modification (Sohlberg et al., 2005; Sohlberg & Mateer, 2010). This process of selecting targets and setting task parameters (e.g., difficulty level) is likened to a physician prescribing medicine, as it "requires some trial and error" and will need to be adjusted based on client performance (Sohlberg et al., 2005, p. 12). Attention targets will vary based on the version of APT and its associated theoretical model/attention framework (e.g., APT II targets versus APT III targets), but in all cases treatment begins with basic areas of attention that are challenging for the client (Haskins et al., 2012). As the client experiences success, these tasks progressively become more difficult (Haskins et al., 2012).

In the execution of APT tasks, there is a general approach applied within each APT version. Before each task, the clinician instructs the patient on requirements and demonstrates the task. Once the client indicates understanding, the task begins. Feedback about accuracy and speed of performance (if measured) is also provided following each exercise (Sohlberg et al., 2005). The APT III program, while distinctly different in its implementation method (i.e., via computer), also utilizes this general construct.

Along with the appropriate scoring and documentation forms, APT employs both quantitative and qualitative measures for tracking client performance on training tasks. Quantitative measures assess task completion parameters such as accuracy, speed, or level of cueing, while qualitative measures assess error patterns and patient and environmental factors that may impact performance (Haskins et al., 2012, p. 77).

Generalization tasks are also initiated during this stage. Those tasks identified in the evaluation stage are used as probes that allow the clinician to monitor performance on different levels of functioning (i.e., impairment level and functional level) (Sohlberg & Mateer, 2010). As the patient progresses through APT, and improvements in attentional processing have been

realized, generalization tasks are adjusted. Therefore, the clinician should engage in periodic probing of attentional performance in naturalistic settings (Sohlberg & Mateer, 2001b, p. 367).

## Generalization

The final stage of APT is that of a "formal training phase to actively facilitate generalization" (Sohlberg & Mateer, 2005, p. 83). In APT treatment manuals, authors offer suggestions for designing generalization activities. As above, these activities are initially established in the evaluation stage and have been practiced and possibly modified throughout the training stage. During the generalization stage, the client and clinician establish a plan and schedule for carrying out generalization exercises outside of the treatment setting (Sohlberg et al., 2005). A data collection plan for monitoring performance on these activities is also established, using a modified version of the *Attention Lapse Log* and/or *Attention Success Log*, and other APT data tools (available in the APT manual). At the end of treatment, attention abilities are reevaluated through the use of questionnaires, formalized measures, attention logs implemented during the final weeks of treatment, and recorded data for the last trials of generalization activities. APT III also measures treatment progress utilizing a specialized *Goal Attainment Scale*.

## d. Dual-Task Training (DTT)

## Candidacy Recommendations

Based on a composite of research in this area (Couillet et al., 2010; Evans, Greenfield, Wilson, & Bateman, 2009; Fritz & Basso, 2013), dual-task training (DTT) is recommended in the post-acute stages after TBI for:

1. **Individuals who evidence difficulty on divided attention (dual-task) performance measures.** Examples of recommended measures in the area of divided attention and dual-task performance are listed in Table 7–14. In general, assessment first involves baseline assessment of performance parameters (speed, accuracy, error rate) during single-function tasks, such as clicking a

---

**Table 7–14.** Dual-Task/Divided Attention Measures

Test for Attentional Performance (TAP; Divided Attention Subtest) (Zimmermann & Fimm, 2017)

Brief Test of Attention (Auditory Divided Attention)

Paced Auditory Serial Addition Test

Trail Making Test, Part B

Test for Divided Attention

The Walking and Remembering Test (WAR), (McCulloch, Mercer Guiliani, & Marshall 2009)

---

hand-held mechanical counter (single-function motor task) or repeating the months of the year backward (single-function cognitive task) (Weightman & McCulloch, 2014). Performance is then compared with performance while completing two of these tasks simultaneously (dual-task condition). A reduction in performance or "dual-task cost" can then be calculated using the formula in Figure 7–9 for each condition.

It should be noted, however, that non-neurologically impaired individuals also show a cost reduction during dual-task performance. For example, on a walking and digit-span dual task, McCulloch and colleagues reported that non-neurologically impaired young adults had a digit-span cost reduction of 9% to 10% (walking speed cost reduction of 2%–3%), while older adults in a similar paradigm had a digit-span cost reduction of 15% (walking speed cost reduction of 4%) (McCulloch, Mercer, Giuliani, & Marshall, 2009). As such, normative data in this area are valuable.

2. **Individuals who report difficulties with divided attention (dual-tasking) in everyday activities.** The *Dual-Tasking Questionnaire* (Appendix 7–7)

---

Dual-Task Cost Reduction Calculation:

$$\frac{Dual\text{-}Task\ Performance - Single\text{-}Function\ Task\ Performance}{Single\text{-}Function\ Task\ Performance} \times 100 = \%\ \begin{array}{l} Dual\text{-}Task \\ Cost\ Reduction \end{array}$$

Sample: Digit-Span Dual-Task Cost Reduction

$$\frac{50\%\ Digit\text{-}Span\ Dual\text{-}Task - 90\%\ Digit\text{-}Span\ Single\text{-}Function}{90\%\ Digit\text{-}Span\ Single\text{-}Function} \times 100 = 44\%\ \begin{array}{l} Dual\text{-}Task \\ Cost\ Reduction \end{array}$$

**Figure 7–9.** Calculation used to show dual-task costs reduction and a sample for digit-span accuracy cost reduction.

can be used for this purpose (Evans et al., 2009). Similarly, the *Rating Scale of Attentional Behaviour* (Ponsford & Kinsella, 1991) contains one question in the area of divided attention. Clinicians can also conduct structured interviews with the client (and significant others) regarding instances of difficulty doing two things at the same time in relevant home, work, recreation, and educational environments.

3. **Individuals with sufficient motor and visual spatial abilities to perform dual-task motor and cognitive tasks recommended within the approach.** It should be noted, however, that cognitive and motor tasks of this approach can be modified and adapted to meet the specific abilities and needs of an individual with TBI.

## Treatment Evidence

There is Level A evidence to support training using DTT with individuals with TBI, in order to improve dual task performance on tasks similar to those trained (Figure 7–10;

Ponsford, Bayley, Wiseman-Hakes, Togher, Velikonja, & McIntyre, 2014, p. 325).

## Theoretical Frame

DTT combines the use of calibration and restoration treatment techniques (Figure 7–11). Similar to Attention Processing

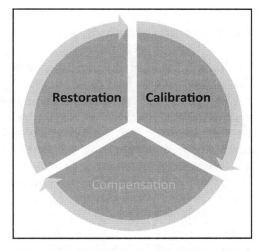

**Figure 7–11.** Theoretical framework of dual-task training. Treatment approaches evident in contemporary versions of DTT.

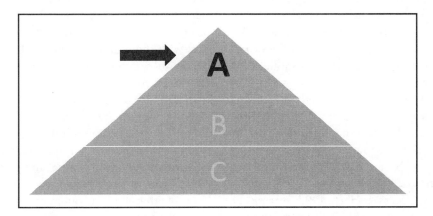

**Figure 7–10.** Level A evidence for the use of DTT. Level A consists of "recommendation supported by at least one meta-analysis, systematic review, or randomized controlled trial study of appropriate size and relevant control group" (Bayley et al., 2014, p. 295).

Training (APT), restorative aspects of DTT seek to address attention system deficits through training specific aspects of attention performance, in a hierarchical manner. More recent aspects of DTT also address metacognition (calibration), through self-reflection, performance feedback, and other instructional tasks that seek to enhance attentional awareness (Couillet et al., 2010; Evans et al., 2009).

## Background Introduction

Dual-tasking is the ability to perform two things at once (Posner & Peterson, 1990). It is also referred to as divided attention. It is closely related to executive function and working memory and requires complex strategic allocation of attention, task switching, and attention synchronization (Couillet et al., 2010, p. 322). Two examples of dual tasks in daily activities are "two cognitive tasks (e.g., monitoring a cooking pot while listening to the news), or a cognitive task and a motor task (e.g., walking and holding a conversation)" (Evans et al., 2009, p. 112). Dual-tasking and divided attention are frequently impaired in individuals with TBI (Azouvi et al., 2004; Haggard & Cockburn, 1998). DTT seeks to address deficits in this area and to generalize those skills to situations requiring a similar level of performance in daily activities (Couillet et al., 2010; Evans et al., 2009).

DTT was initially based on research in the area of attention, which noted that specific-skills training improved performance of trained tasks requiring attention, including those of divided attention (Park & Ingles, 2001; Ponsford, 2008; Sturm, Wilmes, Orgass, & Hartj, 1997; Sturm et al., 2002). Similar to APT, its initial premise was that attention deficits benefited from training that targets specific aspects of the attentional system, progressing hierarchically from simple and relatively automatic to complex and resource-demanding (Couillet et al., 2010; Evans et al., 2009).

Early work in the area of DTT for individuals with TBI noted that dual-task learning was generally task specific (Evans et al., 2009)—meaning that the ability to generalize from one type of novel dual task to a dissimilar dual task, or to a real-life untrained dual task, was not consistently evident. As such, current recommendations in the area of DTT (Ponsford et al., 2014) suggest that tasks be selected to mirror the cognitive and/or motor demands for which performance outside treatment is desired.

## Treatment in Action

### Establishing Treatment Tasks and Hierarchy

After assessment for candidacy, the first step in DTT is selection and organization of treatment tasks (Weightman & McCulloch, 2014). The goal in this stage of planning is to identify *real-world* dual tasks that are important to the client and his/her family and are currently challenging to perform due to divided attention deficits. This is done through reflection and collaboration with the individual with TBI and his/her family members. The *Dual-Tasking Questionnaire* (Appendix 7–7) combined with structured interviews can be used as a starting point in these efforts. This conversation can also begin with description and examples of divided attention and dual-task performance, both in general and given the client's performance on standardized measures of attention. The outcome of this discussion should be the creation of a list of *real-world* dual-task activities, relevant to that client and his/her environment.

Once established, the activities on this list should be organized and sorted based on importance for the client and his/her family, and based on complexity of task demands. One possible approach to accomplishing this task is to have the client and significant others rate each activity from greatest importance to least importance. The clinician can also rate each activity from the highest complexity/demand to lowest complexity/demand. These two ratings can then be combined so that activities are placed in order, as noted in Figure 7–12. As can be seen, activities of high importance are given top priority (and ranked from low complexity/demand to high complexity/demand). As time permits, activities of lower importance would also be addressed, similarly from low complexity/demand to high complexity/demand.

This framework will serve as the foundation for the next step in the planning stage, which is to develop the DTT tasks and hierarchy. Starting with the highest importance and least complex/demanding real-world dual-task activity, the team establishes a DTT task progression that accounts for the core motor, manual, visual-spatial, and cognitive function in each of the elements of the real-world dual-task activity to be targeted. This will be the starting point for implementing treatment.

DTT utilizes discrete tasks addressing specific core functions of increasing complexity. As a point of reference, Table 7–15 contains several sample tasks used in DTT research. These are not exhaustive of all possible tasks but do offer a sample of the types of discrete tasks that serve as the building blocks for a DTT progression "ladder." This progression ladder should modulate aspects of difficulty relevant to the client's performance, such as time pressure, executive demands, working memory, motor complexity, and so forth, starting with lower complexity/demand and increasing to higher complexity/demand (Couillet et al., 2010). Figure 7–13 contains a sample

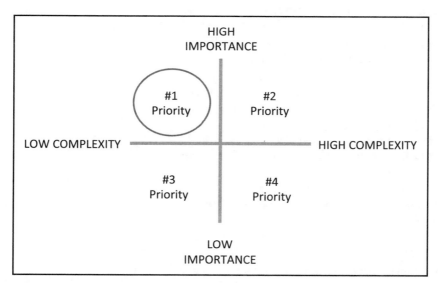

**Figure 7–12.** Hierarchical organization of dual-task goals (importance and complexity). The potential sorting of real-life dual-task treatment targets, given importance and complexity.

**Table 7–15.** Sample DTT Tasks: Cognitive and Motor

| Sample DTT Cognitive Tasks[1] | Sample DTT Motor Tasks |
|---|---|
| **Auditory discrimination tasks:** Patient asked to identify the noises or voices from a compact disc such as: (1) Identifying voices (man, woman, child) (2) Identifying noises (hand clap, door close, dog bark, cat meow) | **Hand Activity[2]**<br>Clicking a hand-held mechanical counter with the thumb of the dominant hand. |
| **Name things/words:** Patient asked to name things such as types of flower, states, and men's names. | **Stance Activities[3]**<br>Semi-tandem, eyes open, arm alteration |
| **Visual discrimination tasks:** Patient shown the pictures before and after performing the balance tasks. They were asked to memorize the pictures and to respond if the pictures were the same. They were required to say "yes" if the pictures were the same and "no" if they were different. | Semi-tandem, eyes closed, arm alteration<br>Draw letter with right foot<br>Draw letters with left foot |
| **Random digit generation:** Patient asked to randomly name the numbers between 0 and 300. | Perturbed standing, holding a ball |
| **Counting backward:** (e.g., by twos, threes). | **Gait Activities[3]**<br>Walk, narrow base of support |
| **Visual spatial task:** Patient asked to place numbers, objects, or letters in the imagined matrixes. Then they were required to name the numbers, objects, or letters in the specific matrix cell. | Walk, narrow base of support, step sideways, backward avoiding the obstacles (holding a basket) |
| **Visual imaginary spatial tasks:** Patient asked to imagine and tell the road direction (e.g., the road direction from their home to the post office). | Walk and kick a ball to hit the cans direction of the ball<br>Walk and reach and trunk twisting |
| **N-Back task:** Patient asked to recite numbers, days, or months backward (e.g., December, November, . . . January). | |
| **Subtract or add number to letter:** Patient asked to give the letter as a result of the equation (e.g., k–1 = j). | |
| **Remembering things:** Patient asked to memorize telephone numbers, prices, objects, or words. | |
| **Tell story:** Patient asked to tell any story such as what they did in the morning, what they did on their vacation, and so on. | |
| **Tell opposite direction of action:** Patient asked to name the opposite direction of their actions. For example, they were required to name "left" when they move their right leg. | |
| **Spell the word backward:** Patients asked to spell a word backward such as "apple," "bird," and "television." | |
| **Say any complete sentence:** Patient asked to say any complete sentence. | |
| **Stroop task:** Patient asked to name the color of the ink while ignoring the meaning of the word | |

*Source:* [1]Silsupadol, Siu, Shumway-Cook,& Woollacott (2006, Appendix 2, p. 281); [2]Evans, Greenfield, Wilson, & Bateman (2009, p. 114); [3]Silsupadol, Siu, Shumway-Cook, & Woollacott (2006, Appendix 3, p 281).

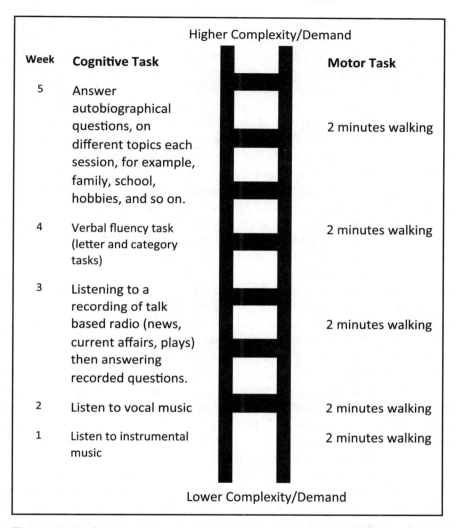

**Figure 7–13.** Sample DTT progression ladder. Task progression from Evans, Greenfield, Wilson, and Bateman (2009), displayed within the visual frame of a progression ladder.

DTT progression. As can be seen, within this progression ladder, the researchers kept the motor tasks consistent but modulated the cognitive tasks. Within DTT, progression can be modulated in any pattern applicable to the individual client. This is where coordinated care and interdisciplinary teams are extremely valuable, as team members can collaborate given specific areas of expertise to establish an effective DTT progression ladder for each individual client. Once established, the next step is treatment implementation.

## Implementing Treatment

The general construct of DTT is to first target each component within a dual task separately (within a single-function task), in order to ensure that the client is able to complete the task efficiently (Couillet et al., 2010). Then, both tasks are addressed simultaneously, within the dual-task paradigm. Couillet and colleagues recommend that as soon as a client achieves approximately 90% accuracy on a dual task, a higher-level task should be addressed (Couillet et al., 2010). As such, accurate data collection across tasks within the progression ladder is important in determining when task progression can occur. This can be done in a variety of ways, including using a modified version of the data collection sheet in Appendix 7–7.

An important part of DTT is frequent practice of DTT tasks (Evans et al., 2009). Clients are asked to practice specific dual tasks on the DTT ladder outside of treatment. Evans and colleagues recommend task completion at least twice per day, five days per week (Evans et al., 2009). Treatment sessions with the clinician entail discussion about performance on the previous week's DTT task and introduction and practice on the upcoming week's DTT task (Evans et al., 2009).

An additional aspect of DTT treatment is metacognitive instruction and reflection on task performance (Weightman & McCulloch, 2014). During tasks, clients are instructed to be conscious of their attentional processing, such as encouraging clients to "try to consciously dual-task, that is to keep listening to the music (or other task depending on week of intervention)

while walking" (Evans et al., 2009, p. 115). To bring additional awareness to attentional performance, during treatment sessions the clinician also instructs the client to shift attention from one task to the other, using cues such as, "This time really focus on the balance task," then, "This time really concentrate on getting the cognitive task correct" (Weightman & McCulloch, 2014, p. 332).

Evans and colleagues also recommend using a metaphor to help the client visualize dual-task processing. They suggest the image of wheels of a wagon running along railway lines, to highlight the importance of the client focusing his/her attention *equally* on both tasks, noting that like the wheels of a wagon, attention on both tasks must be going at the same speed and equally aligned for there to be task success. This is represented visually in Figure 7–14 and can be used as a reminder throughout treatment to recall this aspect of dual-task performance.

Lastly, self- and clinician-guided reflection is also used within DTT, to increase awareness of attentional performance (Evans et al., 2009). This can be done through questions at the end of each task that require the client to rate his/her performance. Questions and ratings similar to those in Table 7–16 can be used for this purpose. Direct feedback on performance accuracy from the clinician can also be provided as a point of reference to the client's self-reflection (Couillet et al., 2010; Weightman & McCulloch, 2014).

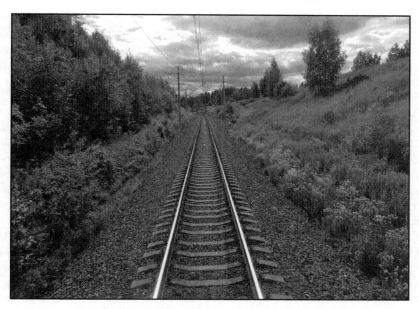

**Figure 7–14.** Dual-task metaphor. The metaphor of dual-task performance as a wagon running along railway lines, to highlight the importance of the client focusing his/her attention equally on both tasks.

| **Table 7–16.** DTT Self-Reflection Questions |
| --- |
| Did you manage to dual-task? |
| *Almost none of the time*................*Almost all of the time* |
| Where was your attention most of the time? |
| *Equally divided*................*All over the place* |
| How difficult did you find this task? |
| *Very difficult*................*Very easy* |

*Source:* Evans, Greenfield, Wilson, & Bateman (2009, p. 115).

## References

American Speech-Language-Hearing Association. (2003). *Evaluating and treating communication and cognitive disorders: approaches to referral and collaboration for speech-language pathology and clinical neuropsychology* [Technical report]. Retrieved from http://www.asha.org/policy

Azouvi, P., Couillet, J., Leclercq, M., Martin, M., Asloun, S., & Rousseaux, M. (2004). Divided attention and mental effort after severe traumatic brain injury. *Neuropsychologia, 42,* 1260–1268.

Bayley, M., Tate, R., Douglas, J. M., Turkstra, L. S., Ponsford, J., Stergiou-Kita, M., . . . INCOG Expert Panel. (2014). INCOG guidelines for cognitive rehabilitation following traumatic brain injury: Methods and overview.

*Journal of Head Trauma Rehabilitation, 29*(4), 290–306.

Bergquist, T. F., & Jacket, M. P. (1993). Programme methodology: Awareness and goal setting with the traumatically brain injured. *Brain Injury, 7*, 275–282.

Brookshire, R. H. (2015). Traumatic brain injury. In M. R. McNeil (Ed.), *Introduction to neurogenic communication disorders* (8th ed., pp. 287–344). St. Louis, MO: Mosby.

Cicerone, K., Dahlberg, C., Kalmar, K., Langenbahn, D., Malec, J., Bergquist, T.F., . . . Morse, P. A. (2000). Evidence-based cognitive rehabilitation: Recommendations for clinical practice. *Archives of Physical Medicine and Rehabilitation, 81*(12), 1596–1615.

Cicerone, K., Dahlberg, C., Malec, J., Langenbahn, D., Felicetti, T., Kneipp, S., . . . Catanese, J. (2005). Evidence-based cognitive rehabilitation: Updated review of the literature from 1998 through 2002. *Archives of Physical Medicine and Rehabilitation, 86*(8), 1681–1692.

Cicerone, K. D., Langenbahn, D. M., Braden, C., Malec, J. F., Kalmar, K., Fraas, M., . . . Ashman, T. (2011). Evidence-based cognitive rehabilitation: Updated review of the literature from 2003 through 2008. *Archives of Physical Medicine and Rehabilitation, 92*(4), 519–530.

Couillet, J., Soury, S., Lebornec, G., Asloun, S., Joseph, P., Mazaux, J. M., & Azouvi, P. (2010). Rehabilitation of divided attention after severe traumatic brain injury: A randomised trial. *Neuropsychological Rehabilitation, 20*(3), 321–339.

Evans, J. J., Greenfield, E., Wilson, B. A., & Bateman, A. (2009). Walking and talking therapy: Improving cognitive-motor dual-tasking in neurological illness. *Journal of International Neuropsychological Society, 15*, 112–120.

Ezrachi, O., Ben-Yishay, Y., Kay, T., DiUer, L., & Rattok, J. (1991). Predicting employment in traumatic brain injury following neuropsychological rehabilitation. *Journal of Head Trauma Rehabilitation 6*, 71–84.

Fasotti, L., Kovacs, F., Eling, A. T. M., & Brouwer, W. (2000). Time pressure management as a compensatory strategy training after closed head injury. *Neuropsychological Rehabilitation, 10*(1), 47–65.

Flashman, L. A., Amador, X., & McAllister, T. W. (1998). Lack of awareness of deficits in traumatic brain injury. *Seminars in Clinical Neuropsychiatry 3*, 201–210.

Flashman, L., & McAllister, T. (2002). Lack of awareness and its impact in traumatic brain injury. *NeuroRehabilitation, 17*(4), 285–296.

Fritz, E., & Basso, M. (2013). Dual-task training for balance and mobility in a person with severe traumatic brain injury: A case study. *Journal of Neurologic Physical Therapy, 37*(1), 37–43.

Haggard, P., & Cockburn, J. (1998). Dividing attention between cognitive and motor tasks in neurological rehabilitation. *Neuropsychological Rehabilitation, 8*, 155–170.

Haskins, E. C., Shapiro-Rosenbaum, A., Dams-O'Connor, K., Eberle, R., Cicerone, K., & Langenbahn, D. (2012). Rehabilitation for impairments of attention. In L. E. Trexler (Ed.), *Cognitive rehabilitation manual: Translating evidence-based recommendations into practice* (pp. 73–87). Reston, VA: American Congress of Rehabilitation Medicine.

Mathias, J., Wheaton, P., & Becker, J. (2007). Changes in attention and information-processing speed following severe traumatic brain injury: A meta-analytic review. *Neuropsychology, 21*(2), 212–223.

McCulloch, K. L., Mercer, V., Giuliani, C., & Marshall, S. (2009). Development of a clinical measure of dual-task performance in walking: Reliability and preliminary validity of the Walking and Remembering Test. *Journal of Geriatric Physical Therapy, 32*(1), 2–9.

Meichenbaum, D. (1977). *Cognitive behavior modification: An integrative approach.* New York, NY: Plenum Press.

Meichenbaum, D. (1980). Self instructional methods. In F. H. Kanfer & A. P. Goldstein (Eds.), *Helping people change.* New York, NY: Pergamon Press.

Ponsford, J., Bayley, M., Wiseman-Hakes, C., Togher, L., Velikonja, D., & McIntyre, A. (2014). INCOG recommendations for management of cognition following traumatic brain injury, part II: Attention and information processing speed. *Journal of Head Trauma Rehabilitation, 29*(4), 321–337.

Ponsford, J., & Kinsella, G. (1991). The use of a rating scale of attentional behaviour. *Neuropsychological Rehabilitation, 1*, 241–257.

Posner, M. I., & Peterson, S. E. (1990). The attention system of the human brain. *Annual Review of Neuroscience, 13*, 25–42.

Prigatano, G. P., Altman, I. M., & O'Brien, K. P. (1990). Behavioral limitations that brain injured patients tend to underestimate. *Clinical Neuropsychologist, 4*, 163–176.

Radomski, M. V., Goo-Yoshino, S., Smith Hammond, C., Isaki, E., Maclennan, D., Manning, K., . . . Zola, J. (n.d.). Cognitive assessment and intervention. In M. Weightman, M. Vining Radomski, P. Mashima, & C. R. Roth (Eds.), *Mild traumatic brain injury rehabilitation toolkit*. Fort Sam Houston, TX: Borden Institute.

Silsupadol, P., Siu, K. C., Shumway-Cook, A., & Woollacott, M. H. (2006). Training of balance under single- and dual-task conditions in older adults with balance impairment. *Physical Therapy, 86*(2), 269–281.

Sohlberg, M. M., Johnson, L., Paule, L., Raskin, S. A., & Mateer, C. A. (2005). *Attention process training II: A program to address attentional deficits for person with mild cognitive dysfunction* (3rd ed.) [Rehabilitation materials]. Youngsville, NC: Lash & Associates.

Sohlberg, M. M., & Mateer, C. A. (1987). Effectiveness of an attention-training program. *Journal of Clinical Experimental Neuropsychology, 9*, 117–130.

Sohlberg, M. M., & Mateer, C. A. (2001). *Cognitive rehabilitation: An integrative neuropsychological approach*. New York, NY: Guilford.

Sohlberg, M. M., & Mateer, C. A. (2001a). *Attention process training I* (2nd ed.) [Rehabilitation materials]. Youngsville, NC: Lash & Associates.

Sohlberg, M. M., & Mateer, C. A. (2001b). Improving attention and managing attentional problems: Adapting rehabilitation techniques to adults with ADD. *Annals New York Academy of Sciences, 931*(1), 359–375.

Sohlberg, M. M., & Mateer, C. A. (2010). *Attention process training III: A direct attention training program for persons with acquired brain injury* (3rd ed.) [Rehabilitation materials]. Youngsville, NC: Lash & Associates.

Sturm, W., Fimm, B., Cantagallo, A., Cremel, N., North, P., Passadori, A., . . . LeClercq, M. (2002). Computerized training of specific attention deficits in stroke and traumatic brain-injured patients: A multicentric efficacy study. In M. Leclercq & P. Zimmermann (Eds.), *Applied neuropsychology of attention* (pp. 365–380). Hove, UK: Psychology Press.

Sturm, W., Willmes, K., Orgass, B., & Hartje, W. (1997). Do specific attention deficits need specific training? *Neuropsychological Rehabilitation, 7*, 81–103.

Weightman, M. M., & McCulloch, K. (2014). Dual-task assessment and intervention. In M. Weightman, M. Vining Radomski, & P. Mashima (Ed.), *Mild traumatic brain injury rehabilitation toolkit*. Fort Sam Houston, TX: Office of The Surgeon General (Borden Institute).

Winkens, I., Van Heugten, C., Fasotti, L., & Wade, D. (2009). Reliability and validity of two new instruments for measuring aspects of mental slowness in the daily lives of stroke patients. *Neuropsychological Rehabilitation, 19*(1), 64–85.

Winkens, I., Van Heugten, C. M., Wade, D. T., & Fasotti, L. (2009). Training patients in time pressure management, a cognitive strategy for mental slowness. *Clinical Rehabilitation, 23*(1), 79–90.

Winkens, I., Van Heugten, C. M., Wade, D. T., Habets, E. J., & Fasotti, L. (2009). Efficacy of time pressure management in stroke patients with slowed information processing: A randomized controlled trial. *Archives of Physical Medicine and Rehabilitation, 90*(10), 1672–1679.

Ylvisaker, M., Hanks, R., & Johnson-Greene, D. (2002). Perspectives on rehabilitation of individuals with cognitive impairment after brain injury: Rationale for reconsideration of theoretical paradigms. *Journal of Head Trauma Rehabilitation, 17*(3), 191–209.

Ylvisaker, M. S., & Holland, A. L. (1985). Coaching, self-coaching, and rehabilitation of head injury. In *Clinical management of neurogenic communicative disorders*. Boston, MA: Little Brown & Company.

## APPENDIX 7-1

## Real-World Task Assessment: Attention

Client: _____

| Task | Date | Type of Attention[1] | Difficulty[2] | Duration | Task Accuracy[3] | Errors/ Opportunities | Type of Error(s) (Describe) | Error Awareness[4] | Additional Notes |
|------|------|----------------------|---------------|----------|------------------|----------------------|----------------------------|--------------------|------------------|
|      |      |                      |               |          |                  |                      |                            |                    |                  |
|      |      |                      |               |          |                  |                      |                            |                    |                  |
|      |      |                      |               |          |                  |                      |                            |                    |                  |
|      |      |                      |               |          |                  |                      |                            |                    |                  |
|      |      |                      |               |          |                  |                      |                            |                    |                  |
|      |      |                      |               |          |                  |                      |                            |                    |                  |
|      |      |                      |               |          |                  |                      |                            |                    |                  |
|      |      |                      |               |          |                  |                      |                            |                    |                  |
|      |      |                      |               |          |                  |                      |                            |                    |                  |
|      |      |                      |               |          |                  |                      |                            |                    |                  |
|      |      |                      |               |          |                  |                      |                            |                    |                  |
|      |      |                      |               |          |                  |                      |                            |                    |                  |

*Notes.* [1]Type of Attention: S = Sustained, SL = Selective, A = Alternating, D = Divided; [2]Level of Difficulty: 1 = Very difficult, 2 = Difficult/3 =Easy, 4 = Very Easy; [3]Accuracy: A = Accurate/Complete, I = Inaccurate/Incomplete. [4]Awareness: F = Fully Aware, P = Partially Aware, U = Unaware

Client: _____

APPENDIX 7–2

## Self-Observation: Attention

| Date/ Time | What did I do that required attention? | What type of attention was needed? | How difficult was the task *overall?* | How was my attention during this task? | Is there anything I would do differently (or remember for next time)? |
|---|---|---|---|---|---|
| | | | | | |
| | | | | | |
| | | | | | |
| | | | | | |

Type of Attention: S = Sustained, SL = Selective, A = Alternating, D = Divided
Level of Difficulty: 1 = Very difficult, 2 = Difficult/3 =Difficult/3 =Easy, 4 = Very Easy

## Self-Reflection:  Attention

Client: _____

| | KNOWLEDGE | | ATTRIBUTE | EMOTION | IMPACT | | |
| --- | --- | --- | --- | --- | --- | --- | --- |
| | *What are my strengths?* | *What are my challenges?* | *What is causing difficulty in this area?* | *How do I feel about this?* | *How does this impact me in my daily life?* | *What things help?* | *What things make it more challenging?* |
| Processing Speed | | | | | | | |
| Sustained Attention | | | | | | | |
| Selective Attention | | | | | | | |
| Divided Attention | | | | | | | |
| Alternating Attention | | | | | | | |

# Mental Slowness Questionnaire

Below you see a list of situations that may happen in daily life. For every situation, could you fill in whether this has become a problem due to the stroke? If a certain situation has always been a bit of a problem for you, circle the number 0. If it has worsened, please circle the number that applies to you. The numbers have the following meaning:

0 = this *never* happens to me

1 = this *rarely* happens to me, less than once a week

2 = this happens to me *now and then*, approximately once a week

3 = this happens to me *frequently*, two or three times a week

4 = this happens to me *often*, more than three times a week

For every question you also fill in how troublesome it is to you when this happens. You can choose between:

not: I do *not* find this troublesome

fairly: I find this *fairly* troublesome

very: I find this *very* troublesome

(Of course, if you fill in that a certain situation never happens to you, you do not have to fill in how troublesome it is to you.)

**Example**

When someone is talking to me, it takes longer before I understand what he/she is saying.
0  1  2  3  4

If it now and then takes longer before you understand what someone if saying, then you circle the number 2.

How troublesome is this to you?     not   fairly   very

Perhaps you find it very troublesome that now and then it takes longer before you understand what someone is saying. If this is the case, you circle the word "very."

0 = *never*   1 = *rarely*   2 = *now and then*   3 = *frequently*   4 = *often*

Since stroke . . .

1. When someone is talking to me, it takes longer before I understand what he/she is saying.
   0  1  2  3  4
   How troublesome if this to you?     not   fairly   very

2. I have trouble keeping up with people (for example, when I am on the phone, or in a meeting).

0 1 2 3 4

How troublesome if this to you?     not   fairly   very

3. When I am reading (the newspaper, a book), it takes longer before I understand what it says.

0 1 2 3 4

How troublesome if this to you?     not   fairly   very

4. When I am listening to the radio, or watching television, I can't keep up with the story.

0 1 2 3 4

How troublesome if this to you?     not   fairly   very

5. It takes longer before I come up with the right phone number or word.

0 1 2 3 4

How troublesome if this to you?     not   fairly   very

6. When I meet someone in the street, it takes a while before I remember who it is.

0 1 2 3 4

How troublesome if this to you?     not   fairly   very

7. I can no longer perform tasks automatically, I have to think more (when doing household tasks or work).

0 1 2 3 4

How troublesome if this to you?     not   fairly   very

8. I need more time for doing my work or household tasks, because I have to think more (NOT because of physical disabilities).

0 1 2 3 4

How troublesome if this to you?     not   fairly   very

9. When I am engaged in a task, I feel I have too little time to do it right.

0 1 2 3 4

How troublesome if this to you?     not   fairly   very

10. If I have to deal with unexpected events, I get restless or agitated.

0 1 2 3 4

How troublesome if this to you?     not   fairly   very

11. If I do something too fast, I make mistakes or forget things.

0 1 2 3 4

How troublesome if this to you?     not   fairly   very

*continues*

12. I find it difficult to do two things at the same time (such as doing household tasks when someone is talking to me, or cooking and making a telephone call at the same time).

0 1 2 3 4

How troublesome if this to you?     not   fairly   very

13. Being in traffic (on foot, by bike, or by car) is difficult for me, because I quickly get overwhelmed.

0 1 2 3 4

How troublesome if this to you?     not   fairly   very

14. When I have to do two things at the same time, I get restless or agitated, or make mistakes.

0 1 2 3 4

How troublesome if this to you?     not   fairly   very

15. When I am busy and I am disturbed, (for example, when the phone rings, or someone speaks to me) I start making mistakes.

0 1 2 3 4

How troublesome if this to you?     not   fairly   very

16. When I am in a noisy room (e.g., a shop or pub) I have difficulty paying attention.

0 1 2 3 4

How troublesome if this to you?     not   fairly   very

17. I get distracted by my own thoughts, and then I make mistakes.

0 1 2 3 4

How troublesome if this to you?     not   fairly   very

18. When several people speak at the same time, (e.g., at a party or in a meeting) I lose track of what they are saying.

0 1 2 3 4

How troublesome if this to you?     not   fairly   very

19. I get tired easily because everything seems to go so fast.

0 1 2 3 4

How troublesome if this to you?     not   fairly   very

20. When I have to do two things at the same time, I get tired easily.

0 1 2 3 4

How troublesome if this to you?     not   fairly   very

21. If I have to concentrate in a noisy room, I get tired easily.

0 1 2 3 4

How troublesome if this to you?     not   fairly   very

*Source:* Winkens, Van Heugten, Fasotti, & Wade (2009). Used with permission.

# Mental Slowness Observation Test

(Pencil and paper is lying in front of the patient.)

General instructions to the subject are as follows:

*"I will ask you to perform five tasks that are very similar to tasks that you may encounter in daily life. For example following a route description, making a telephone call, or looking up telephone numbers. I will observe how well you perform the task and I will be timing you. For all the tasks there is one general rule: you are allowed to do anything you would do in normal life to make these tasks easier for yourself."*

**Subtask 1: Following a route description**

Instruction:

*"Imagine you are in an unfamiliar city, and would like to know where the nearest bakery is. Let's pretend I am a pedestrian, and you decide to ask me. In a minute I will give you a route description. Afterwards, I would like you to draw the route on a map, and tell me where the bakery is* [the map will be handed to the patient after the route description is given]. *So please make sure that you'll know how to get to the bakery."*

Read the following route description to the patient:

*"You walk straight on and then take the second turn on your right. When you reach the Bank you go left. Then you take the second turn on your right. You will pass an ancient gate. Keep on walking until you reach a pub, there you turn left. Keep on walking and the bakery will be on your right."*

Hand the map to the patient:

*"Now try to draw the route on this map. When you are ready, please tell me where the bakery must be."*

Time starts when you start reading the route description until the patient shows you on the map where the bakery is. If the patient gets lost and asks for a new route description, take away the map while you read the route description again.

Task materials: paper and pencil, stopwatch, a map, score form.

*continues*

**Subtask 2: Making a telephone call**

Instruction:

*"Imagine you would like to visit someone in the University hospital in Maastricht. The visiting hour starts at three o'clock. You leave from the train station in Den Bosch, and travel by public transport. You are now going to call the public transport information service to find out what time you have to leave and which train you have to take. This is the telephone number, and this is the question you can ask* [hand out paper with information]. *Please wait until you can speak to an operator. When you have made the phone call, I will ask you to tell me how you will travel. So make sure you can tell me afterwards. Are you ready? Then you can make the phone call* [the patient can read the question from a piece of paper].

Time starts when the operator starts speaking until the patient has reported the information.

Task materials: Piece of paper with the question and phone number, stopwatch, paper and pencil, phone, score form.

**Subtask 3: Sorting money**

Instruction:

*"In a minute I will ask you to sort from this pile of money 10 precise amounts. The amounts I'm asking for are on this piece of paper* [show the paper to the patient]. *Every time you have sorted out one amount, please put the money back on the pile. Try to do it as fast as possible. I'll give you five minutes to do this, so try to be ready in time. This watch will keep track of time. The alarm goes off whenever 60 seconds have passed, and every time I will tell you how much time is left. Let's start, shall we?"*

Time limit: 5 minutes. Time starts when the patient picks up the first coin until he has sorted out the last amount.

Task materials: change, stopwatch, timer, score form, piece of paper with the requested amounts.

**Subtask 4: Listening to the radio news (this subtask has been excluded from the final version of the MSOT)**

Instruction:

*"Imagine you have plans for going to Zandvoort, to the coast, this Saturday and Sunday. You decide to listen to the radio news to find out whether you can expect heavy traffic, what the weather will be like and so forth, so you can decide what you will do and what you have to take with you. In a minute you will listen to a part of the radio news. Afterwards I will ask you some questions. The questions I will ask you are on this piece of paper* [show it to the patient]. *Listen carefully so you will be able to answer the questions. Do you understand this task? Are you ready to begin?"*

Time starts when the radio news starts to play until the patient answers the last question.

Task materials: tape recorder and tape, pen and paper, paper with questions, stopwatch, score form.

## Subtask 5: Looking up telephone numbers

Instruction:

*"I will ask you to look up several phone numbers in this phone book. These are the people of whom I'd like to know their phone numbers* [show names on a piece of paper]. *You can write the numbers down. You have 10 minutes. While you are looking up the phone numbers, I will also ask you several questions you have to answer. At the end of the task I would like you to give me all phone numbers. Do you understand what you have to do? Then you may begin with the first phone number."*

Time limit: 10 minutes. Time starts when the patient opens the phone book until he/she gives the last phone number.

Task materials: phone book, list of names, list of questions, paper and pencil, stopwatch, score form.

*Source:* Winkens, Van Heugten, Fasotti, & Wade (2009). Used with permission.

# TPM Pressure Data Collection and Clinician Rating Form[1]

Date: _____ Task: _____ Client: _____

---

| Analyze the Task | **Identifying time pressure(s)** rating |
|---|---|

1         2         3         4         5

Nature/# of prompts:

Time pressure(s) identified by client (describe):

**Prevention Plan**

**Prevention planning** rating

1         2         3         4         5

Nature/# of prompts:

Prevention plan identified by client (describe):

**Emergency Plan**

**Emergency plan** rating

1         2         3         4         5

Nature/# of prompts:

Emergency plan identified by client (describe):

**Implement/Monitor**

Accuracy of **task completed**:

Accurate/Complete       Inaccurate/Incomplete

Task error(s):

PREVENTION PLAN:

**Prevention plan implementation** rating

1         2         3         4         5

Nature/# of prompts:

Notes:

EMERGENCY PLAN:

Emergency plan required?   Y/N

**Emergency plan implementation** rating

1         2         3         4         5         N A

Nature/# of prompts

Notes:

---

*Note.* Accuracy: 1 = accurate and independent; 2 = accurate with minimal prompt; 3 = accurate with moderate prompts, 4 = accurate with significant prompts, 5 = inaccurate despite prompts.

# Dual-Tasking Questionnaire

*The following questions are about problems which everyone experiences from time to time, but some of which happen more often than others. We want to know how often these things have happened to you in the past few weeks. There are five options, ranging from never to very often (or not applicable, N/A). Please circle the appropriate option to your circumstances.*

**How often do you have difficulty with . . .**

1. Paying attention to more than one thing at once.
   *Never (0)     Rarely (1)     Occasionally (2)     Often (3)     Very Often (4)     N/A*

2. Needing to stop an activity to talk.
   *Never (0)     Rarely (1)     Occasionally (2)     Often (3)     Very Often (4)     N/A*

3. Being unaware of others speaking to you when doing another activity.
   *Never (0)     Rarely (1)     Occasionally (2)     Often (3)     Very Often (4)     N/A*

4. Following or taking part in a conversation where several people are speaking at once.
   *Never (0)     Rarely (1)     Occasionally (2)     Often (3)     Very Often (4)     N/A*

5. Walking deteriorating when you are talking or listening to someone.
   *Never (0)     Rarely (1)     Occasionally (2)     Often (3)     Very Often (4)     N/A*

6. Busy thinking your own thoughts, so not noticing what is going on around you.
   *Never (0)     Rarely (1)     Occasionally (2)     Often (3)     Very Often (4)     N/A*

7. Spilling a drink when carrying it.
   *Never (0)     Rarely (1)     Occasionally (2)     Often (3)     Very Often (4)     N/A*

8. Spilling a drink when carrying it and talking at the same time.
   *Never (0)     Rarely (1)     Occasionally (2)     Often (3)     Very Often (4)     N/A*

9. Bumping into people or dropping things if doing something else as well.
   *Never (0)     Rarely (1)     Occasionally (2)     Often (3)     Very Often (4)     N/A*

10. Difficulty eating and watching television or listening to the radio at the same time.
    *Never (0)     Rarely (1)     Occasionally (2)     Often (3)     Very Often (4)     N/A*

*Source:* Evans, Greenfield, Wilson, & Bateman (2009, p.120). Adapted with permission.

# 8 Memory

| a. Introduction |
| b. Memory Compensation (Internal and External) |
| *Jennifer A. Ostergren and Carley B. Crandall* |

## a. Introduction

International Cognitive (INCOG) treatment recommendations in the area of memory include (Velikonja et al., 2014, pp. 372–375):

1. Teaching internal compensatory strategies may be used for traumatic brain injury (TBI) patients who have memory impairments. These strategies include instructional and/or metacognitive strategies (e.g., visualization/visual imagery, repeated practice, retrieval practice, PQRST (preview, question, read, study, test), self-cueing, self-generation, self-talk, etc.). Their use tends to be most effective with patients who have mild to moderate range impairments and/or some preserved executive cognitive skills. Utilizing multiple strategies is considered effective and strategies can be taught individually or in a group format.

2. For TBI patients who have memory impairment and especially for those who have severe memory impairment, environmental supports and reminders are recommended (e.g., NeuroPage, mobile/smartphones, Siris, personal digital assistants, notebooks, whiteboards). Patients with TBI and their caregivers/support staff must be trained in how to use these external supports.

3. The selection of external memory aids should take into account the following considerations regarding the person with a traumatic brain injury: age, severity of impairment, premorbid use of electronic and other memory devices, cognitive strengths and weaknesses, and physical comorbidities.

4. There are a number of key instructional practices that can promote learning for individuals with memory impairments, which include:

   a. Clearly define intervention goals and integrate methodologies that allow for breaking down tasks into smaller components such as task analysis when training multi-step procedures.

   b. Allow sufficient time and opportunity for practice.

   c. Use principles of distributed practice.

d. Promote strategies that allow for more effortful processing of information/stimuli (e.g., verbal elaboration, visual imagery).

e. Select and train to goals that are relevant to the patient (i.e., ecologically valid).

f. Teach strategies using variations in the stimuli/information being presented (e.g., multiple exemplars, practical tasks).

g. Use teaching strategies that constrain errors (e.g., errorless, spaced retrieval) when acquiring new or relearning information and procedures.

5. Group-based interventions may be considered for remediation of mild to moderate memory deficits following TBI.

6. Restorative techniques such as computer-based training show no evidence of enhancing sustained memory performance. Guidelines in using such techniques indicate that it should only be considered to develop adjunct memory rehabilitation strategies with evidence-based instructional and compensatory strategies, and only if developed in conjunction with a therapist with a focus on strategy development and transfer to functional tasks.

Similarly, the American Congress of Rehabilitation Medicine (ACRM), given multiple meta-analyses in this area (Cicerone et al., 2000, 2005; Cicerone et al., 2011, p. 523), recommends:

1. Memory strategy training is recommended for mild memory impairments from TBI, including the use of internalized strategies (e.g., visual imagery) and external memory compensations (e.g., notebooks) (Practice Standard).

2. Use of external compensations with direct application to functional activities is recommended for people with severe memory deficits after TBI or stroke (Practice Guideline).

3. For people with severe memory impairments after TBI, errorless learning techniques may be effective for learning specific skills or knowledge, with limited transfer to novel tasks or reduction in overall functional memory problems (Practice Option).

4. Group-based interventions may be considered for remediation of memory deficits after TBI (Practice Option).

Memory treatment approaches are addressed within this chapter using the hierarchical diagram in Figure 8–1. Internal and external memory compensation is recommended for those individuals for whom posttraumatic amnesia has resolved (Velikonja et al., 2014).

## Assessment

Table 8–1 contains examples of common assessment measures in the area of memory, including direct measures and questionnaires/rating scales. These are helpful measures in identifying particular strengths and weaknesses, and in the case of standardized assessment, comparison to a normative data set. The rehabilitative process also benefits from ongoing structured evaluation of performance in real-world tasks (Sohlberg & Mateer, 2001). Table 8–2 contains examples of real-world tasks, stratified by types of memory. These can be individualized to the client's home, recreational, vocational, and educational experiences. Important factors applicable to each client, such as delay, accuracy, difficulty of task, type of memory, and nature and awareness of errors, can be assessed during these structured activities before, during, and after inter-

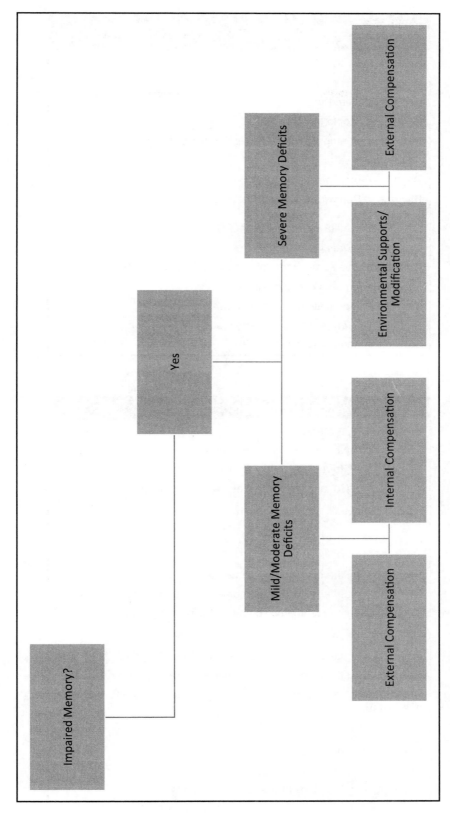

**Figure 8–1.** Memory treatment in action hierarchy. Suggested treatment approaches in the area of memory processing, given severity of memory impairments.

**Table 8–1.** Common Memory Measures: Direct Measures and Questionnaires/Rating Scales

DIRECT MEASURES

California Auditory Verbal Learning Test

Contextual Memory Test

Doors and People Memory Test

Prospective Memory Training Screening (PROMS)

Rey Auditory Verbal Learning Test

Rey-Osterrieth Complex Figure

Rivermead Behavioral Memory Test

QUESTIONNAIRES/RATING SCALES

Cognitive Failures Questionnaire

Comprehensive Assessment of Prospective Memory (CAPM)

Everyday Memory Questionnaire

Memory Compensation Questionnaire

Prospective-Retrospective Memory Questionnaire

Subjective Memory Questionnaire

---

**Table 8–2.** Examples of Real-World Memory Tasks

PROSPECTIVE MEMORY

Remembering to schedule an appointment for a haircut

Remembering to reply to an email from a friend

Remembering to take medication at a specific time of day

RETROSPECTIVE MEMORY

Declarative

*Episodic*

Remembering the events from dinner the night before

Remembering the day you came home from the hospital after the TBI

Remembering a recent family gathering at Thanksgiving

*Semantic*

Remembering the name of the current and past President

Remembering the types of birds or native plants in your local area

Remembering the formula for calculating the appropriate tip/gratuity at a restaurant

Non-Declarative (Procedural)

Remembering how to tie your shoe

Remembering how to prune a rose bush

Remembering the steps of a favorite line-dance

vention, regardless of the approach utilized. Appendix 8–1 is an example of a data recording sheet that can be modified for this purpose.

Engaging the client in an ongoing self-assessment can be a valuable exercise in the rehabilitation process. Several authors have noted awareness after a brain injury to be an important factor across a variety of rehabilitation approaches (Bergquist & Jacket, 1993; Ezrachi Ben-Yishay, Kay, DiUer, & Rattok, 1991; Prigatano, Altman, & O'Brien, 1990). A helpful first step in this process is self-observation. This can be done by asking the client to keep a structured journal or log about memory performance during daily tasks. The speech-language pathologist (SLP) can collaborate with the client to identify good times for this observation (during specific periods of the day, while performing specific tasks, etc.). This could be done by alternating observation periods (one day of tracking success in memory / one day of tracking lapses in memory) or by requesting that the client record memory successes and lapses, in a given time period of observation. Appendix 8–2 shows a sample data collection sheet that can be modified for this purpose. As with all aspects of self-reflection, this would begin with and include ongoing conversations with the client about types of memory and what they mean specifically to the client's daily tasks and his/her unique needs/skills.

Overall self-assessment after self-observation is also valuable. Using a framework based on levels of awareness (Flashman, Amador, & McAllister, 1998), this self-assessment could include reflection on: (1) the nature of a specific deficit (knowledge); (2) the source of the deficit/difficulty (attributes); (3) how the individual feels about that deficit/difficulty (emotion); and (4) how that deficit/difficulty affects daily tasks (impact). Appendix 8–3 shows a sample worksheet for overall reflection and discussion between the SLP and the client in the area of memory. This should be tailored to meet each individual's needs and abilities and pursued after an effective and trusting therapeutic relationship has been established between the client and the SLP (Flashman & McAllister, 2002). Individuals with ongoing strong negative emotions in this area should be referred to a psychologist or neuropsychologist team member for additional support (American Speech-Language-Hearing Association, 2003).

## b. Memory Compensation (Internal and External)

## Candidacy Recommendations

The use of compensation for memory impairments is applicable to many individuals with TBI in the post-acute phases of recovery (Velikonja et al., 2014). Compensation approaches are classified into either internal strategies (internal compensation) or external aids (external compensation) (Sohlberg & Mateer, 1989). Candidacy recommendations for each vary slightly, as below. It is also important to note that the compensation itself, its purpose, and the context and level of support in implementation also play key roles in candidacy recommendations in this area.

### Internal Strategies

1. **Individuals who evidence mild-to-moderate memory impairments** (Velikonja et al., 2014). It should be noted, however, that O'Neil-Pirozzi, Kennedy, and Sohlberg (2016) concluded that due to insufficiently defined participation

profiles of past studies, there appears to be "no clear indication that only those with mild memory impairment benefit from these strategies" (p. E9).

2. **Individuals who experience memory failures in everyday activities.**

3. **Individuals who have awareness and preserved executive function skills (Velikonja et al., 2014) sufficient to benefit from and generalize internal compensation techniques to real-world tasks.** Ylvisaker and Holland's (1985) recommendations relative to successful compensatory training characteristics (patient and strategy) (Table 8–3) are helpful in this area.

### External Aids and Devices

1. **Individuals who evidence memory impairments (mild, moderate, or severe)** (Velikonja et al., 2014). As above, these can be assessed given the memory measures listed at the start of this chapter (see Table 8–1).

2. **Individuals who experience memory failures in everyday activities.**

3. **Individuals who have sufficient awareness (or support in their envi-** ronment) **to generalize strategies to real-world tasks.**

## Treatment Evidence

There is Level A evidence to support each of the following in the treatment of memory impairments in individuals with TBI (Figure 8–2; Velikonja et al., 2014):

1. Internal compensation strategies, including visualization/visual imagery, repeated practice, retrieval practice, self-cueing, and so forth

2. External compensation aids and devices, such as diaries, notebooks, customized memory books, organizers, planners, and pagers

3. The use of the key instructional practices listed in Table 8–4

The combination of these approaches (as appropriate to the individual with TBI) has also been shown to further enhance effectiveness of memory intervention (Fleming, Shum, Strong, & Lightbody, 2005; Freeman, Mittenberg, Dicowden, & Bat-Ami, 1992; Sohlberg, Kennedy, & Avery, 2007).

**Table 8–3.** Requisite Patient and Strategy Variable for Successful Compensatory Training

| *Patient* | *Strategy* |
|---|---|
| The patient must recognize the existence of impairments that cannot be alleviated by restitution of underlying problems | The strategy must be fitted to the patient's needs, personality, and abilities |
| The patient must be capable of recognizing problems as they occur or, better yet, anticipate problems before they occur | The strategy must fulfill an obvious and apparent need that personally is felt by the patient |
| The patient must be capable of invoking a strategy based on recognition of a present or potential problem situation | The strategy must fit the personal inclination and the attitudes of patient |
| | The strategy must be easy enough that the patient can invoke it automatically and effortlessly |

*Source:* Ylvisaker & Holland (1985).

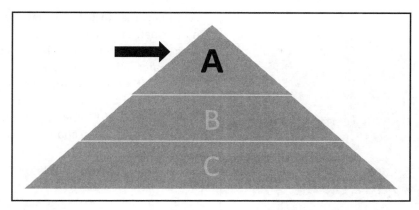

**Figure 8–2.** Level A evidence for the use of memory compensation (internal and external). Level A consists of "recommendation supported by at least one meta-analysis, systematic review or randomized controlled trial study of appropriate size and relevant control group" (Bayley et al., 2014, p. 295).

**Table 8–4.** Key Instructional Practices Shown to Promote Learning in Individuals with Memory Impairments Post TBI

Clearly define intervention goals

Integrate methodologies that allow for breaking down tasks into smaller components such as task analysis when training multistep procedures

Allow sufficient time and opportunity for practice

Use principles of distributed practice

Teach strategies using variations in the stimuli/information being presented (e.g., multiple exemplars, practical tasks)

Promote strategies that allow for more effortful processing of information/stimuli (e.g., verbal elaboration; visual imagery, etc)

Selection of and train to goals that are relevant to the patient (i.e., ecologically validity)

Use teaching strategies that constrain errors (e.g., errorless, spaced retrieval, etc) when acquiring new or relearning information and procedures

*Source:* Velikonja, Tate, Ponsford, et al. (2014, p. 379).

## Theoretical Frame

Internal and external compensation techniques used in memory intervention are classically defined as compensation approaches. In recent years, some researchers have also suggested the importance of including metacognitive strategies (calibration) to improve metamemory in individuals with TBI (Kennedy, 2006). Both of these approaches (compensation and calibration) are listed in Figure 8–3.

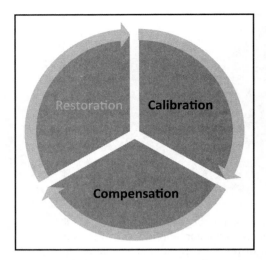

**Figure 8–3.** Theoretical frames of treatment approaches for memory which utilize internal compensation, external compensation, and metamemory approaches.

Of note, restorative techniques in the area of memory "show no evidence in enhancing sustained memory performance" beyond trained tasks (Velikonja et al., 2014, p. 382). This includes paper-and-pencil tasks and those executed via computer-based repetitive drills and practice. Guidelines in this area recommend that restorative approaches "only be considered to develop adjunct memory rehabilitation strategies with evidence-based instructional and compensatory strategies, and only if developed in conjunction with a clinician with a focus on strategy development and transfer to functional tasks" (p. 382).

## Background Information

Compensation for memory impairments has a long history in the research literature (Sohlberg & Mateer, 1989). Internal strategy compensation approaches comprise primarily mnemonic or imagery techniques that foster new ways of taking in information or making that information more salient for future recall. Internal strategy compensation techniques can be classified as either association techniques or organizational and elaboration techniques (Haskins et al., 2012). Several examples of internal compensation approaches are listed in Table 8–5.

External compensation aids and devices provide either reminders of the need to recall information or storage and display of the information to be recalled. These can run the gamut of sophistication and complexity, from a simple notepad, used to create written reminders of a specific task, to complex electronic devices, such as smartphones with multiple applications such as calendars, alarms, reminders, detailed list features, and so forth. Many external compensation aids are designed for prospective memory tasks (Velikonja et al., 2014). Table 8–6 contains a list of several common external aids and devices and an example use for memory compensation.

## Treatment in Action

"Training protocols describing specific methods to teach use of compensatory strategies to individuals with brain injuries are limited in the cognitive literature" (Sohlberg & Mateer, 2001, p. 195). As such, clinical implementation of compensatory memory approaches recommended here is based on an amalgamation of research evidence in this area (Haskins et al., 2012; Kaschel et al., 2002; O'Neil-Pirozzi et al., 2016; O'Neil-Pirozzi et al., 2010; Sohlberg & Mateer, 1989, 2001; Velikonja et al., 2014; Wilson, 2009). The procedures described are applicable to both internal and external compensation approaches and are broken

**Table 8–5.** Examples of Internal Compensation Strategies

| Memory Strategy Training | Brief Description of Strategy | Example |
|---|---|---|
| **Association Techniques** | | |
| Face-name recognition/association | A name (verbal information) is linked or associated with either a picture (visual) of the person or the image of a face (visual imagery). | Individual is taught to identify a prominent feature of the person's face (e.g., ears), which could be associated with their name (e.g., Mrs. Crossley). The next step is to transform the name into something meaningful (e.g., Crossley is transformed into "cross leaf"). The final step is to link the feature to the transformed name, so a crossed leaf would be imagined growing out of her ears. |
| Visual peg method | Target items (visual or verbal information) are linked or associated with a standard set of peg words (visual imagery), which are already learned and memorized in a fixed sequence (e.g., rhyming peg method). | Rhyming pegs are memorized (e.g., one-bun; two-shoe; three-tree, four-door, etc.). To remember grocery items (e.g., bread, butter, Gatorade, kiwis, Oreos), the first item, bread, would be linked visually to "bun," butter would be linked to "shoe," Gatorade with "tree," and so on. After associations are made the client can retrieve list by recall of rhyming peg words with the associated visual image.<br><br>1. bun (bread)—slicing bread and placing beside buns<br><br>2. shoe (butter)—a shoe filled with butter<br><br>3. tree (Gatorade)—a tree with Gatorade growing from the branches |
| Method of loci | Target items (verbal or visual information) are linked or associated with locations or places (visual imagery) already known. | Individual makes visual associations between target words and specific places or objects in a familiar room (e.g., bedroom). They are taught to mentally scan room for designated locations/objects to retrieve items to be recalled. |

*continues*

**Table 8–5.** *continued*

| Memory Strategy Training | Brief Description of Strategy | Example |
|---|---|---|
| **Organizational and Elaboration Techniques** | | |
| First-letter mnemonics | Use of the first letter of each of a set of target words to form a single word or pseudoword. | FANBOYS is an acronym for the seven coordinating conjunctions **F**or, **A**nd, **N**or, **B**ut, **O**r, **Y**et, **S**o |
| Semantic Clustering | Target items are broken into informational categories or "clusters" based on meaning of the words. | Individual is taught to group items on a grocery list based on sections of the grocery store or food type. The individual might use the categories "fruits and vegetables," and "ingredients to make brownies" as the two clusters of items. |
| PQRST | A rehearsal strategy, wherein memorization of PQRST steps (i.e., Preview, Question, Read, State, Test) enables self-instruction, promotes active learning, and engages elaboration and review of what has been learned and remembered. | Individuals returning to an academic environment might be taught to use strategy when recalling written information: 1. Preview: Preview information to be recalled 2. Question: Ask key questions about the text ("What is the central theme or may concepts conveyed? In what year did the action take place? How many people were involved") 3. Read: Read the material carefully to answer questions 4. State: State the answers and, if necessary, read the text again until answers can be stated. 5. Test: Test regularly for retention of information. |
| Story telling/use of humor | Information or target items are linked together through interaction in a story or joke. | Target items yacht, box of matches, and rope can be remembered by creating a story: Bill hoisted the box of matches onto the yacht with a line of rope. |

*Source:* Haskins et al., (2012, pp. 62–64) and Wilson (2009, pp. 77–78).

**Table 8–6.** Examples of Common Types of Compensation Aids and Device and Sample Use for Memory Compensation

| Type of External Aid/Device | Sample Use in Memory Compensation |
|---|---|
| Sticky Notes/Note Pad | Used to write reminders or checklist of tasks to be performed (e.g., make a list of items to be purchased at the store) |
| Voice Recorder | Used to record a verbal reminder for replay at a later time (e.g., "Call mom when I get home to wish her a Happy Anniversary"). Available in dedicated form or within applications "apps" on mobile devices. |
| Pagers | Personal messages and reminders placed by caregiver (or individuals with TBI) and send at a specific time (e.g., written message of "TAKE YOUR MEDICATION" sent via pager at 10:00 every day). |
| Timer and Alarms | Used as a reminder to perform a specific task. Available as dedicated devices, such as a kitchen timer, or via apps installed on mobile devices. |
| Calendars and Planner | Either paper/pencil or electronic, used to record and store important events, reminders, and to-do lists. |
| Environmental Organizers | Systems such as mail basket sorters, door-hanging organizers, index card holders, accordion folders, that store information for ready access and retrieval. |
| Object Locators | Wireless sensors that are attached to important objects (e.g., keys, T.V. remote control), with a remote that sounds a signal for location of the object, if lost. Remotes are also available installed on mobile devices. |
| Photographic Phone/Contact List | Specialized phones (or apps on mobile phones) that store and display important numbers with photographs for easy recall and dialing of important numbers. |
| Global Positioning Systems (GPS) | Navigation systems (either dedicated or given apps on mobile devices) that store and display routes to desired location in real-time, given current location. |
| Medication Management | Specialized medication storage and dispensing devices that offer alarms, timed dispensing, voice output, and other reminders for medication management. Mobile apps are also available specific to medication reminders and management. |

down into four phases (assessment/anticipation, acquisition, application, adaptation) (Figure 8–4 and Table 8–7). These phases are based upon a three-stage behavioral training protocol initially outlined by Sohlberg and Mateer (1989), modified to include a preliminary, fourth stage, reflecting refinements made in experimental literature (Schmitter-Edgecombe, Fahy, Whelan, & Long, 1995).

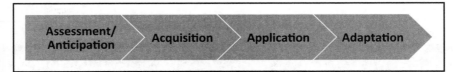

**Figure 8–4.** The four phases of compensation training.

| Table 8–7. Phases of Compensatory Implementation | | |
|---|---|---|
| *Phase* | *Components/Goal* | *Can be achieved by* |
| **Phase 1: Assessment (Anticipation)** | Develop client needs profile<br><br>Identify compensatory strategy(s)<br><br>Establish treatment goals<br><br>Collect baselines | Needs assessment<br>  –Organic Factors<br>  –Personal Factors<br>  –Situational Factors<br>    –Neuropsychological testing<br>    –Questionnaires/ Interview<br>    –Behavioral observation<br>    –Checklist<br>    –Diary/Memory Log |
| **Phase 2: Acquisition** | Introduce strategy and demonstrate strategy utility (i.e., usefulness)<br><br>Teach strategy components/steps<br><br>Client demonstrates understanding of newly learned technique(s)<br><br>Task and situations in which the strategy(s) can be applied are identified | Meaningful and personalized information and examples<br>Learning Strategies:<br>  –Errorless learning<br>  –Spaced retrieval<br>  –Chaining (forward and backward)<br>External compensations |
| **Phase 3: Application** | Client applies strategy(s) across tasks, situations, and participant-reported difficulties<br><br>Promote internalization of strategies<br><br>Monitor progress toward goals | Practice, feedback, and demonstration<br>Learning Strategies:<br>  –Errorless learning<br>  –Spaced retrieval<br>  –Chaining (forward and backward)<br>External compensations<br>Homework assignments<br>Record form |
| **Phase 4: Adaptation** | Client applies strategy(s) in natural task settings<br><br>Promote transfer of training to similar/novel tasks | Observation of performance in naturalistic environments<br>Feedback<br>Homework assignments<br>Elicit help of family and community members |

### *Phase 1: Assessment/Anticipation*

The process of selecting compensatory strategies and devising a plan to implement them begins in Phase 1 (Assessment/Anticipation) through systematic assessment of client needs. In this initial phase, the goals are to:

1. Utilize assessment procedures (i.e., standardized, functional, and behavioral assessments) to develop an accurate picture of an individual's cognitive, emotional, and interpersonal functioning as it relates to memory impairment (Sohlberg & Mateer, 2001)
2. Generate a list of suitable compensatory options that complement client needs, abilities, and activity goals (i.e., tasks that the client currently struggles with but wishes to perform)
3. Establish treatment goals
4. Collect initial measurements of identified problems (i.e., baselines)

A thorough assessment of client functioning, strengths, and needs enables a speech-language pathologist (SLP) to select and/or design the most appropriate compensation (internal or external) consistent with the client's individual profile.

To guide in matching a system to an individual, Sohlberg and Mateer (2001) recommend that clinicians evaluate the individual needs of a client through conducting a *needs assessment*. The needs assessment facilitates collection of information in three broad categories: (1) organic factors (e.g., cognitive and physical ability); (2) personal factors (e.g., system preferences and available resources and support systems); and (3) situational factors (e.g., contexts in which use of strategies are desirable) (Table 8–8). Taking the time to collaborate with the client and other relevant persons during a needs assessment will result in selection of strategies or aids that can be implemented with maximum efficiency and success (Sohlberg & Mateer, 2001, p. 198). It is also recommended that the SLP identify strategies that build upon existing skill sets and directly apply to contexts and areas of need (Sohlberg & Mateer, 2001).

The *Assistive Technology for Cognition Checklist* in Chapter 6, Appendix 6–1, can serve as a helpful resource in the area of needs assessment, especially for external strategies and devices, as it combines Sohlberg and Mateer's (2001) needs assessment with common device assessment information (e.g., ease of use, access, portability, environment, modifications, costs). It can also be modified for assessment in the area of internal compensation.

Information on organic factors that affect the client's ability to learn and remember new skills (i.e., cognitive/learning profile) can be obtained through formal cognitive assessments (Sohlberg & Mateer, 2001, p. 199), using common measures of memory assessment listed in Table 8–1. The majority of information needed to guide treatment goals (i.e., organic [physical profile], personal, and situational factors) comes from additional functional or behavioral assessment procedures (i.e., direct observations, self-report measures, and interviews) (Sohlberg & Mateer, 2001). Appendix 8–2 (*Self-Observation: Memory*) can be used to gather information about current memory success and lapses during real-world tasks in the client's own environment. Appendix 8–3 (*Self-Reflection: Memory*) can be used for discussion in these areas and reflection on the client's level of understanding and awareness of these difficulties. In addition, in some cases, an individual with memory impairment may not be able to recall the skill sets or systems he/she currently uses or previously used prior to injury; likewise,

**Table 8–8.** Needs Assessment: Categories of Assessment

| Factors | Description | Example information |
|---------|-------------|---------------------|
| Organic Factors | Relevant physical and cognitive functions | *Cognitive/learning profile*:<br>−Ability to learn and remember new skills<br><br>*Physical profile*:<br>−Significant disturbances in motor ability or sensory function |
| Personal Factors | Relevant psychosocial and environmental elements | *Spontaneous use of compensation strategies*:<br>−Existing strategies utilized pre-injury, or those currently in place<br><br>*Personal preference*:<br>−Appearance (e.g., color, size, style)<br>−Mode (e.g., electronic versus paper and pencil)<br>−System function (e.g., calendar, orientation, things-to-do)<br><br>*Available support*:<br>−Level of available support in both current environment and projected discharge environment. |
| Situational Factors | Contexts in which use of compensatory strategies is desirable | *Context*:<br>−Where and under what circumstances does the cognitive problem interfere with functioning?<br>−What are the consequences when there is a breakdown?<br>−Are there any contexts where the target cognitive issues is NOT a problem, and if so, why?<br><br>*History*:<br>−Accommodations or strategies that have already been tried<br>−Were aids successful or not? |

*Source:* Sohlberg & Mateer, 2001, pp. 199–201.

he/she may not be able to provide relevant information regarding memory breakdowns. As such, in these instances, directly observing the individual and consulting family members and/or those who interact closely with the client can help to fill in information gaps. Appendix 8–1 (*Real-World Task Assessment: Memory*) can be used for direct observation. Appendix 8–2 can also be modified for completion by significant others. This information will inform the SLP of where compensations can be implemented, allowing the clinician to develop an inventory of applicable compensation.

The next step in Phase 1 is for the SLP to utilize information from assessment procedures to delineate suitable compensation options (internal and/or external) to accommodate that client's ability and directly address personally meaningful tasks. Acceptance of the compensation approach is essential to successful implementation (Sander & van Veldhoven, 2014). Therefore, it is helpful to provide clients and their families with a list of possible compensation options and openly discuss comfort level and any anticipated obstacles in compensatory use (Sander & van Veldhoven, 2014, p. 179). This process might involve:

- Re-evaluating areas of need (i.e., adversely affected memory activities) and current strategies (if any)
- Weighing pros and cons of new systems
- Picking a system to try and evaluating its success
- Choosing alternative solutions if the first one does not work (or is not preferred)

Following collaborative discussion, and any experimental trial runs, the SLP will assist the individual in narrowing down the best compensation options and in setting personally relevant treatment goals. The SLP should negotiate and help formulate both short- and long-term goals that are realistic, measurable, and client centered (Wilson, 2009). Long-term goals reflect anticipated treatment outcomes, or what an individual is expected to accomplish by the end of the rehabilitation program, while short-term goals outline the steps that need to be taken in order to achieve the long-term goal. For example, if a long-term goal

is for the client to use a memory notebook to remember what he or she has to do each day, an initial short-term goal might be for the client to remember to check what day it is. Specific goals often fall under broad life domains, which are outlined by Wilson (2009; Table 8–9).

After goals have been set, the SLP should begin intervention, establishing a system to periodically review the client's progress toward meeting goals. The overall purpose of rehabilitation is to enable individuals to improve day-to-day functioning and achieve personal goals. Therefore, setting goals and assessing whether they are achieved can be viewed as a means of collecting baselines and measuring outcomes (Sohlberg & Mateer, 2001; Wilson, 2009). That is, the SLP should utilize direct observation, interviews, and memory logs to establish goals (i.e., baselines) and use periodic review to monitor progress toward outcomes. When goals are achieved, the SLP should set new ones; however, when goals have been hindered, the clinician should consider possible deficiencies (e.g., Was the goal appropriate? Is more time required? Do other people need to be recruited to ensure consistency throughout the day?) and make efforts to modify goals (Wilson, 2009, p. 153). By the end of Phase 1, the SLP should have established a client-needs profile, selected appropriate compensation (internal and/or external), identified functional and personally meaningful tasks to train the client in compensation use, and established treatment goals.

### Phase 2: Acquisition

In Phase 2 (Acquisition), the agreed upon compensation(s) is/are formally introduced and demonstrated. The goal for training in this phase is for the individual to learn

**Table 8–9.** Sample Memory Goals: Life Domains

| Domain | Examples |
| --- | --- |
| Mobility | Remembering how to safely get in and out of a wheelchair |
| Communication | Remembering information from prior conversations |
| Self-Care activities | Remembering to brush teeth, wash hands |
| | Remembering to take medication |
| | Asking where restrooms are remembering instructions |
| Productivity | Carrying out financial responsibilities (e.g., writing checks, completing tax forms) |
| | Learning the names of work colleagues |
| | Learning way to and around workplace |
| Leisure, hobbies, interests | Learning the way to the shops or around the neighborhood, hospital, school, or workplace |
| | Learning the names of acquaintances |
| Understanding brain injury, mood, and cognitive functioning | Remembering and describing autobiographical details to others (e.g., describing deficits to others, describing emotional responses) |

*Source:* Wilson 2009, p. 158.

methods involved in using compensation and to become familiar with its practicality (i.e., how, when, and why it should be applied). Initially, the SLP begins by educating clients on how "learning the technique can improve their overall effectiveness and independence in performing their current everyday tasks" (Haskins et al., 2012, p. 65). Providing meaningful and personalized stories and examples can help facilitate this process.

Additionally, it may be beneficial to demonstrate usefulness of techniques by offering examples of how an individual might already apply the compensation in his/her own life. For example, in a study implementing visual association techniques, Kaschel et al. (2002) asked clients to remember a past holiday. In doing so, they were shown that they were already using images to recall events and "assured that training would build on their ability to do so" (p. 137). Similar techniques can be applied when introducing external strategies, such as memory notebooks and checklists. For example, the SLP might demonstrate how the individual already uses calendars, things-to-do lists, or logs containing addresses and phone numbers. By introducing compensation in this fashion (i.e., relating the strategy to a skill already utilized), the strategy seems less novel, potentially increasing motivation and acceptance (Haskins et al., 2012).

Once a client sees the need for the compensation, instruction on components and features should begin. The SLP can assist the individual by guiding him/her systematically through the steps involved in implementation. To do so, the clinician may choose to utilize learning strategies such as errorless learning, spaced retrieval, and/or chaining (Table 8–10). Often, the selection

**Table 8–10.** Learning Strategies

| Strategy | Definition/Goal | Example(s) | Guidelines/Tips |
|---|---|---|---|
| Errorless learning (EL) | The most common method of presenting information is to simply make a statement and ask the patient to recall the statement without delay.<br><br>The goal is to not allow a patient to make a mistake on which the patient may perseverate repeatedly. | Simple statements/ commands:<br>1. My name is Dr. Ostergren. "What is my name?"<br>2. Your wife's name is Stacey. "What is your wife's name?"<br><br>Simple command with a conditional clause<br>1. When you pick up the phone, say, "Hello this is Carley." "What should you say when you pick up the phone?"<br>2. Before you sit down, make sure that you feel for the back of the chair. "What should you do before you sit down?" | −Provide cues freely as needed<br>−Frequent repetition is helpful<br>−Train skill or present information in the actual setting or context in which it will be used<br>−Do not allow guessing or trial-and-error learning<br>−Can be used as a standalone procedure to present simple information or in conjunction with more complex techniques. |
| Spaced retrieval (SR) | Identical to errorless learning except that the patient is asked to retain the information for progressively longer periods of time (e.g., immediate, 15-second delay, and 30-second delay) | Immediate retrieval<br>1. "Today we are going to practice remembering my name. My name is _____. What is my name?"<br><br>15-second delay<br>1. "I want to help you see if you can remember my name for a longer period of time. Lets try again and see if you can remember my name after 15 seconds. My name is _____."<br>After 15-second delay, the therapist would then ask, "What is my name?"<br><br>30-second delay (repeat steps for 15-second delay)<br><br>If the client responds incorrectly at a long delay, say, as a short delay: "Actually my name is _____. What is my name?" | −Before beginning SR technique, screen client's ability to remember information using ER<br>−Duration of intervals can be modified and lengthened according to performance and/ or complexity of information to be remembered<br>−Target information can be accompanied by visual information to assist in learning and retrieval<br>−If the patient completes tasks successfully without making three errors at any of the delays, spaced retrieval is appropriate |

*continues*

**Table 8–10.** *continued*

| Strategy | Definition/Goal | Example(s) | Guidelines/Tips |
|----------|-----------------|------------|-----------------|
| Chaining | Used to train patients to perform sequences of steps. The target task (e.g., washing hands) is broken into steps. The therapist will teach steps, linking each step as a cue to initiate the next step. There are two variations to implementation (i.e., Forward and backward chaining [e.g., vanishing cues]) | Washing-hands task steps<br>Step 1: put hands under running water<br>Step 2: rub soap on hands<br>Step 3: put hands under water again to rinse<br>Step 4: dry hands<br><br>*Forward chaining:* the SLP teaches the client to perform Step 1, then Step 2 is introduced and client is guided to perform both together. When successful Step 3 is introduced, and the client must perform all three. This continues until all steps in sequence are complete.<br><br>*Backward chaining* (vanishing cues): the SLP shows all steps in the sequence. After, the SLP performs Steps 1–3 and guides the client in performing Step 4. When successful, the SLP performs Steps 1–2 and guides patient in performing Steps 3 and 4. This continues until all steps in sequence are performed. | —Chaining can be used with either verbal or visual information<br><br>—It is helpful to incorporate motor movements (when appropriate for task) |

*Source:* Haskins et al. (2012 pp. 49–53) and Wilson (2009).

of the most appropriate learning strategies is guided by severity of learning and memory impairments. For example, errorless learning strategies are often suitable for those with severe persisting memory impairment, as the methods involved rely on preserved procedural learning. That is, acquisition and application of target behaviors do not require the client's conscious control, but are instead facilitated through the clinician's active control and frequent repetition. For these reasons, errorless learning is generally the foundation for all information to be presented to patients with severe memory deficits (Haskins et al., 2012). Its use should be screened before beginning slightly more complex techniques such as spaced retrieval. Learning strategies also may be used in conjunction with one another. More often than not, selecting the most appropriate medley of learning strategies will rely on clinical trial and error.

In addition to learning strategies referenced in Table 8–9, external compensations may also be used as additional reinforcements during acquisition and application phases to minimize mistakes and help individuals learn more effectively. For example, when teaching a client to perform a task (e.g., washing hands) using forward chaining, it may be beneficial to incorporate use of an alarm system to cue the client to initiate the next step in a sequence. Alternatively, the clinician may choose to supplement training with use of a checklist to make sure all steps are completed. The individual needs to gain competence in selected compensatory strategies and demonstrate knowledge of how to use them in day-to-day activities. Ultimately, by the end of Phase 2, the client should be able to "describe the methods involved in the technique, identify tasks and situations in which its use can help them, and be able to recite the steps involved in applying the strategy" (Haskins et al., 2012, p. 65).

## Phase 3: Application

In Phase 3 (Application), the individual begins to practice compensation in simple real-life or role-play tasks *in the clinical environment* (Haskins et al., 2012; O'Neil-Pirozzi et al., 2010; Sohlberg & Mateer, 2001). The SLP should work collaboratively with the client to choose personally relevant tasks and activities that reflect client-reported difficulties in daily functioning. Example activities applicable for use in the clinical environment for both internal and external compensation are listed in Table 8–11.

The SLP should provide specific instruction, modeling, and cueing to assist the client in applying the compensation in the clinical setting. High levels of assistance and supervision may be required initially, as well as continued utilization of the teaching/learning strategies mentioned above (i.e., errorless learning, spaced retrieval, and chaining). To maximize success, the therapy staff, caregivers, and family members who regularly interact with the client should be taught to adopt the same cueing and external support methods utilized in therapy. The goal is to provide ample support, structure, and practice until the individual demonstrates the ability to apply compensation independently (Haskins et al., 2012).

Once strategy *application* has become a self-generated process, the subsequent focus of Phase 3 is to improve accuracy of implementation (e.g., accuracy of the information to be recalled using visualization techniques or of information to be retrieved from a memory notebook) with independent use of the strategy (Haskins et al., 2012). This can be facilitated by adjusting the amounts of information to be retrieved and the amount of time that information must be stored or remembered.

The SLP can monitor accuracy by recording data of the client's recall over training trials. Appendix 8–1 contains an example of a record form which can be modified based on the compensations being utilized. For example, when using internal strategies, the SLP might record accuracy of information to be recalled over time (i.e., how long the client can remember target information), increasing task difficulty by extending recall periods (immediate, after 24-hour period, after 48-hour period, etc). Alternatively, when using an external strategy, such as an electronic planner, the SLP might choose to track the amount and/or complexity of information to be retrieved, adjusting task difficulty by requiring more or less information to be stored or retrieved. The SLP should also monitor the level of

**Table 8–11.** Sample Activities for the Application Stage (Within the Clinical Setting)

| Technique | Example Activity |
|---|---|
| **Internal Strategies**[1] | |
| Face/name association | Remembering names of therapists or other patients/clients |
| Visual imagery | Recalling locations, such as how to get to the therapy room; remembering story details |
| Verbal mnemonics | Remembering items on a mock grocery list, to-do list; steps involved in functional activities |
| Organizational strategy | Remembering one's medication schedule by category/ purpose or administration time; organization important details from a short newspaper or magazine article; remembering items from a mock grocery shopping list. |
| PQRST | Remembering information from a newspaper article or brief news program. |
| **External Strategies** | |
| Memory Notebook | Remembering what therapies to attend at what times of day |
| Electronic Devices | Training use of alarms, phones, or times to cue patients to implement internal or external strategies. |

*Source:* [1]Haskins et al. (2012, p. 66).

cueing involved, as this is an additional means to adjust task complexity (e.g., gradually fading cues or level of supports to increase task difficulty).

At the end of each session, the SLP records recall accuracy, the level of cueing required to recall target information, as well as any additional information related to client performance (e.g., disregard versus self-correction of errors) (Haskins et al., 2012). It is also recommended that the clinician allow sufficient time to discuss performance with the client and solicit his/her subjective opinion of success or lack thereof (Haskins et al., 2012). Engaging in self-reflection allows the SLP to provide constructive feedback and encourages the individual to start generating self-instructional questions to address difficulties encountered (e.g., "how am I going to remember this?").

## Phase 4: Adaptation

In Phase 4 (Adaptation), the individual practices strategy application *in naturalistic settings outside of the clinic* (Haskins, et al., 2012; O'Neil-Pirozzi, et al., 2010; Sohlberg & Mateer, 2001; Wilson, 2009). The main focus is to promote generalization through direct transfer of skills learned in the therapy setting to different situations or problems that the client will face in everyday life. During this transfer period, the SLP's role is largely supportive and involves assisting the client in determining which strategies are most useful and in which situations or tasks outside the clinic they can be successfully applied (Haskins et al., 2012). For example, if the individual is highly sociable but frequently forgets the names of acquaintances at social gatherings, the SLP might choose to improve face/name recognition by supporting use of visual imagery techniques during interpersonal exchanges. Any task

or skill that was practiced through in-clinic role-playing can be adapted to and performed in the community (Haskins et al., 2012). Examples of activities for the adaptation stage outside of the clinical setting are listed in Table 8–12.

Generalization of strategy use to community activities most likely will not occur spontaneously or automatically without further assistance or monitoring (e.g., cue-

**Table 8–12.** Sample Activities for the Adaptation Stage

| Technique | Example Activity |
| --- | --- |
| **Internal Strategies[1]** | |
| Face/name association | Remembering names of classmates, co-workers, people at a party or other group gathering |
| Visual imagery | Studying for a test; remembering pending appointments and events; remembering locations; recalling details about new people encountered |
| Verbal mnemonics | To remember items from a grocery list when they go shopping. Also to remember the steps involved in a recipe; lists when studying for tests; to-do lists |
| Visual-verbal associations | Meeting people at a gathering: Clinician presents actual photos graphs of non-familiar faces/people and provides five pieces of demographic information (e.g., first/last name, profession, and city/state). Patient then generates ideas of how to learn, but using the strategies presented. The level of difficulty can be increased by the number of informational elements to be recalled, and the rate in which the information is presented. To determine which strategies are the most successful for a patient, it can be useful to ask the patient to indicate what strategy they are using when performing a given task and compare their performance according to different strategy utilization. |
| Organizational strategies | To help encode essential details from lectures and textbooks; remembering items from a grocery list by category (dairy, meat, frozen). |
| **External Strategies** | |
| Memory Notebook | Training to remember to perform future actions (prospective memory); training in process of periodically removing old and unnecessary pages from memory notebooks. |
| Electronic Devices | Training use of alarms, phones, or times to cue patients to implement internal or external strategies. |

*Source:* [1]Haskins et al. (2012 p. 67).

ing and feedback) (Haskins et al., 2012; Sohlberg & Mateer, 2001; Wilson, 2009). For this reason, it may be beneficial for the SLP to initially accompany the individual and observe the application of compensation outside the clinical setting. This allows the clinician to reinforce implementation, monitor success, provide feedback, and make necessary modifications. Accompanying the individual in daily activities may not always be possible. As such, the clinician can encourage skill development and regularly review and evaluate performance through assigning homework (Brain Injury–Interdisciplinary Special Interest Group [BI-ISIG], 2002). As the individual demonstrates mastery of compensation use, the clinician can gradually fade in involvement in community outings and/or recruit family members and caregivers to support strategy use. Haskins and colleagues also recommend the following to promote transfer of skills outside the therapy environment (Haskins et al., 2012, p. 66):

1. Focus on teaching strategies that the patient used naturally to help maximize the likelihood of generalization to other tasks and settings.

2. Help the patient identify how and when the use of the various techniques will be helpful for them.

3. When teaching patients to use mnemonics in their daily lives, encourage them to generate their own. Information is more likely to be remembered when it is salient and personally meaningful.

4. Incorporate the family into treatment at this stage whenever possible, as they can play an important role in encouraging the patient to use the strategy in the home and community. Thus, even in situations where the patient does not spontaneously initiate using the techniques, family members can remind them to apply and practice it in specific circumstances.

## References

American Speech-Language-Hearing Association. (2003). *Evaluating and treating communication and cognitive disorders: approaches to referral and collaboration for speech-language pathology and clinical neuropsychology* [Technical report]. Available from http://www.asha.org/policy

Bayley, M., Tate, R., Douglas, J., Turkstra, L., Ponsford, J., Stergiou-Kita, M., . . . INGOG Expert Panel. (2014). INCOG guidelines for cognitive rehabilitation following traumatic brain injury: Methods and overview. *Journal of Head Trauma Rehabilitation, 29*(4), 290–306.

Bergquist, T. F., & Jacket, M. P. (1993). Programme methodology: Awareness and goal setting with the traumatically brain injured. *Brain Injury, 7*, 275–282.

Cicerone, K., Dahlberg, C., Kalmar, K., Langenbahn, D., Malec, J., Bergquist, T. F., . . . Morse, P. A. (2000). Evidence-based cognitive rehabilitation: Recommendations for clinical practice. *Archives of Physical Medicine and Rehabilitation, 81*(12), 1596–1615.

Cicerone, K., Dahlberg, C., Malec, J., Langenbahn, D., Felicetti, T., Kneipp, S., . . . Catanese, J. (2005). Evidence-based cognitive rehabilitation: Updated review of the literature from 1998 through 2002. *Archives of Physical Medicine and Rehabilitation, 86*(8), 1681–1692.

Cicerone, K. D., Langenbahn, D. M., Braden, C., Malec, J. F., Kalmar, K., Fraas, M., . . . Ashman, T. (2011). Evidence-based cognitive rehabilitation: Updated review of the literature from 2003 through 2008. *Archives of Physical Medicine and Rehabilitation, 92*(4), 519–530.

Ezrachi, O., Ben-Yishay, Y., Kay, T., DiUer, L., & Rattok, J. (1991). Predicting employment in traumatic brain injury following neuropsychological rehabilitation. *Journal of Head Trauma Rehabilitation, 6*, 71–84.

Flashman, L. A., Amador, X., & McAllister, T. W. (1998). Lack of awareness of deficits in traumatic brain injury. *Seminars in Clinical Neuropsychiatry, 3*, 201–210.

Flashman, L., & McAllister, T. (2002). Lack of awareness and its impact in traumatic brain injury. *NeuroRehabilitation, 17*(4), 285–296.

Fleming, J. M., Shum, D., Strong, J., & Lightbody, S. (2005). Prospective memory rehabilitation for adults with traumatic brain injury: A compensatory training programme. *Brain Injury, 19*(1), 1–10.

Freeman, M. R., Mittenberg, W., Dicowden, M., & Bat-Ami, M. (1992). Executive and compensatory memory retraining in traumatic brain injury. *Brain Injury, 6*(1), 65–70.

Haskins, E. C., Shapiro-Rosenbaum, A., Dams-O'Connor, K., Eberle, R., Cicerone, K., & Langenbahn, D. (2012). Rehabilitation for impairments of memory. In L. E. Trexler (Ed.), *Cognitive rehabilitation manual: Translating evidence-based recommendations into practice* (pp. 43–72). Reston, VA: American Congress of Rehabilitation Medicine.

Kaschel, R., Della Sala, S., Cantagallo, A., Fahlböck, A., Laaksonen, R., & Kazen, M. (2002). Imagery mnemonics for the rehabilitation of memory: A randomised group controlled trial. *Neuropsychological Rehabilitation, 12*(2), 127–153.

Kennedy, M. (2006). Managing memory and metamemory impairments in individuals with traumatic brain injury. *ASHA Leader, 11*(14), 8–9, 34–36.

O'Neil-Pirozzi, T. M., Kennedy, M. R., & Sohlberg, M. M. (2016). Evidence-based practice for the use of internal strategies as a memory compensation technique after brain injury: A systematic review. *Journal of Head Trauma Rehabilitation, 31*(4), E1–E11.

O'Neil-Pirozzi, T. M., Strangman, G. E., Goldstein, R., Katz, D. I., Savage, C. R., Kelkar, K., . . . Glenn, M. B. (2010). A controlled treatment study of internal memory strategies (I-MEMS) following traumatic brain injury.

*Journal of Head Trauma Rehabilitation, 25*(1), 43–51.

Prigatano, G. P., Altman, I. M., & O'Brien, K. P. (1990). Behavioral limitations that brain injured patients tend to underestimate. *Clinical Neuropsychologist 4,* 163–176.

Sander, A. M., & van Veldhoven, L. M. (2014). Rehabilitation of memory problems associated with traumatic brain injury. In M. Sherer & A. Sander (Eds.), *Handbook on the neuropsychology of traumatic brain injury* (pp. 173–190). New York, NY: Springer.

Schmitter-Edgecombe, M., Fahy, J. F., Whelan, J. P., & Long, C. J. (1995). Memory remediation after severe closed head injury: Notebook training versus supportive therapy. *Journal of Consulting and Clinical Psychology, 63*(3), 484–489.

Sohlberg, M. M., & Mateer, C. A. (1989). Training use of compensatory memory books: A three-stage behavioral approach. *Journal of Clinical and Experimental Neuropsychology, 11*(6), 871–891.

Sohlberg, M. M., & Mateer, C. A. (2001). *Cognitive rehabilitation: An integrative neuropsychological approach.* New York, NY: Guilford Press.

Sohlberg, M. M., Kennedy, M., Avery, J., Coelho, C., Turkstra, L., Ylvisaker, M., & Yorkston, K. (2007). Evidence-based practice for the use of external aids as a memory compensation technique. *Journal of Medical Speech-Language Pathology, 15*(1), xv–li.

Velikonja, D., Tate, R., Ponsford, J., McIntyre, A., Janzen, S., Bayley, M., & INCOG Expert Panel (2014). INCOG recommendations for management of cognition following traumatic brain injury, Part v: Memory. *Journal of Head Trauma Rehabilitation, 29*(4), 369–386.

Wilson, B. A. (2009). *Memory rehabilitation: Integrating theory and practice.* New York, NY: Guilford Press.

## APPENDIX 8–1

## Real-World Task Assessment: Memory

Client: _____

| Task | Date | Type of Memory[1] | Difficulty[2] | Delay | Task Accuracy[3] | Errors/ Opportunities | Type of Error(s) (Describe) | Error Awareness[4] | Additional Notes |
|---|---|---|---|---|---|---|---|---|---|
| Remembering to take medication at 10:00 am (Monday) | 3/12/17 | PR | 1 | 2-hours (reminder given at 8:00 am) | A | 0/1 (0% error) | N/A | N/A | |
| | | | | | | | | | |
| | | | | | | | | | |
| | | | | | | | | | |
| | | | | | | | | | |
| | | | | | | | | | |
| | | | | | | | | | |
| | | | | | | | | | |
| | | | | | | | | | |
| | | | | | | | | | |

*Notes.* [1]Type of Memory: RG = Retrograde, AG = Anterograde, PR = Prospective/RR = Retrospective, EP = Episodic, SM = Semantic, PC = Procedural; [2]Level of Difficulty: 1 = Very difficult, 2 = Difficult, 3 = Easy, 4 = Very Easy; [3]Accuracy: A = Accurate/Complete, I = Inaccurate/Incomplete. [4]Error Awareness: F = Fully Aware, P = Partially Aware, U = Unaware

# Self-Observation:  Memory

Client: _____

| Date/ Time | What did I do that required memory? | What type of memory was needed? | How difficult was the task *overall*? | How was my memory like during this task? | Is there anything I would do differently next time? |
|---|---|---|---|---|---|
| | | | | | |
| | | | | | |
| | | | | | |
| | | | | | |

Type of Memory:  Type of Memory: RG = Retrograde, AG = Anterograde, PR = Prospective/RR = Retrospective, EP = Episodic, SM = Semantic, PC = Procedural
Level of Difficulty:  1 = Very easy, 2 = Easy, 3 = Difficult, 4 = Very Difficult

APPENDIX 8–3

## Self-Reflection: Memory

Client: _____

| | KNOWLEDGE | | ATTRIBUTE | EMOTION | IMPACT | | |
|---|---|---|---|---|---|---|---|
| | *What are my strengths?* | *What are my challenges?* | *What is causing difficulty in this area?* | *How do I feel about this?* | *How does this impact me in my daily life?* | *What things help?* | *What things make it more challenging?* |
| *Memory of things before my TBI (Retrograde Memory)* | | | | | | | |
| *Memory for things after my TBI (Anterograde Memory)* | | | | | | | |
| *Memory for things that have already happened (Retrospective Memory)* | | | | | | | |
| *Memory for things to come (Prospective Memory)* | | | | | | | |

| | KNOWLEDGE | | ATTRIBUTE | EMOTION | IMPACT | | |
|---|---|---|---|---|---|---|---|
| | What are my strengths? | What are my challenges? | What is causing difficulty in this area? | How do I feel about this? | How does this impact me in my daily life? | What things help? | What things make it more challenging? |
| Memory for information and facts (Semantic Memory) | | | | | | | |
| Memory for experiences and events (Episodic Memory) | | | | | | | |
| Memory for procedures (Procedural Memory) | | | | | | | |

# 9 Executive Function and Awareness

> a. Introduction
> b. Goal Management Training (GMT)
> c. Strategic Memory Advanced Reasoning Training (SMART)
> d. Constructive Feedback Awareness Training (CFAT)

## a. Introduction

International Cognitive (INCOG) treatment recommendations in the area of executive function and awareness (Tate et al., 2014, p. 343) include:

1. Metacognitive strategy instruction should be used with adults with TBI for difficulty with problem solving, planning, and organization. These strategies should be focused on everyday problems and functional outcomes. Metacognitive strategy instruction is optimized when the patient has awareness of the need to use a strategy and can identify contexts in which the strategy should be used. Common elements of all metacognitive strategies are self-monitoring and incorporation of feedback into future performance.
2. Strategies to improve the capacity to analyze and synthesize information should be used with adults with TBI who have impaired reasoning skills.

3. Direct corrective feedback should be used with adults with TBI who have impaired self-awareness. The feedback should be delivered within the context of a therapeutic, multicontext program to treat awareness deficits.
4. Group-based interventions may be considered for remediation of executive and problem-solving deficits after TBI.

Similarly, the American Congress of Rehabilitation Medicine (ACRM), given multiple meta-analyses in this area (Cicerone et al., 2000, Cicerone et al., 2005; Cicerone et al., 2011, p. 521) recommends:

1. Metacognitive strategy training (self-monitoring and self-regulation) is recommended for deficits in executive functioning after TBI, including impairments of emotional self-regulation, and as a component of interventions for deficits in attention, neglect, and memory (Practice Standard).
2. Training in formal problem-solving strategies and their application to everyday

situations and functional activities is recommended during post-acute rehabilitation after TBI (Practice Guideline).

3. Group-based interventions may be considered for remediation of executive and problem-solving deficits after TBI (Practice Option).

Executive function and awareness treatment approaches are addressed within this chapter using the hierarchical diagram in Figure 9–1, to include sections on:

1. **Metacognitive Treatment.** Goal Management Training (GMT) is discussed in this chapter. Time Pressure Management (TPM) is discussed in Chapter 7b. For details on Multifaceted Treatment of Executive Dysfunction (MTED), the reader is referred to Spikman, Boelen, Lamberts, Brouwer, and Fasotti (2010).

2. **The Strategic Memory Advanced Reasoning Training (SMART)**

3. **Constructive Feedback Awareness Training (CFAT)**

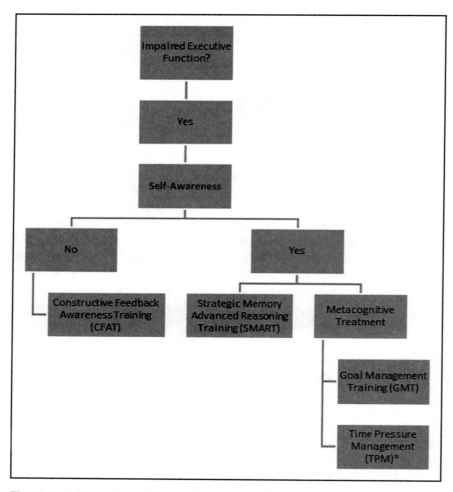

**Figure 9–1.** Executive function and awareness treatment in action hierarchy. Suggested treatment approaches in the area of executive function and awareness. *TPM is discussed in Chapter 7.

Lastly, Sohlberg and Mateer (2001) offer a helpful list of suggestion in the area of environmental modifications and cues in the area of executive function. These are listed in Table 9–1.

## Assessment

Table 9–2 contains examples of several common assessment measures in the area of executive function and related measures (Chan, Sumn, Toulopoulou, & Chen, 2008). This is not an exhaustive list of all possible measures. Rather, it is a sample of some more frequently utilized tests in this area. Given the nature of executive function, some of these tests evaluate a narrowly prescribed aspect of executive function (verbal/non-verbal switching, response inhibition, plan-

ning, executive memory, rule detection, and so forth), while others cross multiple aspects of executive function. Tests of this nature are helpful measures in identifying particular strengths and weaknesses and, in the case of standardized assessment, making comparisons to a normative data set. The rehabilitative process also benefits from ongoing structured evaluation of performance in real-world tasks (Sohlberg & Mateer, 2001). Assessment of individuals' performance in real-world tasks should be individualized to their specific home, recreational, vocational, and educational contexts, performed before, during, and after intervention, regardless of the approach utilized. Appendix 9–1 contains an example of a data recording sheet that can be modified for this purpose.

Engaging the client in an ongoing self-assessment can be a valuable exercise in the

---

**Table 9–1.** Suggested Environmental Modifications and Prompts to Support Executive Function

| Environmental Modifications | Environmental Prompts and Cue |
|---|---|
| • Labeling cupboard contents<br>• Using large bulletin boards with separate labeled sections for different types of information<br>• Designating kitchen shelves (or refrigerator shelves) for special types of foods<br>• Establishing a designated place for clutter—only items that are not critical can go in this bin<br>• Setting up bill-paying systems<br>• Using large family planning calendars<br>• Putting a family message center on the refrigerator<br>• Setting up file cabinets with labeled folders for home management tasks | • Reminders of what to take to school or work each day, posted by the front door (e.g., keys, wallet, lunch, bus card)<br>• Grooming routine, posted on the bathroom mirror<br>• Menus for specific meals, posted on the refrigerator<br>• Before-going-to-bed (or morning-rising) routine, posted on the bedroom closet door (e.g., turn off lights, turn down heater, set alarm medication)<br>• Reminders of operating procedures for laundry machine, dishwasher, computer, and the like, posted next to those appliances<br>• Conservation prompts such as photo albums, placed at suitable locations<br>• Schedules to help with time management, placed wherever necessary. |

*Source:* Solhberg & Mateer (2001, p. 244).

**Table 9–2.** Common Executive Function and Awareness Measures: Direct Measures and Questionnaire/Rating Scales

DIRECT MEASURES

- Behavioral Assessment of the Dysexecutive Syndrome
- Delis–Kaplan Executive Function System
- Five-Point Test
- F-A-S Verbal Fluency Test
- Hotel Test
- Six Element Test
- Stoop
- Tinkertoy Test
- Tower of London
- Tower of Hanoi
- Trail Making Test
- Wisconsin Card Sorting Test

QUESTIONNAIRES/RATING SCALES

- Behavior Rating Inventory of Executive Functions
- Cognitive Failures Questionnaire
- Dysexecutive Questionnaire

pose. As with all aspects of self-reflection, this would begin with and include ongoing conversations with the client about domains of executive function (initiation, inhibition, persistence, organization, generative thinking, awareness) and what they mean specifically to the client's daily tasks and his/her unique needs/skills.

Overall self-assessment after self-observation is also valuable. Appendix 9–3 shows a sample worksheet for overall reflection and discussion between the SLP and the client in the area of executive function. This should be tailored to meet each individual's needs and abilities and should be pursued after an effective and trusting therapeutic relationship has been established between the client and the SLP (Flashman & McAllister, 2002). It can be completed with one or all domains of executive function. Individuals with ongoing strong negative emotions in this area should be referred to a psychologist or neuropsychologist team member for additional support (American Speech-Language-Hearing Association, 2003).

rehabilitation process. Several authors have noted awareness after a brain injury to be an important factor across a variety of rehabilitation approaches (Bergquist & Jacket, 1993; Ezrachi et al., 1991; Prigatano, Altman, & O'Brien, 1990). A helpful first step in this process is that of self-observation. This can be done by asking the client to keep a structured journal or log about executive function performance during daily tasks. The SLP can collaborate with the client to identify good times for this observation (during specific periods of the day, while performing specific tasks, etc.). Appendix 9–2 shows a sample data collection sheet that can be modified for this pur-

## b. Goal Management Training (GMT)

Goal Management Training (GMT) was initially developed in the 1990s by Robertson (1996). It is now commercially marketed by Levine and Manly. SLPs interested in purchasing GMT can do so at: http://goalmanagementtraining.weebly.com/

## Candidacy Recommendations

Based on a composite of research in this area (Fish et al., 2007; Grant, Ponsford, & Bennett, 2012; Levine et al., 2000; Levine et al., 2011; Waid-Ebbs et al., 2014), GMT is recommended in the post-acute stages after TBI for:

1. **Individuals who evidence executive functioning deficits, such as impaired planning, decision making, and self-regulation.** Examples of recommended measures in this area are listed in Table 9–3. Given the difficulties in assessing executive function with traditional measures, evaluation of deficits is also recommended given real-life activities (or reports thereof) (Levine et al., 2011). In terms of measuring performance outcomes of GMT, Levine and colleagues suggest that everyday paper-and-pencil tasks that require "holding goals in mind, subgoal analysis, and monitoring" can be utilized (Levine et al., 2000, pp. 301–302). Examples of these are listed in Table 9–4. Time spent reading the instructions and completing the task, as well as number of errors in performing the task, can be assessed for both the proofreading and grouping tasks (Levine et al., 2000). On the room

**Table 9–3.** GMT-Related Executive Function Measures

Behavior Rating Inventory of Executive Functions - Adult Version[2]

Cognitive Failures Questionnaire

Dysexecutive Questionnaire[1]

Hotel Test[1]

Six Element Test[3]

Tower of London[2]

Tower Test from the Delis–Kaplan Executive Function System (D–KEFS)[1]

*Note.* [1]Recommended by Levine, Schweizer, O'Connor, Turner, et al. (2011); [2]Recommended by Waid-Ebbs, Daly, et al. (2014); [3]Recommended by Bertens, Fasotti, Boelen, & Kessels (2013).

**Table 9–4.** Sample Everyday Tasks for Assessing GMT

**Proofreading**[1]**:** Proofreading a short paragraph, using simple rules, such as underlining, circling, and crossing out certain words.

**Grouping**[1]**:** Given a list with two columns, group items based on specific rules. For example, given a two-column list of the ages and gender of specific individuals, provide instructions to place a "2" by females over age 30, a check mark by males, circle individuals age 65 and up, and so forth.

**Room layout:** Answer questions of varying complexity, given a 5 × 5 grid of information. For example, the grid could be a seating scheme of employees from one of five companies (company A, company B, etc.). Questions could be, "What company has an employee seated first in row 2"? "What company is next to the third company B employee in the second row?" "How many company D employees are in column 5?" and so forth.

*Note.* [1]For proofreading and grouping, rules are presented briefly (maximum 60 seconds) and then removed before tasks completion. Verbal instructions are given to work as quickly and as accurately as possible.

*Source:* Levine, Robertson, Clare, et al. (2000, pp. 301–302).

layout task, time needed to answer questions and the number of correctly answered questions can be assessed (Levine et al., 2000).

2. **Individuals who have sufficient cognitive, sensory, and motor function to engage in therapy and assessment tasks.**

## Treatment Evidence

Multiple meta-analyses and systematic reviews have recommended the use of metacognitive strategy for executive function deficits (Cicerone et al., 2005; Kennedy et al., 2008; Tate et al., 2014). Specific to GMT, there is Level A evidence to support its use for individuals with TBI (Figure 9–2, Tate et al., 2014).

## Theoretical Frame

As per Levine and colleagues, GMT comprises "metacognitive intervention that combines education, narrative, task performance and feedback, and incorporation

of participants' own personal task failures and successes" (Levine et al., 2011, p. 6). As such, as a metacognitive approach, GMT is classified as a calibration approach within this text (Figure 9–3). It should be noted, however, that aspects of GMT, such as behavioral practice and training in a specific set of steps for task performance, could also be considered compensation, based on the

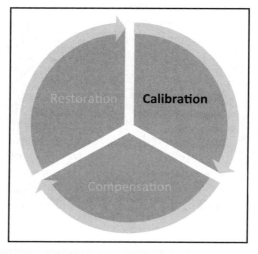

**Figure 9–3.** Theoretical framework of GMT. The predominant treatment approach present in GMT.

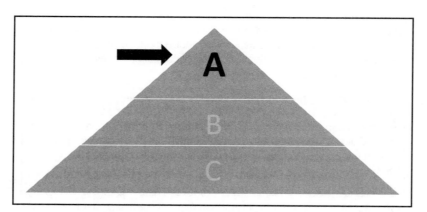

**Figure 9–2.** Level A evidence for the use of GMT in addressing executive function deficits post TBI. Level A consists of "recommendation supported by at least one meta-analysis, systematic review or randomized controlled trial study of appropriate size and relevant control group" (Bayley et al., 2014, p. 295).

nature of treatment and execution of cognitive rehabilitation therapy (CRT).

## Background

GMT is based on theories of sustained attention as integral to supporting executive function (Stuss & Levine, 2002; Stuss & Alexander, 2007), such that lapses in sustained attention result in "slips of intention" that impair executive function and task performance. Levine and colleagues postulate that sustained attention comprises habits that "may oppose and displace higher order goals, resulting in . . . distracted behavior that is a hallmark of patients with attentional and executive deficits" (Levine et al., 2011, p. 2). For example, an individual who needs to drive a different route to work one day to deliver a package, must deviate from the regular (habituated) route he normally takes by actively maintaining this new goal (a new route) in working memory. This prevents this new goal from being displaced by the habitual route. To achieve the new goal, several steps need to be coordinated (Waid-Ebbs et al., 2014, p. 1556):

1. The difference between the current state and the desired state must be detected.
2. There must be formulation of the steps needed to reach that desired state.
3. The desired state must be kept in mind while resisting distractions.
4. The barriers that occur along the way must be overcome until finally the goal is achieved.

Duncan and colleagues refer to the inability to actively maintain this new goal as goal neglect (Duncan, Emslie, Williams, Johnson, & Freer, 1996). GMT seeks to prevent goal neglect, thereby enabling accurate task execution.

## Treatment in Action

GMT teaches individuals to monitor performance, identify slips in intention that could lead to goal neglect, and implement strategies to reduce them. It incorporates metacognitive awareness and implementation of the five GMT strategies in task execution: Stop, Define, List, Learn, and Check (Figure 9–4). Within the Stop stage, the client is taught to ask him/herself, "What am I doing?," which serves as grounding and a reminder for the task at hand. This allows for orienting of mental efforts to the "current state of affairs" and any relevant goals of the task to be completed (Levine et al., 2000, p. 300). In the Define stage, clients are instructed to think about and outline the main goal of the task to be completed. In the List stage, the client learns to identify and outline the steps needed to complete the desired goal. This is followed by the Learn stage, where the client seeks to retain goals and subgoals outlined in the previous stages. This is also the stage where clients use self-reflection to ensure that they understand steps and actions needed to achieve their goal. If in the Learn stage the goal (or its specific steps) are unclear, the client is asked to return to the initial stages of Define and List, in order to recalibrate the task at hand (Define) and re-establish the needed steps (List), before proceeding again to the Learn stage for self-assessment. If in the Learn stage the task and steps are clear to the client, the client is instructed to proceed to task implementation, continually engaging in the Check stage at each step of the task, asking, "Am I doing it as planned?" The bookends of Stop and Check (and each of the steps between) create a continual process of mental calibration to ensure successful goal attainment.

GMT sessions are designed to guide the client through educational, narrative, and

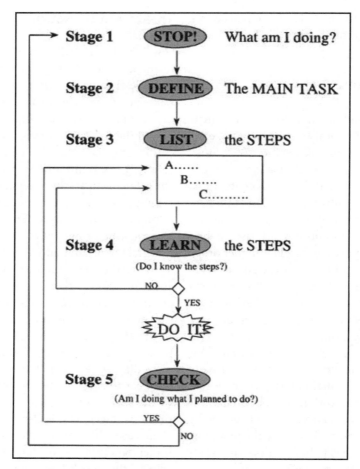

**Figure 9–4.** The five stages of GMT. *Source:* Levine et al. (2000, p. 300). Copyright © Cambridge University Press. Used with permission.

experiential learning tasks, for the express purpose of bringing metacognitive awareness to the process of executive function, the impacts of lapses in attention on executive function, and the importance and use of the above cycle in mindful decision making in execution of daily tasks.

Levine et al. (2011) recommend the session progress as highlighted in Table 9–5. This progression can also be modified to address the unique educational needs of specific individuals with TBI. For example, Waid-Ebbs and colleagues (2014) included

additional sessions designed to provide education to military personnel on blast injury, concussion, and posttraumatic stress disorder (PTSD) as it relates to executive function and GMT. Within each session, the clinician can provide examples and narration to explain concepts important to GMT, drawing as much as possible from the client's own real-life experiences (Waid-Ebbs, 2014). Experiential learning tasks and hypothetical scenarios can also be used to illustrate concepts important to GMT. For example, Grant, Ponsford, and Bennett (2012) had clients practice applying the five stages of the GMT model to hypothetical everyday activities, such as "making a drink, preparing a sandwich, doing the laundry, returning books to a library," as a way to identify specific strengths and weaknesses in task execution using the GMT cycle (p. 862).

Sohlberg and Turkstra (2011) also provide a helpful framework in training metacognitive strategies use, within the three phases highlighted in Figure 9–5: Acquisition, Mastery/Generalization, and Maintenance. This can be applied to GMT and the other strategies discussed in this chapter.

### Phase 1: Acquisition

In the acquisition phase of this framework, the purpose of training is to "establish the client's conceptual knowledge about how

**Table 9–5.** GMT Session Progress and Objectives

| Session | General Purpose/Objective |
|---|---|
| Session 1 | The clinician defines absentmindedness, giving examples of absentminded errors in daily life. |
| Session 2 | The clinician frames absentminded errors as the by product of habit (e.g., "automatic pilot"), which can be altered by redirecting attention to the task at hand. In this stage the concept of Stop (Stage 1) is introduced. |
| Session 3 | The clinician explains the concept of working memory as a "mental blackboard," where the goals and steps to be accomplished are stored, but easily disrupted without the active process of stopping and checking goals. |
| Session 4 | The clinician describes methods that can be used to redirect thoughts to the goal |
| Session 5 | The clinician describes the process of completing goals using the act of to-do lists for step completion |
| Session 6 | The clinician provides opportunities for the client to practice parsing goals into subgoals and steps. |
| Session 7 | The clinician provides opportunities for stopping/checking for the purposes of interrupting ongoing behavior to monitor performance. |

*Source:* Levine, Schweizer, O'Connor, Turner, et al. (2011, p. 3).

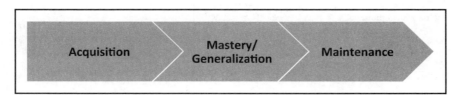

**Figure 9–5.** Suggested strategy training phases applicable to GMT.

and when to use the target strategy" (Sohlberg & Turkstra, 2001, p. 205). Success in this phase results in the client demonstrating: (1) understanding of the basic components of the strategy, and (2) performance of the strategy successfully in a structured and favorable context (e.g., in the therapy setting, without distractions, during basic tasks). In this phase, the strategy is first practiced with clinician support and modeling. As the client gains success with this support, gradually cues are faded. A variety of cues and supports can be used to aid in learning during this phase, such as checklist of the steps (Figure 9–6), visual reminders of the strategy (Figure 9–7), and environmental supports like alarms to initiate the strategy. Errorless learning principles can

---

**Stop:** What am I doing?
_____

**Define:** What is my main purpose/goal?
_____

**List:** What are the steps to my goal?

1. _____
2. _____
3. _____
4. _____

**Learn:** Do I know my goal and steps?
_____

**Check:** Am I doing what I planned to do?
_____

---

**Figure 9–6.** A checklist of GMT steps that can be used in the acquisition phase of training to teach this strategy.

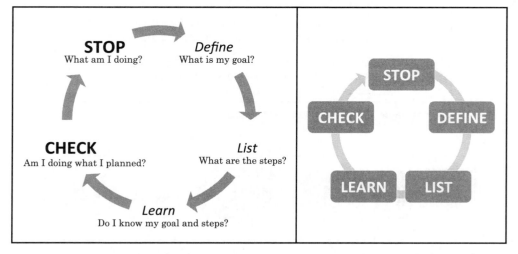

**Figure 9–7.** Examples of visual reminders that can be used in the acquisition phase of strategy training.

also be utilized in this phase of training. In doing so, the clinician prevents error or guessing in strategy development by the provision of prompts and cues after each stage in the strategy. Bertens and colleagues reported that the use of errorless learning within GMT for individuals with TBI and stroke contributed to more effective training of daily activities than conventional GMT (Bertens et al., 2013; Bertens, Kessels, Boelen, & Fasotti, 2016; Bertens, Kessels, Fiorenzato, Boelen, & Fasotti, 2015).

To assess comprehension of the strategy within this phase, the SLP can ask a variety of questions about the strategy at the beginning and end of therapy sessions (What are the steps in the cycle? When would you use it?, etc.). To assess performance of the strategy, the clinician can measure aspects of strategy execution, such as number of strategy steps demonstrated with and without prompting.

## Phase 2: Mastery/ Generalization Phase

In the mastery/generalization phase, strategy use is extended to more complex and less structured circumstances (within and outside the therapy setting) (Sohlberg & Turkstra, 2011). In this phase, the goal of training is to make the strategy as automatic as possible and to ensure its use in real-world tasks in the client's everyday context. Sohlberg and Turkstra (2011) recommend that the principles listed in Table 9–6 be utilized in this phase. Waid-Ebbs et al. (2014) recommend that homework be provided at the end of each session, in order to reinforce the concept during activities in the client's home environment. These authors also suggest that significant others in the client's home environment be asked to observe homework and report back on any particular challenges or difficulty.

## Phase 3: Maintenance Phase

Lastly, in the maintenance phase the clinician seeks to "increase the likelihood that a rehabilitation target will be retained after therapy ends" (Sohlberg & Turkstra, 2011, p. 209). To accomplish this task, the clinician should facilitate high frequency practice of the technique and identify people in the client's environments who can serve as

**Table 9–6.** Important Mastery/Generalization Phase Principles

| | |
|---|---|
| Fading Learning Supports | The clinician systematically fades the prompts and cues used in the acquisition phase, such as removing the visual reminders and checklists or transitioning from the client stating the steps aloud to verbalizing them internally |
| Incorporating or Increasing Stimulus Variability | The clinician creates opportunities for practice of the strategy in different contexts and given different circumstances, such as in response to different circumstances, while interacting with different people, and in different environments, including the client's everyday context |
| Increasing Engagement | The clinician maintains the client's motivation for the use of the strategy by customizing its use to meet the client's needs, discussing with the client potential barriers in implementation, and highlighting client successes for strategy use. |

*Source:* Sohlberg & Tukrstra (2011, pp. 208–209).

ongoing supports to encourage continued strategy use. It is also important that the clinician plan for reevaluation and periodic clinician support, via follow-up visits and phone support over time.

## c. Strategic Memory Advanced Reasoning Training (SMART)

## Candidacy Recommendations

Based on a composite of research in this area (Cook, Chapman, Elliott, Evenson, & Vinton, 2014; Vas, Chapman, Cook, Elliott, & Keebler, 2011; Vas et al., 2016), the use of gist reasoning techniques, and specifically Strategic Memory Advanced Reasoning Training (SMART), is recommended in the post-acute stages after TBI for:

1. **Individuals who have moderate-to-significant difficulties accomplishing complex tasks involving flexible and innovative thinking and problem solving** (Vas et al., 2016, p. 504).

2. **Individuals with sufficient information processing capacity to complete SMART tasks.** Traditional versions of SMART require reading of lengthy information. As such, Vas et al. (2016) recommend that individuals have reading comprehension, vision, and hearing capacities sufficient to participate in SMART tasks (modified as needed). In addition, these researchers note that processing speed could confound gist reasoning performance. As such, they recommend that individuals who participate in SMART not have significantly impaired processing speed. Recommended assessment of

processing speed includes the Delis–Kaplan Executive Function System (Color–Word Interference Tasks 1 and 2), the Trail Making Test (Part A), or the Hayling Sentence Completion Test (Vas et al., 2016, p. 154). Chapter 7b (Time Pressure Management) contains additional measures in the area of processing speed.

SMART outcomes have been assessed using measures of gist reasoning, questionnaires and ratings of daily function, and related measures of executive function deficits (e.g., working memory, inhibition, cognitive flexibility). Several examples of measures in this area are listed in Table 9–7.

**Table 9–7.** SMART-Related Outcome Measures

*Gist Reasoning*

- Test of Strategic Learning

*Daily Functioning (Measures and Questionnaires)*

- Functional Status Examination
- Community Integration Questionnaire
- Awareness Questionnaire (Sherer, 2004) (Appendix 9–4, 9–5, and 9–6)

*Executive Function Related Measures*

- Delis–Kaplan Executive Function System (The Color–Word Interference and Category Switching)
- Listening Span Task (Controlled Oral Word Association Test, Daneman & Carpenter, 1980)
- Wechsler Adult Intelligence Scale III (Letter Number-Sequence Task, Digits Forward, Digits Backwards, Matrix Reasoning)
- Trail Making Test (Part B)

*Source:* Vas, Chapman, Cook, Elliott, & Keebler (2011) and Vas et al. (2016).

## Treatment Evidence

There is Level A evidence to support the use of "strategies to improve the capacity to analyze and synthesize information" with individuals with TBI who have impaired reasoning (Figure 9–8; Tate et al., 2014, p. 343). At the time of these recommendations, INCOG reviewers noted that work by Vas and colleagues specific to SMART (Vas et al., 2011) had the strongest evidence in this area (p. 344). Since then, additional studies of SMART with individuals with TBI (Cook et al., 2014; Vas et al., 2016) have also demonstrated similar positive results.

## Theoretical Frame

As per Vas and colleagues, the stated goals of SMART are to "teach metacognitive strategies to improve cognitive control functions of strategic attention, integrative reasoning, and innovation" (Vas, 2016, p. 509). As such, as a metacognitive approach, SMART is classified as calibration within the context of this text (Figure 9–9).

## Background

Gist reasoning is defined as "the ability to synthesize complex information, whether written, auditorily presented, or visually depicted, into abstracted meanings that are not explicitly stated" (Chapman, 1995, as

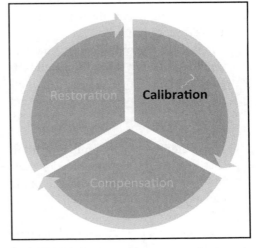

**Figure 9–9.** Theoretical framework of SMART. The predominant treatment approaches present in SMART.

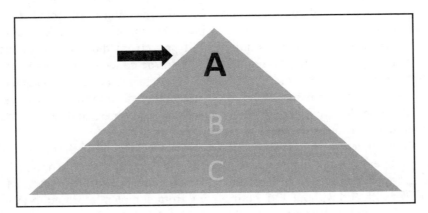

**Figure 9–8.** Level A evidence for the use of SMART in addressing executive function deficits post TBI. Level A consists of "recommendation supported by at least one meta-analysis, systematic review or randomized controlled trial study of appropriate size and relevant control group" (Bayley et al., 2014, p. 295).

cited in Vas, Spence, & Chapman, 2015). It is based on the premise that "the whole is more than the sum of its parts" (Chapman & Mudar, 2015, p. 521). Chapman and Mudar (2015, pp. 521–522) described it as comprising the following core cognitive capacities:

1. Strategic attention which allows for direction of the cognitive processes to focus on important details (and suppress irrelevant ones)
2. Integrated reasoning skills that are deployed in connecting the stated facts to world knowledge, in order to generate higher level and novel meanings not explicitly present in what is heard, read, and/or seen
3. Elaborated reasoning and innovation that results in the generation of multiple meanings, rather than a single convergent response

Gist reasoning is a crucial skill in communication and daily activities, across a wide variety of contexts. Deficits in the ability to engage in gist reasoning can impact any number of daily activities, such as face-to-face conversations, listening to the radio, watching movies, and reading for pleasure or employment.

Numerous researchers have studied this construct across a variety of populations, both in healthy adults and in those with neurologic impairments. A small number of studies have implicated frontal regions in gist processing (Nichelli et al., 1995; Robertson et al., 2000; Wong et al., 2006). Vas, Spence, and Chapman (2015) studied group differences in gist reasoning in adults with and without TBI, noting that individuals with TBI performed significantly poorer than those without TBI on measures of gist reasoning (e.g., fewer number of details recalled and less ability to

construct gist meanings from lengthy text-based information). This was true even after these researchers adjusted for variables such as education, IQ, reading comprehension, and speed of processing. These researchers also reported that executive function was positively associated with gist reasoning and that gist reasoning predicted daily functioning measures better than executive function measures alone. Other researchers have also noted a connection between gist reasoning ability and executive function related processes, such as attention, inhibition, working memory, switching, and goal maintenance (Brookshire, Chapman Song, & Levine, 2000; Chapman et al., 2006).

Vas, Spence, and Chapman (2015) provided a helpful example to illustrate differences in gist reasoning between those with TBI and those without TBI in their study (Table 9–8). Column A contains a narrative from an individual with TBI, while column B contains a narrative from an individual without TBI (control group). Participants in this example are similar age, IQ, and education. In this sample the researchers highlighted the ideas not specifically stated in the original text. They note that while the narratives share commonalities, they differ in "how meaning is extracted from complex information" (p. 161). For example, the TBI participant did not convey meaning beyond the concrete facts, while the control participant's narrative contained information not stated in the original text, such as, "values, kindness, and societal contributions" (p. 161).

SMART is based on the theoretical principles and stages of gist reasoning, designed to train individuals to abstract novel meaning from complex information (Vas et al., 2011). As above, its goals are to "teach metacognitive strategies to improve cognitive control functions of strategic attention, integrative reasoning, and innovation"

(Vas et al., 2016, p. 509). In general, studies regarding outcomes of SMART with individuals with TBI have shown positive gains in gist reasoning, executive functions, and real life participation, which have persisted after treatment discontinuance.

## Treatment in Action

SMART is implemented in the three phases of Strategic Attention, Integrated Reasoning, and Innovation/Cognitive Flexibility (Figure 9–10). Within the Strategic Atten-

tion Phase, the primary goal is to "reduce the load of incoming details by inhibiting less relevant information" (Vas et al., 2011, p. 227). This is done with the strategy of Filter, such that clients are taught to identify and discard irrelevant information. For example, the client could be asked to read information from a newspaper article a few times to understand the big picture, and then identify and "discard" (e.g., filter) irrelevant information.

In the Integrated Reasoning phase, the main purposes is to instruct the client in the process of combining "important facts . . .

**Table 9–8.** Example of Difference in Gist Reasoning

| Column A | Column B |
|---|---|
| **TBI participant** | **Control participant** |
| John started his career as a schoolteacher and went on to becoming a professor. He was considered a failure at these professions, as he was too easy on his students. He then decided to focus his attention on the legal world. He failed as a lawyer as he did not take on big cases that brought in more money. He then became a storeowner, but failed at it as he gave too much credit to his customers and did not make profit. He also worked as a file clerk in his seventies, but did not enjoy his job. Many years after his death, ***it was realized that he helped the society***. | One may think of John as a failure. He was a ***kind and generous man*** who ***thought of others' welfare*** rather than bringing in more money at all his careers such as teaching, practicing law and so on. ***He wanted to improve the system at every job***. But, those ideas did not go well with the bosses and John could not keep any job for long. Therefore, he was thought of as a ***failure both by himself and by the society***. However, when we look back, ***John is considered very successful as his ideas that are used even today helped the society over the years.*** |

*Source:* Vas, Spence, & Chapman (2015).

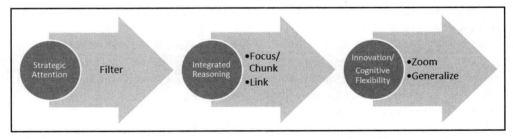

**Figure 9–10.** The three phases of SMART and their associated strategies. *Source:* Cook, Chapman, Elliott, Evenson, and Vinton (2014) and Vas et al. (2016).

by integrating the explicit content with pre-existing knowledge to form more global, gist-based representations" (Vas et al., 2011, p. 227). This is done through the strategies of: (1) Focus/Chunk and (2) Link. These strategies teach the client to combine (e.g., "chunk") information by similar ideas and then link it to information they already know from personal experience and world knowledge. Cook et al. (2014) recommend the use of inferencing and paraphrasing during this process, such as asking the client to read a passage and then write sentences in his/her own words that contain the main idea/gist concepts (Focus/Chuck) or having the client write a summary that communicates new ideas about the content (Link).

Lastly, the Innovation/Cognitive Flexibility phase seeks to teach the client the process of "evaluating the information from different perspectives" (Vas et al., 2011, p. 227). Within this phase, the strategy of Zoom is used to encourage the client to evaluate the information from different perspectives, such as describing meaning from a larger-picture perspective (zooming out) and from a more detailed and narrow perspective (zooming in). This phase also uses the strategy of Generalize, to encourage clients to expand their evaluation to other information and extend their interpretation to more than one perspective, outside of the immediate context.

SMART can be deployed in individual or group format, but Vas and colleagues note that group format has the potential advantage of group discussions, further reinforcing SMART strategies (Vas et al., 2011). Each of the phases within SMART is implemented in a similar fashion. First, the applicable phase (and each of the associated strategies) is explained using visual supports and written materials, with the goals of: (1) helping the client understand the phases/strategies, and (2) connecting those

strategies to how the frontal lobe processes information, and the concepts of executive function and gist reasoning. Importantly, the clinician also describes the concepts as they relate to everyday activities, providing relevant materials and real-world examples within each phase/strategy description. Next, the client is given an opportunity to practice the applicable strategies during the treatment session (reading an article and filtering it for irrelevant information, taking that information and chunking it into similar ideas, and so forth). At the end of each session, the client is given homework that requires completion of one or more of the strategies with pre-selected reading materials. As part of homework, the client is also asked to identify a specific activity(s) in his/her daily life that applies SMART concepts. A helpful illustration of this real-world SMART application is provided by Vas et al. (2011) (Figure 9–11). This is based on a participant's application of SMART principles to resumé writing.

## d. Constructive Feedback Awareness Training (CFAT)

## Candidacy Recommendations

Based on a composite of research in this area (Cheng & Man, 2006; McGraw-Hunter, Faw, & Davis, 2006; Ownsworth, Fleming, Desbois, Strong, & Kuipers, 2006; Ownsworth, Quinn, Fleming, Kendall, & Shum, 2010; Schmidt, Fleming, Ownsworth, & Lannin, 2013), Constructive Feedback Awareness Training (CFAT) is recommended in the post-acute stages after TBI for:

1. **Individuals who demonstrate impaired self-awareness following TBI.** The Awareness Questionnaire (Appendix

9–4, Sherer, Berg-loff, Boake, High, & Levin, 1998; Sherer, 2014) can be used for evaluating awareness in implementation of CFAT. This questionnaire contains rating forms for the client, family/significant other, and clinician (Appendices 9–5 and 9–6). Richardson, McKay, and Ponsford (2015) recommend evaluating the Awareness Questionnaire responses using a modified discrepancy analysis (Figure 9–12). Since the Awareness Questionnaire contains parallel rating forms for both the clinician and family/significant other, this analysis can be conducted comparing the client's awareness to the clinician and/or a significant other's ratings. Using this calculation, a positive discrepancy score is suggestive of unawareness, as it represents an individual who is reporting fewer symptoms than ratings of a clinician or significant other. In contrast, a negative discrepancy score suggests "hyper-vigilance of deficits as the individual with TBI is reporting a greater level of impairment" compared with a

The first step of strategic attention (ie, strategy of filter) involved deleting information that would not be relevant to include in the individual's resume. In addition, the individual had to selectively identify the most important information related to his/her own skills and strengths. The second step of integration (ie, strategies of focus and link) involved categorizing the individual's skills and strengths into academic accomplishments, leadership qualities, professional or personal characteristics, and work experience including volunteer work that related to the job requirements. These categories were then supported with relevant details to help the employer/interviewer capture the breadth and depth of that particular category. The third step of innovation (ie, strategies of zoom and generalize) involved summarizing the qualifications and abilities at a higher/broader level, into 2 or 3 succinct statements to provide the resume "objective" statement. Innovation also involved flexibility in preparing the resume in multiple formats and revising the objectives statements to adapt to the different employers needs and job requirements.

**Figure 9–11.** A narrative in the use of SMART applied to resumé development. *Source:* Vas, Chapman, Cook, Elliott, and Keebler (2011, p. 231).

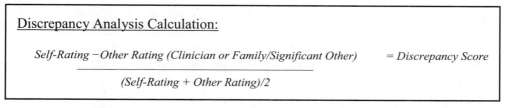

Discrepancy Analysis Calculation:

$$\frac{\textit{Self-Rating} - \textit{Other Rating (Clinician or Family/Significant Other)}}{\textit{(Self-Rating} + \textit{Other Rating)/2}} = \textit{Discrepancy Score}$$

**Figure 9–12.** Calculation for discrepancy ratings. *Source:* Richardson, McKay, and Ponsford (2015, p. 238).

clinician or family member/significant other (Richardson et al., 2015, p. 238). For CFAT, Schmidt and colleague recommend that individuals demonstrate at least a 2-point positive discrepancy score (Schmidt et al., 2013). Of note, discrepancy analysis can also be performed on domain-specific awareness (e.g., social competence, memory, attention) or given the difference between a client's own predicted and actual performance ratings. For example, Rebmann, Hannon, and Eisenberg (1995) measured unawareness for memory in CFAT implementation, given a discrepancy analysis between predicted test scores and actual test scores on the *Brief Multiparametric Memory Test.*

2. **Individuals who have sufficient cognitive, sensory, and motor function to engage in therapy and assessment tasks.** This will be largely determined by the tasks used during awareness training. For example, researchers have utilized a variety of real-world and experimental tasks for implementation of CFAT, such as meal preparation and volunteer work activities. Inclusion criteria in these studies was based on ability to participate in these treatment tasks, but clinically, tasks can be tailored to the individual and modified to address and client's cognitive, sensory, and motor functions.

Table 9–9 contains a sample of CFAT-related measures. Research in this area has also included measures of depression and distress within CFAT studies, such as the Hospital Anxiety and Depression Scale. This is due in part to the fact that depression and anxiety can lead to "heightened and in some cases exaggerated awareness of limitations" (Richardson et al., p. 234). Increased self-awareness (and awareness of

| **Table 9–9.** CFAT Related Measures |
|---|
| ***Awareness and Perception Measures*** |
| Awareness Questionnaire (Sherer et al., 1998) |
| Self-Perceptions in Rehabilitation Questionnaire (Ownsworth, Stewart, Fleming, & Griffin, 2013) |
| The Self-Awareness of Deficits Interview (Fleming, Strong, & Ashton, 1996) |
| ***Executive Function–Related Measures*** |
| Behavioral Assessment of the Dysexecutive Syndrome |
| Wisconsin Card Sorting Test |
| Wechsler Memory Scale - III |
| Trail Making Test (A and B) |
| Tinker Toy Test (Lezak, 1993) |
| Five-Point Test (Figural Fluency) |
| F-A-S Test (Verbal Fluency, Spreen & Strauss, 1998). |

change in function) has also been associated with greater anxiety and depression in individuals with TBI (Richardson et al., 2015). As such, it is important that clinicians work closely with neuropsychologists and other relevant team members, prior to and during implementation of CFAT, in order to both assess the presence of related psychological factors and monitor changes in this area during CFAT implementation. Relative to this, International Cognitive (INCOG) researchers recommend that clinicians targeting awareness in treatment: (1) develop a trusting therapeutic relationship, (2) use the client's emotional status to guide treatment, (3) engage the client in goal-setting and selection of relevant activities and tasks, and (4) use treatment tasks that are emotionally neutral and adaptable for strategy use (Tate et al., p. 344).

## Treatment Evidence

There is Level A evidence to recommend use of direct feedback (verbal, audiovisual, experiential) within the context of an awareness-specific therapeutic program (Figure 9–13; Tate et al., 2014, p. 343).

## Theoretical Frame

The majority of recent studies in the area of direct feedback specific to self-awareness "draw extensively on metacognitive strategy instruction procedures, the distinction being that the outcomes of interest focus on self-awareness, rather than cognitive aspects of executive performance" (see Figure 9–13; Tate et al., 2014, p. 345). As such, the principles of CFAT described in this chapter are classified as calibration (Figure 9–14).

## Background

Self-awareness is described as a "person's understanding of [his/her] own strengths

and limitations and how these affect every day functioning" (Schmidt et al., 2013, p. 316). It includes the ability to perceive one's self relatively objectively while maintaining a sense of subjectivity (Cheng & Man, 2006). The terms "self-awareness deficit" and "anosognosia" are often used

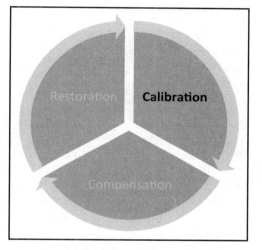

**Figure 9–14.** Theoretical framework of CFAT. This figure illustrates the predominant treatment approach present in treatment using corrective feedback for self-awareness.

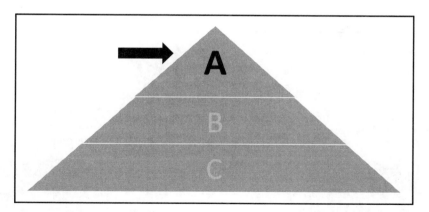

**Figure 9–13.** Level of evidence: Constructive Feedback Awareness Training (CFAT). Level A evidence for the use of direct feedback in addressing executive function deficits post TBI. Level A consists of "recommendation supported by at least one meta-analysis, systematic review or randomized controlled trial study of appropriate size and relevant control group" (Bayley et al., 2014, p. 295).

interchangeably, defined as a phenomenon in which a patient "does not appear to be aware of impaired neurological or neuropsychological function, which is obvious to the clinician and other reasonably attentive individuals" (Cheng & Man, 2006, p. 622).

As was described in Chapter 6 (Cognitive Rehabilitation Therapy Principles), self-awareness comprises both offline and online awareness (Toglia & Kirk, 2000), including *anticipatory awareness* (how an individual conceptualizes and evaluates the task), *error recognition* (self-monitoring skills to recognize errors in performance), and *self-regulation* (adjusting performance accordingly).

CFAT employs metacognitive strategy training through structured opportunities that help individuals with TBI evaluate their performance, discover errors, and compensate for deficits (Ownsworth & Fleming, 2006). A core aspect of CFAT includes training directed at online and offline awareness, as both are crucial to self-awareness in real-world contexts. As Richardson et al. (2015) note, even if an individual with TBI is given feedback about an error during task performance, this does not automatically translate into "enhanced 'metacognitive' understanding of [his/her] deficits" (offline awareness) (p. 245). The same can be said for metacognition (offline awareness), in that even if an individual has offline awareness, that does not necessarily mean he/she will implement online awareness during task performance.

## Treatment in Action

CFAT is implemented in the steps of pre-task analysis, task feedback, and post-task reflection, in order to address all three aspects of awareness (anticipatory awareness, error recognition, and self-regulation) (Figure 9–15). The core components used to target self-awareness in CFAT are: (1) education about the nature and characteristics of deficits and their impact, (2) feedback about performance within experiential and functional exercises, and (3) opportunities for self-reflection and self-prediction relative to performance.

### Step 1: Pre-Task Analysis

After assessment for candidacy, the first step in CFAT is selection and organization

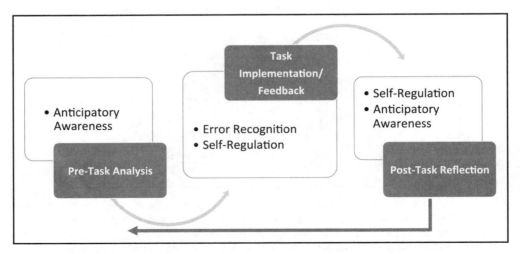

**Figure 9–15.** Core features and awareness aspects targeted within CFAT.

of treatment tasks. The goal in this stage of planning is to identify *real-world* tasks to use during the feedback stage of training. This is done through reflection and collaboration with the individual with TBI and his/her family members. Many of the studies conducted in this area thus far have conducted CFAT within tasks such as meal preparation and volunteer duties (Tate et al., 2014). Of note for speech-language pathologists, this method of training can also be easily applied to targets specific to communication, particularly for use in awareness and training on a specific communication skill (e.g., listening, starting conversation, maintaining conversation, repairing conversation, turn-taking, verbal organization, ending conversation), either alone or in conjunction with the group-based Social Communication Training (SCT) discussed in Chapter 10.

Once a CFAT task is selected with client input, the clinician then carefully evaluates performance parameters for that task, in order to identify the nature of the task and potential errors (both in general and unique to the client). This information will serve as the foundation for discussion with the client before and after task completion (offline awareness training). This information also guides the nature of feedback provided during task completion (online awareness training).

Response analysis can be a helpful framework in task/error analysis. This frame of analysis considers the dimensions of correctness (response accuracy), delay (response latency), and assistance needed (response independence). For example, within the designated CFAT task, the clinician can identify what types of errors are possible (response accuracy), what elements of time or delay are relevant to task performance (response latency), and what types of prompts or assistance may be needed,

both in general and when an error is present (response independence). This should be tailored to the individual and the nature of a specific CFAT task.

An example of response analysis within CFAT implementation is by Ownsworth et al. (2010), who conducted CFAT during meal preparation and defined errors for that task as those that compromise: (1) the participant's own or others' safety, (2) the outcome of the meal, or (3) time efficiency (p. 67). Although more operant than current CFAT approaches, the error analysis hierarchy developed by Gajar, Schloss, Schloss, and Thompson (1984) is shown in Figure 9–16 for error analysis used in participant feedback during group conversation activities (p. 354).

More structured task/error analysis can also be developed and utilized within CFAT, given the parameters of a specific domain: executive function, attention, memory, social communication, and so forth. For example, the *Executive Functional Performance Task* (Baum et al., 2008) could be modified to specific tasks and utilized for task/error analysis in the area of executive function. The EFPT is free and developed by an occupational therapist to provide a performance-based assessment of cognitive function during the execution of four basic tasks: simple cooking, telephone use, medication management, and bill payment. Appendix 9–7 contains samples of scoring for the medication management and telephone tasks within the EFPT. Schmidt et al. (2013) developed a meal independence rating system based on EFPT. Similarly, clinicians can create an EFPT-like data sheet for any CFAT-specific task, given any area targeted: memory, attention, social communication, and so forth. Categories of cues (Table 9–10) and common Likert scaling (Table 9–11) can be helpful for this purpose.

| +/Correct | −/Incorrect |
|---|---|
| ❏ Adding to a group members' conversation | ❏ No response to a fellow group members' question |
| ❏ Making a relevant statement | ❏ Off-topic response |
| ❏ Agreeing/disagreeing and providing a rationale | ❏ Response that is less than 3 words |
| | ❏ Response that is mumbled (unintelligible) |
| ❏ Asking a relevant question | ❏ Interrupting another group member |

**Figure 9–16.** Error analysis utilized for establishing feedback during a group conversation task.

**Table 9–10.** Sample Categories of Cues

| | |
|---|---|
| No Cues Required: | The participant requires no help or reassurance, does not ask questions for clarification, goes directly to the task and does it. Self-cueing is acceptable. Example: speaking to oneself. |
| Indirect Verbal Guidance: | The person requires verbal prompting, such as an open-ended question or an affirmation that will help them move on. Indirect verbal guidance should come in the form of a question, not a direct instruction, e.g.: "What should you do now?"; "What is the next step?"; "What else do you need?" Avoid direct phrases such as "read the instructions" or "turn on the stove." |
| Gestural Guidance: | The person requires gestural prompting. At this level, you are not physically involved with any portion of the task. Instead, you should make a gesticulation that mimics the action that is necessary to complete the subtask, or make a movement that guides the participant, e.g., you may move your hands in a stirring motion, point to where the participant may find the item, point to the appropriate level on the measuring cup, etc. You may not physically participate, such as handing the participant an item. |
| Direct Verbal Assistance: | You are required to deliver a one-step command, so that you are cueing the participant to take an action. For example, say, "pick up the pen" or "pour the water into the pan." |
| Physical Assistance: | You are physically assisting the participant with the step, but you are not doing it for him/her. You may hold the cup while he/she pours, hold the check book while he/she writes, loosen the cap on the medicine container, etc., but the participant is still attending to and participating in the task. |
| Do for the Participant: | You are required to do the step for the participant. |

*Source:* Baum, Connor, Morrison, Hahn, Dromerick, & Edwards (2008).

**Table 9–11.** Common Likert Scales

**Independence**

Complete Independence
Modified Independence (Device use)
Supervision
Minimum Assistance
Moderate Assistance
Maximum Assistance
Total Assistance

**Occurrence**

Never
Seldom
About half the time
Usually
Always

**Importance**

Not important
Moderately important
Very important

**Quality/Accuracy**

Poor
Fair
Average
Good
Excellent

**Satisfaction**

Not at all satisfied
Slightly satisfied
Somewhat satisfied
Very much satisfied

Once a CFAT task has been analyzed, the clinician should engage the client in self-analysis for the purpose of self-assessment and self-prediction of task performance (offline awareness). According to Cheng and Man (2006), in "this question-answer-feedback exercise, the patients' knowledge of and information about their own situations [are reinforced and] . . . the patients are able to obtain objective information about their deficits" (p. 624). This should be initiated with a review of the tasks to be performed, followed by questions from the client and prompts from the clinician for the client to identify potential errors and predict difficulty in task completion. Clinicians can make a list of items identified by the client for comparison with the clinician's pre-task analysis (as above).

This is also an excellent opportunity to discuss any specific cognitive and communication deficits unique to the client. Cheng and Man (2006) used this portion of the session to discuss and explain the "patient's knowledge of [his/her] own disease, the resultant deficits and the patient's present physical, cognitive and functional conditions" (p. 624). These researchers also gave immediate feedback during this discussion to reinforce accurate interpretations. Handouts, checklists, and other supporting material can be used, as needed.

Clients can also be asked to predict their own performance of a functional task before performing the task (Cheng & Man, 2006; Schmidt et al., 2013). This prediction can come in many forms, from a simplistic binary rating (e.g., successful/unsuccessful) to something more elaborate like utilizing the structured error analysis conducted by the clinician and having the client estimate performance for each step of the task. Visual Likert scales such as those in Figure 9–17 can be helpful for this purpose and modified to meet the client's individual cognitive, communicative, and awareness needs.

### Step 2: Task Implementation and Feedback

After task selection and a pre-task analysis, the next stage is task implementation. As the name of this approach suggests, provision of constructive feedback during and after task

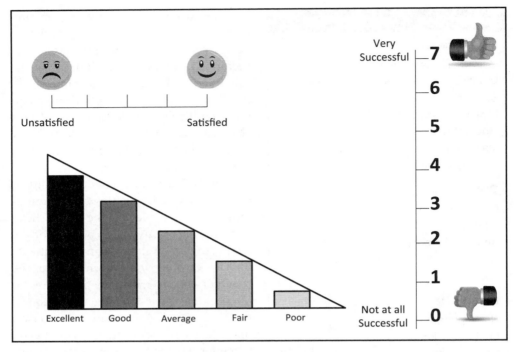

**Figure 9–17.** Examples of visual Likert scales. Visual rating scales that can be utilized in task prediction.

completion (either verbal, videotaped, or a combination thereof) is a cornerstone of CFAT (Richardson et al., 2015). Table 9–12 contains an example of the types of feedback common to CFAT(Schmidt et al., 2013). Peer feedback has also been utilized (McGraw-Hunter et al., 2006). The most recent randomized control study in this area (Schmidt et al., 2013) found that combining video and verbal feedback resulted in improved online awareness (fewer errors in task performance) compared with verbal or experiential feedback alone. As such, the use of combined feedback methods is recommended. The use of video monitoring will depend on the task and environment, but with the increase in mobile technology recording options and associated portable mounts (Figure 9–18), this is now a readily available option within most treatment settings.

The use of "close-other" (parent, spouse, sibling, child, or friend) feedback is also an area of consideration in augmenting CFAT for feedback outside the clinical setting, during real-world tasks. Richardson et al. (2015) reported that most close-others provided feedback to individuals with TBI, *at least sometimes*, but close-others reported low rates of client acceptance/agreement in response to this feedback. Close-others also reported reasons for not providing feedback, including: (1) not wanting to hurt the feelings of the injured individual and (2) believing that pointing out errors would be detrimental to the individual's rehabilitation. Enlisting the help of additional team members, such as neuropsychologists, in discussing these topics and identifying effective strategies and context for close-other feedback is key. Training close-others in the feedback strategy discussed below

**Table 9–12.** Common CFAT Feedback Procedures

| | |
|---|---|
| Video Plus Verbal Feedback | Participants in the video feed-back group watched their videotaped performance with the therapist. While viewing, the therapist encouraged the participant to retrospectively identify errors in task performance, observe areas of strength, and suggest compensatory strategies that could be used in future sessions. The therapist and the participant then verbally discussed any discrepancies in their ratings of the task performance |
| Verbal Feedback | For participants in the verbal feedback group, the therapist followed the same guidelines for verbal discussion of discrepancies between ratings without viewing the videotape. |
| Experiential Feedback | For participants in the experiential feedback group, no direct feedback was provided following the task. The participant and treating therapist separately completed task evaluations and discrepancies and ratings were not discussed. |

*Source:* Schmidt, Fleming, Ownsworth, & Lannin (2013, p. 318).

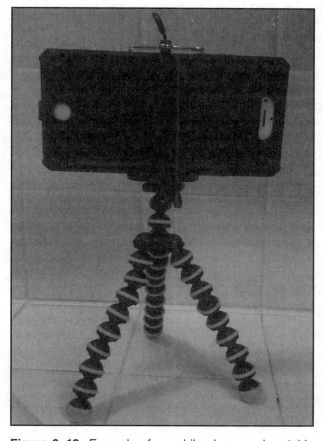

**Figure 9–18.** Example of a mobile phone and portable tripod applicable to CFAT video-recording for feedback on task performance.

(Pause-Prompt-Praise) can also be utilized to best structure close-other feedback outside the clinical setting. Once trained, homework can be assigned for completion of similar tasks with close-others using constructive feedback during task completion.

Special attention is given within CFAT to the nature of feedback provided during task completion. Several researchers have recommended the use of Pause-Prompt-Praise for this purpose (Figure 9–19; Schmidt et al., 2013; Ownsworth et al., 2006). This is an approach initially developed by McNaughton, Glynn, and Robinson (1987) for use in remedial reading instruction.

When using Pause-Prompt-Praise, the clinician does not initially provide prompts when the client makes an error (Wheldall, Merrett, & Colmar, 1987). Rather, the clinician pauses anywhere between 2 and 5 seconds (Schmidt et al., 2013) after an error in task performance. This allows the client time to self-correct. If the client does not correct the error, then the clinician provides a nonspecific prompt, such as, "Is there something you should check?" (Schmidt et al., 2013). Figure 9–20 contains a sample of verbal prompts developed by the *Executive Functional Performance Task* (Baum et al., 2008) which can be used for this purpose. Visual prompts such as gestures can also be used.

After a prompt, the clinician pauses to allow the client to correct the error. If the client does not correct the error, the clinician then provides a more specific prompt, such as, "You should check the _____" (Schmidt et al., 2013). Positive verbal reinforcement is provided when the client corrects an error after a prompt and when he/she uses strategies that enhance task performance. In Pause-Prompt-Praise, Wheldall et al. (1987) recommend that praise be constructive and specific (rather than generic). An example of this would be instead of saying "good work" or "nice job," the clinician

---

Sample Verbal Prompt-Questions

❑ Do you need anything else?

❑ Is there anything you need to do first?

❑ Do you need another item?

❑ What do you need to do next?

❑ Is there another way to do that?

❑ Is there anything you forgot?

❑ Anything else you need to consider?

**Figure 9–20.** Examples of generic verbal prompt questions that can be utilized within Pause-Prompt-Praise. *Source:* Baum et al., 2008.

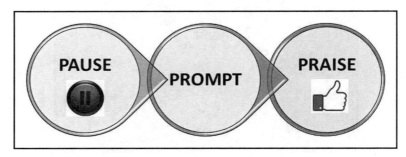

**Figure 9–19.** The stages of Pause-Prompt-Praise during CFAT feedback implementation.

could say something specific about what was effective, such as, "That was a good idea to cross off your steps on the checklist," "It was helpful that you asked Eric for his opinion," and so forth.

### Step 3: Post-Task Reflection

Upon task completion, the clinician and client engage in a similar question-and-answer session to that conducted in the pre-task analysis step, but this time targeted toward analysis of the completed task. This will depend on the nature of the conversation during the pre-task completion step as to what is discussed and in what depth. For example, if a visual Likert scale was used to predict performance, this can be reintroduced for discussion as to whether the prediction was correct and if not, why. Similarly, any checklists or forms for error analysis discussed with the client prior to task completion can also be reintroduced for discussion as to any errors noted by the client and the clinician (Ownsworth et al., 2010; Schmidt et al., 2013).

Video feedback of task completion can also be shown. Schmidt et al. (2013) recommend that while viewing the video, the clinician encourage the participant to "retrospectively identify errors in task performance, observe areas of strength, and suggest compensatory strategies that could be used in future sessions" (p. 318). In discussion of video feedback, it is important to allow opportunities to pause the video and discuss specific aspects of performance, prompting the client to first provide his/her analysis before feedback from the clinician is provided. Clinician feedback should be informational and non-confrontational, with the goal of facilitating self-identification of areas of strength and limitation (Ownsworth et al., 2010; Schmidt et al.,

2013). Cheng and Man (2006) also recommend that clients be asked to set short-term goals based on their performance in the future task completion.

## References

American Speech-Language-Hearing Association. (2003). *Evaluating and treating communication and cognitive disorders: Approaches to referral and collaboration for speech-language pathology and clinical neuropsychology* [Technical report]. Retrieved from http://www.asha.org/policy

Baum, C. M., Connor, L. T., Morrison, T., Hahn, M., Dromerick, A. W., & Edwards, D. F. (2008). Reliability, validity, and clinical utility of the executive function performance test: A measure of executive function in a sample of people with stroke. *American Journal of Occupational Therapy, 62,* 446–455.

Bayley, M., Tate, R., Douglas, J., Turkstra, L., Ponsford, J., Stergiou-Kita, M. . . . INGOG Expert Panel. (2014). INCOG guidelines for cognitive rehabilitation following traumatic brain injury: Methods and overview. *Journal of Head Trauma Rehabilitation, 29*(4), 290–306.

Bergquist, T. F., & Jacket, M. P. (1993). Programme methodology: Awareness and goal setting with the traumatically brain injured. *Brain Injury 7,* 275–282.

Bertens, D., Fasotti, L., Boelen, D. H. E., & Kessels, R. P. C. (2013). A randomized controlled trial on errorless learning in goal management training: Study rationale and protocol. *BMC Neurology, 13,* 64.

Bertens, D., Kessels, R., Boelen, D., & Fasotti, L. (2016). Transfer effects of errorless goal management training on cognitive function and quality of life in brain-injured persons. *NeuroRehabilitation, 38,* 79–84.

Bertens, D., Kessels, R. P. C., Fiorenzato, E., Boelen, D. H. E., & Fasotti, L. (2015). Do old errors always lead to new truths? A randomized controlled trial of errorless goal management training in brain-injured patients. *Journal of the International Neuropsychological Society, 21*, 639–649.

Brookshire, B. L., Chapman, S. B., Song, J., & Levin, H. S. (2000) Cognitive and linguistic correlates of children's discourse after closed head injury: A three-year follow-up. *Journal of the International Neuropsychological Society 6*(7), 741–751.

Chan, R., Shum, D., Toulopoulou, T., & Chen, E. (2008). Assessment of executive functions: Review of instruments and identification of critical issues. *Archives of Clinical Neuropsychology, 23*(2), 201–216.

Chapman, S. B., Gamino, J. F., Cook, L. G. Hanten, G., Li, X., & Levin, H. S. (2006) Impaired discourse gist and working memory in children after brain injury. *Brain and Language 97*(2), 178–188.

Chapman, S., & Mudar, R. (2013). Discourse gist: A window into the brain's complex cognitive capacity. *Discourse Studies, 15*(5), 519–533.

Cheng, S. K., & Man, D. W. (2006). Management of impaired self-awareness in persons with traumatic brain injury. *Brain Injury, 20*(6), 621–628.

Cicerone, K., Dahlberg, C., Kalmar, K., Langenbahn, D., Malec, J., Bergquist, T. F., . . . Morse, P. A. (2000). Evidence-based cognitive rehabilitation: Recommendations for clinical practice. *Archives of Physical Medicine and Rehabilitation, 81*(12), 1596–1615.

Cicerone, K., Dahlberg, C., Malec, J., Langenbahn, D., Felicetti, T., Kneipp, S., . . . Catanese, J. (2005). Evidence-based cognitive rehabilitation: Updated review of the literature from 1998 through 2002. *Archives of Physical Medicine and Rehabilitation, 86*(8), 1681–1692.

Cicerone, K. D., Langenbahn, D. M., Braden, C., Malec, J. F., Kalmar, K., Fraas, M., . . . Ashman, T. (2011). Evidence-based cognitive rehabilitation: Updated review of the literature from 2003 through 2008. *Archives of Physical Medicine and Rehabilitation, 92*(4), 519–530.

Cook, L., Chapman, S., Elliott, A., Evenson, N., & Vinton, K. (2014). Cognitive gains from

gist reasoning training in adolescents with chronic-stage traumatic brain injury. *Frontiers in Neurology, 5*, 87.

Daneman, M., & Carpenter, P. A. (1980). Individual differences in working memory and reading. *Journal of Verbal Learning and Verbal Behavior, 19*(4), 450–466.

Duncan, J., Emslie, H., Williams, P., Johnson, R., & Freer, C. (1996). Intelligence and the frontal lobe: The organization of goal-directed behavior. *Cognitive Psychology, 30*(3), 257–303.

Ezrachi, O., Ben-Yishay, Y., Kay, T., DiUer, L., & Rattok, J. (1991). Predicting employment in traumatic brain injury following neuropsychological rehabilitation. *Journal of Head Trauma Rehabilitation 6*, 71–84.

Fasotti, L., Kovacs, F., Eling, A. T. M., & Brouwer, W. (2000). Time pressure management as a compensatory strategy training after closed head injury. *Neuropsychological Rehabilitation, 10*(1), 47–65.

Fish, J., Evans, J. J., Nimmo, M., Martin, E., Kersel, D., Bateman, A., . . . Manly, T. (2007). Rehabilitation of executive dysfunction following brain injury: "Content-free" cueing improves everyday prospective memory performance. *Neuropsychologia, 45*, 1318–1330.

Flashman, L. A., Amador, X., & McAllister, T. W. (1998). Lack of awareness of deficits in traumatic brain injury. *Seminars in Clinical Neuropsychiatry 3*, 201–210.

Fleming, J. M., Strong, J., & Ashton, R. (1996). Self-awareness of deficits in adults with traumatic brain injury: How best to measure? *Brain Injury, 10*, 1–15.

Gajar, A., Schloss, P. J., Schloss, C. N., & Thompson, C. K. (1984). Effects of feedback and self-monitoring on head trauma youths' conversation skills. *Journal of Applied Behavior Analysis, 17*(3), 353–358.

Grant, M., Ponsford, J., & Bennett, P. (2012). The application of goal management training to aspects of financial management in individuals with traumatic brain injury. *Neuropsychological Rehabilitation, 22*(6), 852–873.

Kennedy, M. R., Coelho, C., Turkstra, L., Ylvisaker, M., Sohlberg, M. M., Yorkston, K., . . . Kan, P. F. (2008). Intervention for executive functions after traumatic brain injury: A systematic review, meta-analysis and clinical recommendations. *Neuropsychological Rehabilitation, 18*(3), 257–299.

Levine, B., Robertson, I. H., Clare, L., Carter, G., Hong, J., Wilson, B. A., . . . Stuss, D. T. (2000). Rehabilitation of executive functioning: An experimental-clinical validation of goal management training. *Journal of the International Neuropsychological Society, 6*, 299–312.

Levine, B., Schweizer, T., O'Connor, C., Turner, G. Gillingham, S., Stuss, D. T., . . . Robertson, I. H. (2011). Rehabilitation of executive functioning in patients with frontal lobe brain damage with goal management training. *Frontiers in Human Neuroscience, 5*(9), 1–9.

McGraw-Hunter, M., Faw, G. D., & Davis, P. K. (2006). The use of video self-modelling and feedback to teach cooking skills to individuals with traumatic brain injury: A pilot study. *Brain Injury, 20*(10), 1061–1068.

McNaughton, S. S., Glynn, T., & Robinson, V. (1987). *Pause, prompt, and praise: Effective tutoring for remedial reading.* Birmingham, UK: Positive Products.

Nichelli, P., Grafman, J., Pietrini, P., Clark, K., Lee, K. Y., & Miletich, R. (1995). Where the brain appreciates the moral of a story. *Neuro-Report, 6*(17), 2309–2313.

Ownsworth, T., Fleming, J., Desbois, J., Strong, J., & Kuipers, P. A. (2006). Metacognitive contextual intervention to enhance error awareness and functional outcome following traumatic brain injury: A single-case experimental design. *Journal of the International Neuropsychological Society, 12*(1), 54–63.

Ownsworth, T., Quinn, H., Fleming, J., Kendall, M., & Shum, D. (2010). Error self-regulation following traumatic brain injury: A single case study evaluation of metacognitive skills training and behavioural practice interventions. *Neuropsychological Rehabilitation, 20*(1), 59–80.

Ownsworth, T., Stewart, E., Fleming, J., Griffin, J., Collier, A. M., & Schmidt, J. (2013). Development and preliminary psychometric evaluation of the self-perceptions in rehabilitation questionnaire for brain injury rehabilitation.

*AJOT: American Journal of Occupational Therapy, 67*(3), 336–344.

Prigatano, G. P., Altman, I. M. & O'Brien, K. P. (1990). Behavioral limitations that brain injured patients tend to underestimate. *Clinical Neuropsychologist, 4*, 163–176.

Rebmann, M., Hannon, R., & Eisenberg, M. (1995). Treatment of unawareness of memory deficits in adults with brain injury: Three case studies. *Rehabilitation Psychology, 40*(4), 279–287.

Richardson, C., McKay, A., & Ponsford, J. (2014). Does feedback influence awareness following traumatic brain injury? *Neuropsychological Rehabilitation, 25*(2), 233–253.

Robertson, D. A., Gernsbacher, M. A., Guidotti, S. J., Robertson, R. R., Irwin. W., & Mock, B. J. (2000). Functional neuroanatomy of the cognitive process of mapping during discourse comprehension. *Psychological Science, 11*, 255–260.

Robertson, I. (1996). *Goal management training: A clinical manual.* Cambridge, UK: Psy Consult.

Schmidt, J., Fleming, J., Ownsworth, T., & Lannin, N. (2013). Video feedback on functional task performance improves self-awareness after traumatic brain injury. *Neurorehabilitation and Neural Repair, 27*(4), 316–324.

Sherer, M. (2004). *The Awareness Questionnaire.* The Center for Outcome Measurement in Brain Injury. Retrieved from http://www .tbims.org/combi/aq

Sherer, M., Bergloff, P., Boake, C., High, W., & Levin, E. (1998). The Awareness Questionnaire: Factor structure and internal consistency. *Brain Injury, 12*, 63– 68.

Sohlberg, M. M., & Mateer, C. A. (2001). *Cognitive rehabilitation: An integrative neuropsychological approach.* New York, NY: Guilford Press.

Sohlberg, M. M. & Turkstra, L. S. (2001). *Optimizing cognitive rehabilitation: Effective instructional methods.* New York, NY: Guilford Press.

Spikman, J. M., Boelen, D. H. E., Lamberts, K. F., Brouwer, W. H., & Fasotti, L. (2010). Effects of a multifaceted treatment program for executive dysfunction after acquired brain injury on indications of executive functioning in daily life. *Journal of the International Neuropsychological Society, 16*(1), 118–129.

Stuss, D., & Alexander, M. (2007). Is there a dysexecutive syndrome? *Philosophical Transactions: Biological Sciences, 362*(1481), 901–915.

Stuss, D. T., & Levine, B. (2002). Adult clinical neuropsychology: Lessons from studies of the frontal lobes. *Annual Review of Psychology, 53*, 401–433.

Tate, R., Kennedy, M., Ponsford, J., Douglas, J., Velikonja, D., Bayley, M., & Stergiou-Kita, M. (2014). INCOG recommendations for management of cognition following traumatic brain injury, Part iii: Executive function and self-awareness. *Journal of Head Trauma Rehabilitation, 29*(4), 338–352.

Toglia, J., & Kirk, U. (2000). Understanding awareness deficits following brain injury. *NeuroRehabilitation, 15*, 57–70.

Vas, A., Chapman, S., Aslan, S., Spence, J., Keebler, M., Rodriguez-Larrain, G., . . . Krawczyk, D. (2016) Reasoning training in veteran and civilian traumatic brain injury with persistent mild impairment. *Neuropsychological Rehabilitation, 26*(4), 502–531.

Vas, A., Chapman, S., Cook, L., Elliott, A., & Keebler, M. (2011). Higher-order reasoning training years after traumatic brain injury in adults. *Journal of Head Trauma Rehabilitation, 26*(3), 224–239.

Vas, A., Spence, J., & Chapman, S. (2015). Abstracting meaning from complex information (gist reasoning) in adult traumatic brain injury. *Journal of Clinical and Experimental Neuropsychology, 1–10.

Waid-Ebbs, J., Daly, J., Wu, S., Berg, W., Bauer, R. M., Perlstein, W. M., & Crosson, B. (2014). Response to goal management training in veterans with blast-related mild traumatic brain injury. *Journal of Rehabilitation Research & Development, 51*(10), 1555–1566.

Wheldall, K., Merrett, F., & Colmar, S. (1987). 'Pause, prompt and praise' for parents and peers: Effective tutoring of low progress readers. *Support for Learning, 2*(1), 5–12.

Winkens, I., Van Heugten, C. M., Wade, D. T., & Fasotti, L. (2009). Training patients in time pressure management, a cognitive strategy for mental slowness. *Clinical Rehabilitation, 23*(1), 79–90.

Winkens, I., Van Heugten, C. M., Wade, D. T., Habets, E. J., & Fasotti, L. (2009). Efficacy of time pressure management in stroke patients with slowed information processing: A randomized controlled trial. *Archives of Physical Medicine and Rehabilitation, 90*(10), 1672–1679.

Wong S., Chapman, S. B., Cook, L. G., Anand, R., Gamino, J. F., & Devous, M. D. (2006). A SPECT study of language and brain reorganization three years after pediatric brain injury. *Progress in Brain Research 157*, 73–185.

## Real-World Task Assessment: Executive Function

Client: _____

| Task | Task/Accuracy Analysis | | Performance Analysis: Executive Function | | | | | | |
|------|------|------|------|------|------|------|------|------|------|
| | Date | Task Difficulty[1] | Task Accuracy[2] | Initiation and Drive (+/−) | Response Inhibition (+/−) | Task Persistence (+/−) | Organization (+/−) | Generative Thinking (+/−) | Error Awareness[3] | Notes/Error Description |
| Grocery shopping for 3 items (clinician initiated) | 3/12/17 | 2 | I | N/A | + | − | + | N/A | U | Left store with 2/3 items. Initiated and inhibited other purchases (generally organized). Became distracted by another shopper and did not persist in task completion. |
| | | | | | | | | | | |
| | | | | | | | | | | |
| | | | | | | | | | | |
| | | | | | | | | | | |
| | | | | | | | | | | |

*Notes.* [1] Level of Difficulty: 1 = Very easy, 2 = Easy, 3 = Difficult, 4 = Very Difficult. [2] Accuracy: A = Accurate/Complete, I = Inaccurate/Incomplete. [3] Error Awareness: F = Fully Aware, P = Partially Aware, U = Unaware.

APPENDIX 9–2

## Self-Observation: Executive Function

Client: _____

| Date/ Time | What did I do that required executive function? | How difficult what the task overall? | How was my . . . • Initiation? • Inhibition? • Persistence? • Organization? • Creative Problem Solving? • Awareness of Errors? | Is there anything I would do differently (or remember for next time)? |
|---|---|---|---|---|
| | | | | |
| | | | | |
| | | | | |
| | | | | |

Level of Difficulty: 1 = Very difficult, 2 = Difficult, 3 = Easy, 4 = Very Easy

## Self-Reflection: Executive Function

Client: _____

| | KNOWLEDGE | | ATTRIBUTE | EMOTION | IMPACT | | |
|---|---|---|---|---|---|---|---|
| | *What are my strengths?* | *What are my challenges?* | *What is causing difficulty in this area?* | *How do I feel about this?* | *How does this impact me in my daily life?* | *What things help?* | *What things make it more challenging?* |
| Initiation | | | | | | | |
| Inhibition | | | | | | | |
| Task Persistence | | | | | | | |
| Organization | | | | | | | |
| Generative/ Creative Thinking | | | | | | | |
| Awareness | | | | | | | |

# APPENDIX 9-4

## Awareness Questionnaire:  Patient Form

Name: _____ Patient #: _____ Date: _____

1 much worse   2 a little worse   3 about the same   4 a little better   5 much better

_____  1. How good is your ability to live independently now compared with before your injury?

_____  2. How good is your ability to manage your money now compared with before your injury?

_____  3. How well do you get along with people now compared with before your injury?

_____  4. How well can you do on tests that measure thinking and memory skills now compared with before your injury?

_____  5. How well can you do the things you want to do in life now compared with before your injury?

_____  6. How well are you able to see now compared with before your injury?

_____  7. How well can you hear now compared with before your injury?

_____  8. How well can you move your arms and legs now compared with before your injury?

_____  9. How good is your coordination now compared with before your injury?

_____  10. How good are you at keeping up with the time and date and where you are now compared with before your injury?

_____  11. How well can you concentrate now compared with before your injury?

_____  12. How well can you express your thoughts to others now compared with before your injury?

_____  13. How good is your memory for recent events now compared with before your injury?

_____  14. How good are you at planning things now compared with before your injury?

_____  15. How well organized are you now compared with before your injury?

_____ 16. How well can you keep your feelings in control now compared with before your injury?

_____ 17. How well adjusted emotionally are you now compared with before your injury?

*Source:* Sherer (2014). Used with permission. Original source: Sherer, Bergloff, Boake, High, & Levin (1998).

# Awareness Questionnaire: Clinician Form

Clinician Name: _____     Date: _____

Patient: _____     Patient #: _____

1 much worse    2 a little worse    3 about the same    4 a little better    5 much better

_____ 1. How good is the patient's ability to live independently now compared with before his/her injury?

_____ 2. How good is the patient's ability to manage his/her money now compared with before his/her injury?

_____ 3. How well does the patient get along with people now compared with before his/her injury?

_____ 4. How well can the patient do on tests that measure thinking and memory skills now compared with before his/her injury?

_____ 5. How well can the patient do the things he/she wants to do in life now compared with before his/her injury?

_____ 6. How well is the patient able to see now compared with before his/her injury?

_____ 7. How well can the patient hear now compared with before his/her injury?

_____ 8. How well can the patient move his/her arms and legs now compared with before his/her injury?

_____ 9. How good is the patient's coordination now compared with before his/her injury?

_____ 10. How good is the patient at keeping up with the time and date and where he/she is now compared with before his/her injury?

_____ 11. How well can the patient concentrate now compared with before his/her injury?

_____ 12. How well can the patient express his/her thoughts to others now compared with before his/her injury?

_____ 13. How good is the patient's memory for recent events now compared with before his/her injury?

_____ 14. How good is the patient at planning things now compared with before his/her injury?

_____ 15. How well organized is the patient now compared with before his/her injury?

_____ 16. How well can the patient keep his/her feelings in control now compared with before his/her injury?

_____ 17. How well adjusted emotionally is the patient now compared with before his/her injury?

1 completely   2 severely   3 moderately   4 minimally   5 not at all

_____ 18. To what extent is the patient's accurate self-awareness impaired by his/her brain injury?

_Source:_ Sherer (2014). Used with permission. Original source: Sherer, Bergloff, Boake, High, & Levin (1998).

# Awareness Questionnaire:  Family/Significant Other Form

Name: _____  Relationship to patient: _____

Patient: _____  Patient #: _____  Date: _____

    1 much worse   2 a little worse   3 about the same   4 a little better   5 much better

_____   1. How good is the patient's ability to live independently now compared with before his/her injury?

_____   2. How good is the patient's ability to manage his/her money now compared with before his/her injury?

_____   3. How well does the patient get along with people now compared with before his/her injury?

_____   4. How well can the patient do on tests that measure thinking and memory skills now compared with before his/her injury?

_____   5. How well can the patient do the things he/she wants to do in life now compared with before his/her injury?

_____   6. How well is the patient able to see now compared with before his/her injury?

_____   7. How well can the patient hear now compared with before his/her injury?

_____   8. How well can the patient move his/her arms and legs now compared with before his/her injury?

_____   9. How good is the patient's coordination now compared with before his/her injury?

_____  10. How good is the patient at keeping up with the time and date and where he/she is now compared with before his/her injury?

_____  11. How well can the patient concentrate now compared with before his/her injury?

_____  12. How well can the patient express his/her thoughts to others now compared with before his/her injury?

_____  13. How good is the patient's memory for recent events now compared with before his/her injury?

_____ 14. How good is the patient at planning things now compared with before his/her injury?

_____ 15. How well organized is the patient now compared with before his/her injury?

_____ 16. How well can the patient keep his/her feelings in control now compared with before his/her injury?

_____ 17. How well adjusted emotionally is the patient now compared with before his/her injury?

*Source:* Sherer (2014). Used with permission. Original source: Sherer, Bergloff, Boake, High, & Levin (1998).

## APPENDIX 9–7

## Executive Function Performance Test

**Using the Telephone**

| TASK: Using the Telephone  Time for completion of task: ____ | Independent  0 | Verbal Guidance  1 | Gestural Guidance  2 | Verbal Direct Instruction  3 | Physical Assistance  4 | Do For Participant  5 | Score |
|---|---|---|---|---|---|---|---|
| INITIATION: *beginning the task* | | | | | | | |
| Upon your request to start, participant moves to table to gather tools/ materials for making a phone call. | | | | | | | – |
| EXECUTION: *carrying out the actions of the task through the use of organization, sequencing, and judgment* | | | | | | | |
| **Organization:** *arrangement of the tools/ materials to complete the task.* Participant retrieves the items needed (phone book, paper, pencil). | | | | | | | – |

| | | | | | | |
|---|---|---|---|---|---|---|
| **Sequencing:** *execution of steps in appropriate order.* Participant performs steps in an appropriate sequence, e.g., looks up number, lifts receiver, reaches the correct number, and tells you the correct answer. Participant does not confuse steps, e.g., dials number before looking it up, hangs up receiver in middle of dialing, puts away phone book instead of looking number up, etc. | – | | | | | |
| **Judgment & Safety:** *avoidance of dangerous situation.* Participant prevents or avoids danger, e.g., dials number correctly, reports information accurately, etc. | – | | | | | |
| COMPLETION: *termination of task* | | | | | | |
| Participant knows he/she is finished, e.g., hangs up phone and does not continue pushing buttons. | – | | | | | |

*continues*

**Appendix 9–7.** *continued*

**Medication Management**

| TASK: Medication Sorting<br>Time for completion of task: ___ | Independent<br>0 | Verbal<br>Guidance<br>1 | Gestural<br>Guidance<br>2 | Verbal Direct<br>Instruction<br>3 | Physical<br>Assistance<br>4 | Do For<br>Participant<br>5 | Score |
|---|---|---|---|---|---|---|---|
| INITIATION: *beginning the task* | | | | | | | |
| Upon your request to start, participant moves to table to gather tools/ materials for sorting medications. | | | | | | | – |
| EXECUTION: *carrying out the actions of the task through the use of organization, sequencing, and judgment* | | | | | | | |
| **Organization:** *arrangement of the tools/ materials to complete the task.* Participant retrieves the items needed (pill sorter, medicine bottles). | | | | | | | – |

| | | | | | | | |
|---|---|---|---|---|---|---|---|
| | | | | | | | – |
| | | | | | | | |
| | | | | | | | |
| | | | | | | | |
| | | | | | | | |
| | | | | | | | |
| | | | | | | | |
| **Sequencing:** *execution of steps in appropriate order.* Participant performs steps in an appropriate sequence, e.g., reads the direction on pill bottle, opens pill bottle, pours pills into hand or on table, chooses correct number of pills according to prescription, puts unused pills back into bottle, and places pills into correct location of pill sorter, puts cap back on bottles. Participant does not confuse steps, e.g., uses appropriate steps, e.g., places pills in correct slot for all 7 days. | | | | | | | |
| **Judgment & Safety:** *avoidance of dangerous situation.* Participant prevents or avoids danger, e.g., uses correct pills, counts correct number of pills, places them in appropriate location in pill sorter. | | | | | | | – |
| COMPLETION: *termination of task* | | | | | | | |
| Participant knows he/she is finished, e.g., moves away from task, doesn't continue playing with pills, etc. | | | | | | | – |

*Source:* Baum, C. M., Connor, L. T., Morrison, T., Hahn, M., Dromerick, A. W., & Edwards, D. F. (2008). Reliability, validity, and clinical utility of the executive function performance test: A measure of executive function in a sample of people with stroke. *American Journal of Occupational Therapy, 62,* 446–455.

# 10 Social Communication

a. Introduction
b. Social Communication Training (SCT)
   *Carley B. Crandall and Jennifer A. Ostergren*

## a. Introduction

International Cognitive (INCOG) treatment recommendations in the area of cognitive communication (Togher et al., 2014, pp. 356–357) include:

1. Rehabilitation staff should recognize that levels of communication competence and communication characteristics may vary as a function of communication partner, environment, communication demands, communication priorities, fatigue, and other personal factors.
2. A person with TBI who has a cognitive-communication disorder should be offered an appropriate treatment program by an SLP.
3. A cognitive-communication rehabilitation program should take into account the person's premorbid native language, literacy, and language proficiency; cognitive abilities; and communication style, including communication standards and expectations in that individual's culture.
4. A cognitive-communication rehabilitation program should provide the opportunity to rehearse communication skills in situations appropriate to the context in which the individual will live, work, study, and socialize.
5. A cognitive-communication rehabilitation program should provide education and training of communication partners.
6. Individuals with severe communication disability should be assessed for, provided with, and trained in the use of appropriate alternative and augmentative communication aids by suitably accredited clinicians: speech language pathologists (for communication) and occupational therapists (for access to devices, writing aids, seating, etc.).
7. Interventions to address patient-identified goals for social communication deficits are recommended after TBI, with outcomes measured at the level of participation in everyday social life. These interventions can be provided in either group or individual settings; however, published evidence is strongest for group-based interventions.

As was discussed in Chapter 4 (Cognition and Communication), *social* communication is defined as an "amalgamation of verbal and nonverbal skills that enable individuals to express themselves and understand the meanings intended by others in a diverse array of environments and with varying communication partners" (Finch, Copley, Cornwell, & Kelly, 2016, p. 1353). In a recent systematic review specific to intervention for social communication following TBI, researchers (Finch et al., 2016) categorized treatment approaches as either context-sensitive or impairment-specific. Context-sensitive approaches are those that combine "impairment-based interventions, functional activities, and context-supported participation to enable individuals to participate in their desired everyday activities" (p. 1353). In contrast, impairment-specific approaches focus on restoring a specific function, such as emotion perception, verbal interaction skills, or negative social behaviors. Finch and colleagues noted that both context-sensitive and impairment-specific approaches can positively affect social communication behaviors in individuals with TBI, but evidence is greatest to support context-sensitive approaches, delivered predominantly in group-based service models. As such, this chapter will describe group-based context-sensitive Social Communication Training (SCT). Some of the approaches in this area have manuals available for purchase, as below. The content discussed in the sections that follow is a composite of these and other context-sensitive approaches.

1. TBI Express Communication Training (Togher, McDonald, Tate, Power, & Rietdijk, 2013). Available for purchase at http://www.assbi.com.au/tbi%20 express.html. Within the treatment manual, two separate programs are described (i.e., the program for Every-day Communication Partners [ECP] and the communication skills training program for people with TBI who attend treatment without a communication partner).

2. Group-Interactive Structured Treatment (GIST) Social Competency Training (Dahlberg et al., 2007). Available for purchase at http://www.braininjury socialcompetence.com/

## Assessment

Table 10–1 contains examples of common assessment measures in the area of social communication. These are helpful measures in identifying particular strengths and weaknesses, and in the case of standardized assessment, comparison to a normative data set. The rehabilitative process also benefits from ongoing structured evaluation of performance in real-world tasks (Sohlberg & Mateer, 2001).

Engaging the client in an ongoing self-assessment can be a valuable exercise in the rehabilitation process. Several authors have noted awareness after a brain injury to be an important factor across a variety of rehabilitation approaches (Bergquist & Jacket, 1993; Ezrachi et al., 1991; Prigatano, Altman, & O'Brien, 1990). Awareness specific to social communication is also a key area of focus of SCT (Dahlberg et al., 2007). Approaches for incorporating self-awareness and self-reflection are discussed in the sections that follow, but a helpful first step in the process of self-awareness is self-observation. This can be challenging in the context of social communication, given varied and nuanced aspects of self-reflection during conversation. One approach to this is to limit that scope of self-observation to specific targeted aspects. For example, any of the measures listed in Table 10–1 could be utilized

**Table 10–1.** Social Communication Measures

| Measure | Description |
|---|---|
| **Self-report questionnaires** | |
| La Trobe Communication Questionnaire (LCQ) | 30-item, self- and other-report questionnaire specifically designed to address communication problems after TBI. Good internal and test-retest reliability have been demonstrated. |
| The Social Communication Skills Questionnaire (SCSQ) | Self-report questionnaire designed to address communication and social skills problems after TBI. Information on psychometric properties is unavailable. |
| **Social problem-solving measures** | |
| Assessment of Interpersonal Problem-Solving Skills (AIPSS) | 13 video vignettes, 10 of which depict a social problem situation, are viewed with evaluation of problem identification, generation of alternative responses, and performance of response. |
| Social Problem-Solving Inventory (SPSI) | 70-item measure of social problem solving comprised of two scales: problem orientation and problem-solving skills. Items are self-statements depicting either positive (facilitative) or negative (inhibitive) responses to real-life problem-solving situations. Adequate reliability and validity demonstrated. |
| **Measures of receptive communication skills** | |
| Florida Affect Battery (FAB) | The battery consists of 10 subtests (5 facial, 3 prosodic, and 2 cross-modal), assessing perception of five different emotions (happiness, sadness, anger, fear, neutral) |
| The Awareness of Social Inference Test (TASIT) | Three subtests composed of audiovisual vignettes which measure one's ability to name 7 basic emotions, to interpret conversational remarks that are either sincere or sarcastic, and to interpret conversational remarks in which speaker is either lying to be kind or is being sarcastic. Good test-retest reliability and validity. Austrailan actors perform vignettes, thus language accent may impact performance of U.S. respondents. |
| **Behavioral rating scales:** | |
| Profile of Pragmatic Impairments in Communication (PPIC) | 10 feature summary scales along with 84 specific behavior items that assess the frequency of various communication behaviors. The feature summary scales have been found to have acceptable inter-rater reliabilities, high internal consistency, and high concurrent validity. |

*continues*

| **Table 10–1.** *continued* | |
|---|---|
| Behaviorally-Referenced Rating System of Intermediate Social Skills-Revised (BRISS-R) | The BRISS-R provides an intermediate level coding system of social skills provides qualitative ratings of specific behavioral components of social skill, each of which are rated on a 7-point scale ranging from "very appropriate" to "very inappropriate." Behaviors are both verbal and nonverbal in nature. |
| Behavioral rating scales for TBI interactions[a]: | |
| Measure of Support in Conversation (MSC)[a] | A measure of communication partner's ability to acknowledge and reveal communicative competence in the individual with TBI |
| Measure of Participation in Conversation (MPC)[a] | A measure of the individual with TBI's ability to participation in interactional and transactional elements of conversation |

*Sources:* Strutchen (n.d., p. 5) [a]Adapted Kagan Scales (Kagen et al., 2004); Togher, Power, Tate, et al., 2010).

first to glean areas of strengths and potential challenge in social communication for the client. Then some of those areas can be targeted for reflection within a communication journal or log. Appendix 10–1 shows a sample data collection sheet that can be modified for this purpose. The SLP can collaborate with the client to identify good times for this self-observation (during specific periods of the day, while performing specific tasks, etc.). As with all aspects of self-reflection, this would begin with and include ongoing conversations with the client about the nature of social communication in general and specific to the client's daily tasks and unique needs/skills.

Overall self-assessment after self-observation is also valuable. Using a framework based on levels of awareness (Flashman, Amador, & McAllister, 1998), this self-assessment could include reflection on: (1) the nature of a specific deficit (knowledge); (2) the source of the deficit/difficulty (attributes); (3) how the individual feels about that deficit/difficulty (emotion); and (4) how that deficit/difficulty affects daily

tasks (impact). Appendix 10–2 contains a sample worksheet for overall reflection and discussion between the SLP and the client in the area of social communication. As above, this could also be tailored to specific areas of reflection, applicable to the client's needs and abilities, and pursued after an effective and trusting therapeutic relationship has been established between the client and the SLP (Flashman & McAllister, 2002). Individuals with ongoing strong negative emotions in this area should be referred to a psychologist or neuropsychologist team member for additional support (American Speech-Language-Hearing Association, 2003).

## b. Social Communication Training (SCT)

## Candidacy Recommendations

Recommendations within this chapter are tailored to *group-based* applications of Social Communication Training (SCT). This is where the strongest evidence exists (Finch, Copley, Cornwell, & Kelly, 2016; Togher, Wiseman-Hakes, et al., 2014); however, where applicable, it may be beneficial to also incorporate individual sessions as a means of monitoring personalized goals and reinforcing information and strategies taught in group sessions. In these cases, many of the same principles can be applied in a one-on-one session. Techniques discussed relative to Constructive Feedback Awareness Training (CFAT, Chapter 9d, Executive Function and Awareness) may also apply.

Based on a composite of research in this area (Dahlberg et al., 2007; Togher et al., 2009, 2013; Togher, McDonald, Tate, Rietdijk, et al., 2016), group-based SCT is recommended in the post-acute stages after TBI for:

1. **Individuals who experience difficulties in social communication in real-world contexts.** Table 10–1 contains a list of suggested measures in the area of social communication, including self-report questionnaires, receptive communication and social problem-solving measures, and behavioral rating scales. In addition, an adapted version of the Kagan scales for use with individuals with TBI is available in Appendix 10–3 for this purpose. It is recommended that assessment be conducted from a variety of perspectives (self-report, direct observation, communication partner rating) and given communication requiring different communication acts, in different communication environments (Braden, 2014). Dahlberg and colleagues (2007) suggest that SCT is applicable for individuals with some aspect of difficulty in social communication (either self-report or given reports of a significant other), while

Togher and colleagues recommends training be completed with individuals with "significant and chronic social skills deficits including any of the following criteria: awkwardness in social interactions, apparent disregard or lack of awareness of social cues and inappropriate responding, and [those] which were judged to be interfering with the person's everyday communication by the person who was referring the participant or by themselves or their family member" (2013, p. 639).

2. **For treatment that will focus on the communication partner, individuals who have a regular communication partner with whom they interact on a daily basis is recommended** (Togher, 2013).

3. **Individuals whose memory/cognition, speech/language, and behavior are sufficient for successful participation in a group context.** Recommendations in these areas include:

   a. *Memory/Cognition:* Dahlberg and colleagues (2007) recommend that individuals demonstrate "recall of day-to-day events sufficient for learning in the group setting" (p. 1563). These researchers also suggest individuals who are at or above Rancho Los Amigos Level VI.

   b. *Speech/Communication:* In the area of communication, Dahlberg et al. (2007) recommended individuals who have receptive and expressive communication skills equivalent to a 5 or higher on the comprehension and expression items of the Functional Independence Measure (FIM) instrument. Individuals with sufficient speech intelligibility and language processing for group context is also recommended (Dahlberg et al., 2007; Togher, McDonald, Tate, Power, et al., 2009, 2013; Togher, McDonald, Tate, Rietdijk, et al., 2016).

c. *Behavior:* Individuals without behavioral concerns (e.g., frustration tolerance, behavioral/anger control) that would impact successful group participation are recommended.

## Treatment Evidence

There is Level A evidence to support the use of "interventions to address patient-identified goals for social communication deficits . . . measured at the level of participation in everyday social life" (Figure 10–1; Togher, McDonald, Tate, Power, & Rietdijk, 2014, p. 357).

## Theoretical Frame

Theoretical frames within SCT vary, but in general, more recent group-based, context-

sensitive SCT employs predominantly calibration and compensation techniques (Figure 10–2). In a comprehensive review of approaches specific to SCT, Struchen noted commonalities among SCT techniques, such as "feedback, self-monitoring, modeling, behavioral rehearsal, role-play, and social reinforcement" (2014, p. 216). The initial aspects of this description (feedback and self-monitoring) are consistent with

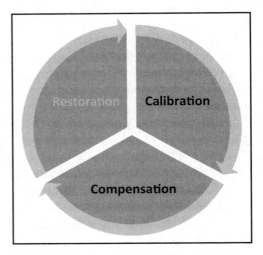

**Figure 10–2.** Theoretical frames of treatment approaches using SCT.

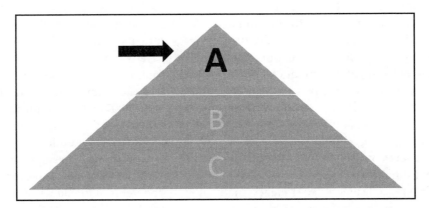

**Figure 10–1.** Level A evidence for the use of group Social Communication Training. Level A consists of "recommendation supported by at least one meta-analysis, systematic review or randomized controlled trial study of appropriate size and relevant control group" (Bayley et al., 2014, p. 295).

metacognitive approaches and are thereby described as calibration within this text. SCT approaches also target communication strategy (compensation), through the latter components of Strutchen's description above (modeling, behavioral rehearsal, role-play, and social reinforcement). This is also a key facet of SCT for both communication partners and individuals with TBI.

## Background Introduction

MacDonald and Wiseman-Hakes (2010) defined social communication intervention as "treatments that target discourse, pragmatics, conversation, social communication, non-verbal communications (eye contact, facial expression, proxemics or personal space, gesture) social perception (theory of mind, listener's perspective etc.). Interventions which target self-regulation or regulation of communication behaviours." (p. 490)

Initial efforts in this area utilized social skills training approaches, which primarily sought to teach social skills in a decontextualized manner, with the assumption that those skills would transfer and generalize to real-world settings (Ylvisaker, Turkstra, & Coelho, 2005). More recent research, however, has addressed the needs of individuals with TBI relative to self-regulation, self-awareness, and social perception deficits (rather than knowledge deficits), by focusing more on self-control strategies and opportunities for guided communication practice in more real-world settings (MacDonald & Wiseman-Hakes, 2010). In general, current approaches in this area include two basic avenues of training: (1) teaching people with TBI with the skills necessary for successful social interaction and (2) teaching the communication partners of people with TBI to use strategies for promoting

more successful interactions (Togher et al., 2009, p. 109).

Although many forms of communication exist, the communications addressed in SCT are conversational in nature (versus narrative or procedural) (Togher, 2014). As such, the core foundations of SCT are those inherent in the definition of conversation as "a two-way process where sharing of information takes place based as an interactionally negotiated achievement" (Togher, 2014, p. 337). This bears a moment of reflection. Conversation is fluid and determined by three key facets: the partners in the conversation, the setting in which the conversation takes place, and the meaning of the information conveyed within the conversation (Togher, 2014). SCT seeks to address all three aspects. This is perhaps why group approaches in this area have shown the strongest evidence, as they offer the potential to address each of these aspects. It is also perhaps why in recent years the role of the communication partner has received greater attention in the research literature, as an informant about the nature and scope of communication with an individual with TBI, but also, importantly, as a partner in the intervention process, either via direct communication partner training (Togher et al., 2009, 2013, 2016) or given an active and collaborative role with the clinician and client when SCT is directed toward the individual with TBI (Dahlberg et al., 2007).

## Treatment in Action

The discussion of group SCT, described here, will be formatted according to training steps outlined in *TBI Express* (Togher, McDonald, Tate, et al., 2010); however, the content of this section will focus on a general framework for SCT that includes other SCT models, such as *Group-Interactive*

*Structured Treatment (GIST) Social Competency Training* (Dahlberg et al., 2007). It contains parallel discussion of group-based SCT sessions, directed at either the communication partner or the individual with TBI, as similar principles apply. Procedures are broken down into four steps, illustrated in Figure 10–3. Their applicable components/ goals and procedures are listed in Table 10–2 and coincide with training specific to the individual with TBI or that targeted at the communication partner. In addition, Dahlberg and colleagues (2007) recommend that SCT comprise *in general* the following key elements:

1. The use of co-group leaders from different clinical backgrounds (i.e., social work and speech pathology), to allow different clinical perspectives, role models, and collaboration between clinicians with different expertise.

2. An emphasis on self-awareness and self-assessment, leading to individual goal setting.
3. Use of the group process to foster interaction, feedback, problem solving, a social support system, and awareness that one is not alone (p. 1564).

### Step 1: Establish Baselines

The first step of training (Establishing Baseline) focuses on thorough assessment of the social communication skills and interpersonal relationship between the individual with TBI and his/her communication partners. The goal of this step is to utilize assessment procedures to establish data that will: (1) be used in measuring treatment outcomes, and (2) serve as a tool to help promote client awareness of conversational contributions and potential inadequacies (verbal and nonverbal). Both are critical for

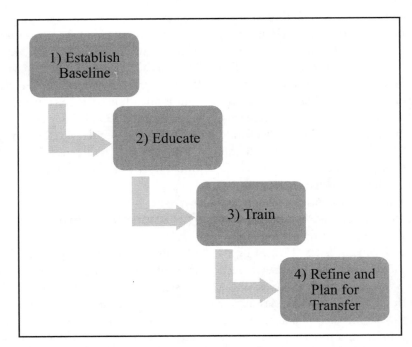

**Figure 10–3.** The essential steps in Social Communication Training.

**Table 10–2.** Steps and Components in Social Communication Training

| Step | Components/Goal(s) | Applicable Procedures |
|------|--------------------|-----------------------|
| **Step 1: Establish Baselines** | Assess | Discourse analysis<br>Questionnaires/interview<br>Observation |
| | Promote awareness | Self-predictions<br>Review testing results<br>Video/audio feedback |
| | Set goals | Collaborative and parallel goal setting |
| **Step 2: Educate** | Introduce aims of training and group guidelines<br>Establish home practice expectations | Handouts and group discussion<br>Set up audio/video recorders |
| | Education on TBI, cognition & communication | Handouts and group discussion |
| | Education on communication roles & rules as well as general communication strategies<br>Identifying barriers to successful communication in everyday life | Handouts and group discussion<br>Video examples<br>Group discussion and self-reflection |
| **Step 3: Train** | Social skills training | Practice and repetition<br>Feedback and discussion |
| | Treatment of emotional perception deficits | Videotaping interactions<br>Self-monitoring<br>Generalization of skills<br>   –Homework<br>   –Community outings |
| | Partner communication training<br>   Collaboration<br>   Elaboration<br>   Helpful Questions | Scaffolding and discussion<br>   –Memory log<br>   –Photographs |
| **Step 4: Refine and Plan for Transfer** | Refresh and reinforce information learnt | Practice of each technique<br>Group feedback and discussion<br>Homework |

the purposes of collaboratively generating treatment goals and measuring their attainment throughout SCT.

Prior to SCT, it is important for the individual with TBI to have completed a comprehensive battery of neuropsychological assessments in the area of cognition (Braden, 2014; Strutchen, n.d.). This provides for clear understanding of the client's cognitive-communication profile (i.e., deficits in attention, memory, executive function, and social cognition). Appendix 10–4 contains a list of suggested neuropsychological assessments in the area of cognition for this purpose.

Once the SLP has obtained baseline measures of cognitive abilities, assessment of specific social communication skills and perceptions of communicative ability can commence. Assessment can involve self-report questionnaires, social problem-solving measures, measures of receptive communication skills, and behavioral rating scales (Braden, 2014). Performance ratings of interactions with everyday communication partners should also be obtained across a variety of partners and contexts. Appendix 10–3 contains the Adapted Kagan scales (i.e., Measure of Support in Conversation [MSC] and Measure of Participation in Conversation [MPC]) (Kagan et al., 2004; Togher, Power, Tate, McDonald, & Rietdijk, 2010). This is a valuable tool for this purpose. These scales, originally developed to capture elements of conversation between adults with aphasia and speaking partners (Kagen et al., 2004), have been modified to specifically focus on the skills of communication partners in providing conversational support to individuals with TBI (Togher, Power, Tate, et al., 2010, p. 922). The Adapted Kagan MPC and MSC scales focus on the contributions of *both* participants in a conversational interaction and are sensitive to detecting change following social communication training (Togher, Power, Tate, et al., 2010; Togher et al., 2013). Other measures in this area are listed at the start of this chapter (see Table 10–1). Finally, in addition to measures listed thus far, it is recommended that the SLP incorporate additional systematic observation, conversational analysis, and use of elicitation tasks to "illuminate specific pragmatic behaviors of interest" (Sohlberg & Mateer, 2001, p. 312).

An important aspect of SCT is that of raising the client's awareness of his or her social communication difficulties (Dahlberg et al., 2007). Eventually, the individual will be taught to monitor the behavior of *others* as a means to regulate his or her own communication. As such, fostering awareness of one's *own* behaviors (verbal and nonverbal) is an important prerequisite skill to be developed within SCT. As Keohane and Prince (2017) note, "for some clients, increasing their awareness of their communication behavior is enough to prompt a change in that behavior. For others, the process of building awareness will allow clearer goals for intervention and therefore clarity about the desired outcomes." (p. 145) One way the clinician can promote awareness is through assessment. For example, if the SLP explains formal assessments throughout the evaluation process, a review of results may contribute to the development of intellectual awareness (Keohane & Prince, 2017, p. 142). Alternatively, it may be helpful to set up simple tasks wherein clients make predictions about expected performance and receive feedback based on actual performance.

Videotaping client performance may also facilitate this process. In this respect, the principles within Constructive Feedback Awareness Training (CFAT), discussed in Chapter 9 (Executive Function and Awareness), are also relevant. When training communication partners, the support measure, MSC, within the Adapted Kagan scales (Appendix 10–3) can be used as a means to provide concrete feedback to the conversation partner and bring about awareness (Kagen et al., 2004, p. 75). Once the individual with TBI and/or communication partners demonstrates some level of awareness, discussions can focus on establishing meaningful goals.

Within SCT, the SLP should dedicate initial sessions to focus on the identification of specific individual goals to work on during treatment (Dahlberg et al, 2007). Goal setting should be a collaborative process between the individual with TBI, the SLP, and/or family members in order to develop goals that are personally relevant and which have the potential to maximize motivation for treatment (Haskins et al., 2012, p. 113). In partner communication training, the goals for participants with TBI and their communication partners should be parallel. For example, if the goal for the individual with TBI is to initiate new topics in conversations, the parallel goal may be for the communication partner to allow the person with TBI to take more turns in conversation (Togher et al., 2009, 2013, 2016). Dahlberg and colleagues (2007) recommend that individuals with TBI formulate two or three specific social communication

skills goals. Samples of SCT goals for training focused on the individual with TBI are listed in Table 10–3.

## Step 2: Educate

The next step in SCT (Educate) includes education directed at learning the aims of training, group guidelines, home practice expectations, and educational lessons on TBI, cognition, and communication (Dahlberg et al., 2007; Togher, McDonald, Tate, et al., 2010). The goal of this step is to provide participants with enough foundational knowledge and awareness to facilitate successful strategy learning in Step 3 and to prime the participant's expectations for parameters of sessions to follow.

In this step, the SLP first provides education on the overarching goals and potential benefits of treatment participation. In training programs focusing solely on the individual with TBI, aims of training are to help the client better understand others and what others mean to communicate, as well as to better express one's own thoughts

| Target Area | Sample Goal |
| --- | --- |
| Cognition | I will remain attentive and participate in the conversation for a 15-minute period |
| Interpersonal | I will be able to name 3 places to meet new people, and will visit 1 of these places |
| Language | I will be able to maintain the topic of conversation for 5 minutes during a group conversation, without jumping to a new topic |
| Speech | I will speak slowly enough to be understood at least 90% of the time |
| Self-awareness | I will be able to name my social skill strengths and weaknesses |

**Table 10–3.** Sample SCT Goals

*Source:* Dahlberg et al., (2007, p. 1564).

and feelings to others in a way that they can understand (Dahlberg et al., 2007; Struchen, n.d.). Alternatively, in partner-training programs, aims are to teach the communication partner how to facilitate interactions with their relative or friend with TBI through use of "positive" communication strategies (Togher, 2014). The SLP will additionally shape expectations for the group session by introducing the general structure and format of the sessions. Dahlberg et al. (2007) recommends that generally, each session proceed as follows (p. 1565):

1. Review of homework
2. Brief introduction of the topic
3. Guided discussion
4. Small group practice
5. Group problem solving and feedback
6. Homework

Opportunities to practice learned strategies in natural environments, with homework embedded in the rehabilitation process, is critical (Haskins et al., 2012). Therefore, during Step 2, it is important for the clinician to outline homework requirements and provide training in any necessary materials needed for successful completion of home tasks. For example, Togher and colleagues recommend homework for communication partners which requires them to audio- or videotape conversations with the person with TBI as a means of practicing skills and strategies (Togher et al., 2016). As such, introductory sessions ensure that participants are provided with or have access to such equipment and other information needed to complete assignments.

Once the SLP has informed participants of treatment protocols and requirements, general education on TBI, cognition, and social communication should begin. A variety of educational methods and formats can be used to facilitate the client learning process. Examples include, but are not limited to, use of PowerPoint presentations, video examples, group discussion, group activity, and handouts. The SLP should dedicate adequate time to introduce concepts related to brain injury, communication, and the impact of brain injury on communication (Dahlberg et al., 2007; Togher et al., 2009). This facilitates understanding about how cognitive profiles and emotional responses can both negatively and positively affect communication (Keohane & Prince, 2017). For example, the SLP might encourage clients to consider how difficulties in attention may make skills such as listening more challenging after brain injury (Keohane & Prince, 2017). The SLP can discuss why listening skills are important when communicating with others (e.g., to obtain and follow directions, to understand and/or follow stories and jokes) and share examples of possible consequences of not utilizing listening skills (e.g., less information retained, faulty interpretation of information or stories, conversation breakdown). Table 10–4 contains samples of suggested topics in this area.

Moreover, it is recommended that special attention be paid to topics of social communication deficits and social and emotional perception deficits, as well as barriers to successful conversations in everyday life. Step 3 will directly address these topics by training group members with the corresponding skills and strategies to overcome these challenges. For example, successful training in *TBI Express* requires communication partners to become aware of *their* role as "communication partners," and how their actions may serve as barriers and/or facilitators to effective communication (Togher, 2014). By providing examples of barriers to successful conversations, and common problems specifically observed in communication partner interactions, partners are more likely to identify patterns in their own behavior

| **Table 10–4.** Suggested Educational Topics and Content | |
|---|---|
| **Topic** | **Content** |
| Brain Injury | • What is TBI? (e.g., define term 'traumatic brain injury') |
| | • Epidemiology of this source so of disability and common causes |
| | • Basic anatomy of the skull and brain |
| | • How trauma impacts upon structures of brain |
| | • The process of recovery and stages of rehabilitation |
| | • The range of cognitive, physical, and behavioral symptoms that may impact social communication |
| | • Life changes associated with TBI (e.g., activities of daily living, work, leisure, marriage, and relationships) |
| | • Psychological reactions (e.g., depression, anxiety, low self-esteem) |
| | • How to observe and compare interaction of individuals with TBI to people who have not sustained brain injury |
| Brain Injury & Communication | • What is social communication? (e.g., define term) |
| | • Social communication deficits (e.g., poor eye contact, inability to take turns, difficult initiating conversation)[a] |
| | • Social and emotional perception deficits (e.g., inability to recognize nonverbal cues) |
| | • Cognitive problems affecting communication (e.g., communication problems resulting from memory deficits and information processing problems) |
| | • Language use within different communication contexts (e.g., different communication settings, and communication partners) |
| | • Different "genres" (e.g., casual conversation, discussion, exposition) |
| Effective Communication | • Different forms of communication (e.g., verbal and nonverbal) |
| | • Importance and purpose of conversation |
| | • Roles in communication and how communication roll affects outcomes of interactions |
| | • Barriers to successful conversations in everyday life[a] |
| | • General communication facilitation strategies (e.g., give the person plenty of time to respond, avoid background noise) |

[a]Important topics to address during education.

*Sources:* Behn, Togher, Power, & Heard, 2012; Togher, McDonald, Code, & Grant, 2004; SELF-STUDY MODULES, 2015.

which interfere with successful interactions. This contributes to an increased level of awareness in future interactions, which will most likely aid in the monitoring and/or changing of such behaviors. Table 10–5 provides examples of social communication deficits observed in individuals with TBI and examples of barriers to successful conversations (i.e., problems observed in communication-partner interactions).

**Table 10–5.** Common Social Communication Problems

| Problems Observed in Individuals After TBI | Problems Observed in Communication Partners' interactions[a] |
|---|---|
| **Verbal** | **Verbal & Nonverbal** |
| • Difficulty starting and ending conversations | • Overcompensating by speaking too slowly/quickly |
| • Difficulty selecting and changing conversation topic (e.g., getting stuck on a topic [perseveration]) | • Not giving individuals with TBI an opportunity to communicate |
| • Difficulty staying on topic (e.g., going off topic without finishing ideas [tangential]) | • Failing to provide natural consequences for communication successes (e.g., showing interest in topics introduced by person with TBI), or failures (e.g., giving non-verbal feedback that the person has been talking for too long) |
| • Difficulty inhibiting inappropriate communication behaviors (e.g., interrupting others; talking too much) | |
| • Difficulty with turn-taking | • Talking for the person |
| • Inappropriate volume or rate of speech | • Questioning the accuracy of responses (i.e., repeatedly checking accuracy of information provided during conversations) |
| • Difficulty using tone of voice to express meaning and feeling | |
| • Asking for clarification | |
| **Nonverbal** | • Asking testing questions (i.e., asking questions that the communication partner already knows that answer to) |
| • Difficulty showing feelings with facial expressions (i.e., flat affect) | • Failing to follow up information given by the person with TBI |
| • Inappropriate use of gestures (i.e., too many or not enough) | |
| • Poor eye contact | |
| • Standing too close to others | |
| • Not listening to others | |
| • Difficulty perceiving emotion through observing facial expressions or tone of voice[b] | |
| • Difficulty observing verbal and nonverbal cues needed to regulate one's own behavior[b] | |

*Note.* [a]Based on previous work of Togher, Hand, & Code, 1997; Togher et al., 2004; Ylvisaker, Feeny, & Urbanczyk, 1993, and Ylvisaker, Sellars, & Edelman, 1998 (as cited by Togher, McDonald, Tate, et al., 2009, 2010, 2013, 2016). [b]Emotion perception problems.

### *Step 3: Train*

The next step in SCT (Train) is communication training wherein participants receive treatment targeting common social communication and emotion perception problems observed in interactions (see Table 10–5).

Social communication skills training can address specific aspects of social behavior such as listening, starting and ending conversations, maintaining conversations, repairing conversations, turn-taking, verbal organizing, and using body language (Keohane & Prince, 2017). Too, it is recommended that social communication training be "enhanced by the inclusion of explicit training in social and emotional perception" (Haskins et al., 2012, p. 110).

Social and emotional perception training includes training in the perception of one's own emotions, in the perception of other's emotions (i.e., observing and interpreting verbal and nonverbal cues), and in regulating behavior based on these perceptions. Readers are referred to Table 10–6 for a description of several approaches or techniques that can be used to structure social communication skills training and emotion perception training. For additional details specific to partner communication training and "positive" communication strategies (i.e., collaboration, elaboration), the reader is referred to Appendix 10–5.

### Social Communication Skills Training.

The approaches listed in Table 10–7, individually and in combination, are implemented to address specific aspects of social behavior. To demonstrate utility of these techniques (e.g., role-play and rehearsal, video feedback), an example in how to teach clients in the identification of verbal and nonverbal behaviors, and use of verification techniques—as means to promote development of pro-social behaviors—is described.

Training in the identification of verbal and nonverbal behaviors enables *better understanding* of others and the meaning of what others intend to communicate (Struchen, n.d.). It is facilitated when communicators adopt an "active" listening style. An active, or *effective*, listening style is characterized by a genuine interest in "understanding what the other person is thinking, feeling, wanting, or what the message means," and involves actively checking or verifying understanding before responding with a new message (Keohane & Prince, 2017, p. 146). The process of verification may involve restating or paraphrasing the other's message to clarify spoken content and/or to ensure correct interpretation. The idea is that when a client is genuinely interested in understanding, he or she is engaged. This leads to observations and verification of social cues, which allow for more effective communication (i.e., to better initiate, maintain, and repair conversations).

The SLP can address concepts of active listening and development of "better understanding" through discussion. For example, the SLP might explain how active engagement, observation, and use of feedback processes (e.g., restating, paraphrasing) are used to facilitate transfer of information, which facilitates effective communication with others. Video examples of conversations between friends and family members are helpful tools that can also be employed to demonstrate what "active" communication styles look like. The SLP may also choose to share videos of passive or combative styles, which contrast with an active style. Together, the SLP and group members can begin to pinpoint verbal and nonverbal behaviors, which appear to show a person is engaged (e.g., laughing, nodding, asking questions) and those which may indicate otherwise (e.g., interrupting, poor eye contact) (Keohane & Prince, 2017, p. 146).

To help group members understand what is meant by "verbal behaviors" and/or "nonverbal behaviors," the SLP can use modeling, group brainstorming activities, role-play, and video examples. For example, in teaching the concept of nonverbal behaviors (e.g., nodding, smiling, eye contact), Keohane and Prince (2017) recommend playing a clip of a soap opera or drama with the sound turned down. While group members watch, the SLP can then ask, "How can we tell some of what the characters are communicating?" (p. 146). Alternatively, the SLP can provide participants with an

**Table 10–6.** Approaches to Treatment of Social Communication Deficits

| Approach | Description/Utility |
|---|---|
| Role-play and rehearsal | Repeated practice of skills in different communication situations can be very helpful. |
| Structured feedback | Receiving information from trusted individuals about what aspects of communicative performance went well and what aspects need to be worked on. Providing feedback immediately after a conversation takes place is most helpful. Feedback should be collaborative, include positive aspects of communication abilities as well as areas that need improvement, and remain oriented on communication goals being worked toward. |
| Use of audio- and videotaped interactions | Recording or videotaping preplanned scenarios or conversations and then playing them back can be very helpful in increasing awareness of communication strengths and weaknesses. |
| Use of observation sheets (self-monitoring) | Use of observation sheets to guide self-monitoring of performance is helpful in developing awareness for one's own communicative behaviors as well as for understanding the behaviors and emotional undertones of others. |
| Modeling | A therapist, group member(s), or communication partner can demonstrate ways to handle different communication situations. |
| Reinforcement | Providing praise and encouragement for positive communication behaviors can help. For some clients, setting up a system for the provision of material rewards may also be useful. For example, a client could earn tokens for each occasion in which he or she engaged in a positive behavior (e.g., initiating a conversation) or failed to exhibit a negative behavior (e.g., interrupting others) that could be collected and used to earn a reward (e.g., an article of clothing or a dinner out at a restaurant). |
| Homework | Exercises given as "homework" extend practice of communication skills learned in daily life, which is especially important for generalization. The more opportunities that a person can work on communication behaviors outside of therapy, the more likely that positive changes will be made. |
| Environmental modifications | Context-specific interventions that address modifications to the person's environment and use of supported relationships to address skill-building in the natural environment may help address problems with generalizing treatment effects to the community. |
| Scaffolding (e.g., scripts, memory logs, photographs) | Scaffolding procedures such as scripts can help individuals with TBI plan what they want to say. Additionally, use of memory logs and photographs can help individuals with TBI and communication partners organize information within a conversational exchange and potentially lighten the "cognitive load" placed on the person with TBI |

*Sources:* Struchen n.d., p. 6; Haskins et al., 2012, pp. 113–114; Sohlberg & Mateer, 2001.s

**Table 10–7.** Sample Activities for Training in Identification of Verbal and Nonverbal Behaviors

| Activity | Description |
|---|---|
| Brainstorming/ Group Discussion | • Have participant(s) brainstorm what they believe is meant by terms "verbal" and "nonverbal behaviors."<br>• Encourage participant(s) to think about family members and other people they know who use lots of nonverbal behavior or who do not use them at all. How does this affect interaction?[a]<br>• Encourage participants(s) to think of examples of people in the community who use lots of nonverbal behavior (e.g., mimes; those with Italian heritage; Teller the silent magician, from Penn and Teller [American entertainers])<br>• Have client's engage in conversation while trying to use nonverbal behaviors. Reflect on how it feels as both a listener and a speaker when these behaviors are used.[a] |
| Silent role-plays and games | • Have two clients silently role-play a preplanned scenario or written prompt, using *only* nonverbal behaviors. Ask group members to guess what was being communicated. Then have client's role-play the same scenario with dialogue and discuss differences.<br>• Set up a game of charades wherein clients take turns pantomiming familiar words or phrases. Have client(s) discuss nonverbal behaviors used. What gestures or actions helped to get the actor's point across? Where more gestures needed? |
| Video Feedback | • Have client(s) video record a conversation at home for homework, or with another group member during a session. Watch video with client(s) and/or group members to identify listening behaviors, what went well, and what could be improved. |
| Contrasting Video Clips | • Gather a collection short video clips demonstrating active listening behaviors (e.g., asking questions, nodding) and unfavorable listening behaviors (e.g., interrupting, disoriented body postures). Have clients practice discriminating between the two.<br>• Gather a collection of unfavorable listening behaviors, and have clients brainstorm alternative or replacement behaviors. What would they do differently? |
| Positive Reinforcement | • Set up a reward or token system. A client can earn tokens for each occasion he or she *uses* active listening styles or behaviors, or each occasion he or she *avoids* using unfavorable or combative listening behaviors (e.g., interrupting) |
| Checklists and Observation Sheets | • Have client(s) watch a video of two people engaged in conversation. Have them tally the number of behaviors (verbal or nonverbal) on an observation sheet. The SLP can simultaneously record observations to compare with the client's. This same activity can be done with a video of the client engaging in conversation (Self-monitoring).<br>• Have client(s) watch a short video clip and use a checklist to identify verbal or nonverbal behaviors. The SLP should watch the clip beforehand to tally the correct number of behaviors to be accounted for.<br>• Have client(s) take home an observation sheet and monitor the verbal and nonverbal behaviors of family members. This activity can be incorporated while the client(s) watches a favorite T.V. show or movie. |

*Note.* Author created/original table except . . . [a]Keohane & Prince, 2017, p. 146.

observation sheet to tally nonverbal or verbal behaviors observed (e.g., using a modified version of the form in Appendix 10–6), comparing observations and providing structured feedback at the video's end. The idea is to bring awareness to the presence of these behaviors in daily communication and to aid in understanding that use of communicative behaviors is not random or arbitrary, but serves a greater purpose; that is, to enhance communication.

The SLP should elaborate on how verbal and nonverbal behaviors can be used as cues, which may help clients pick up signs that a conversation is breaking down or is unbalanced, indicating the need to regulate behavior or "share the floor" (i.e., use better turn-taking). Teaching individuals in identifying verbal and nonverbal behavioral cues should be followed by opportunities to practice using these behaviors in their own conversations. For example, the SLP might engage participants in a role-play activity wherein practice involves ending conversations with others. This skill often combines use of verbal *and* nonverbal behaviors to get the right message across (e.g., getting up while saying, "Well, it was great catching up with you") (Keohane & Prince, 2017, p. 150). Therefore, it may be helpful for the SLP to provide a list of some verbal and nonverbal cues commonly used to end conversations, which participants can reference in role-play. The clinician should follow up with questions asking participants to consider how the use of behaviors in their own conversations feels and/or comes across. See Table 10–7 for more examples of activities to promote use and identification of verbal and nonverbal behaviors.

The ability to actively identify and use communicative behaviors is the first aspect in developing a more effective style of communication. The other component involves verifying understanding of a message by reflecting it back to the sender, which can be done through paraphrasing, asking questions for clarification, and summarizing (Keohane & Prince, 2017). The SLP can explain these concepts (e.g., "paraphrasing" involves repeating information using fewer words to convey the same meaning) and provide opportunities to practice. The SLP should model how to paraphrase or summarize information first before asking clients to practice alone. Example activities might include reading emails or excerpts from books and newspapers. As an alternative, the SLP can ask the client to summarize a TV program or movie that he/she has recently watched (Keohane & Prince, 2017).

When teaching participants to ask questions for clarification, the SLP might provide individuals with scripts or examples of clarifying phrases (e.g., "I beg your pardon?"; "What do you mean by . . . ?"; "Could you give me an example?"), which are to be remembered or kept as external supports (e.g., in the form of a handout or in an easy to access memory notebook). These verification techniques and supports can be used to reinforce communication skills, such as maintaining and repairing conversations. For example, clarifying phrases can be used to keep conversations going or remedy breakdowns in understanding. The SLP can provide clients with specific phrases (e.g., "I'm sorry, I am confused. Would you mind repeating that last part?"), which can be used to avoid or address these situations. Too, the SLP can engage participants in role-play to practice using the clarifying phrases, and provide video feedback so group members can observe how these phrases help the conversation.

**Emotion Perception Training.** Certain individuals with TBI may not benefit from traditional approaches described above because they lack the ability to recognize and interpret emotional cues derived from facial expression, body language, and tone of voice (i.e., nonverbal behaviors); however, "without these abilities, individuals will be unable to adjust their behavior in varying social contexts," and/or apply strategies learned in therapy (Haskins et al., 2012, p. 114). When this is the case, training in social and emotional perception may be an appropriate starting point. Training in social and emotional perception focuses on training the individual to increase judgment accuracy with specific patterns or changes in facial expressions, tone of voice, and body language as they relate to the nonverbal expression of emotion (Bornhofen & McDonald, 2008; Haskins et al., 2012). The SLP should begin by providing basic information on social communication (i.e., Step 2, Educate) with discussions to develop general knowledge of different emotional contexts. This might involve differentiating between various emotionally based scenarios (e.g., attending a funeral versus celebrating a birthday) and identifying or contrasting associated emotions (e.g., sadness and anger versus joy and excitement).

"In learning and practicing emotional perception skills, cues are hierarchically organized so that participants might be asked to judge static emotional cues from line drawings, then photographs, and then in videotapes" (Haskins et al., 2012, pp. 114–115). Too, practice activities should be graduated based on level of difficulty. For example, it may be more appropriate for the SLP to begin presenting emotional cues in one modality (e.g., visual), before presenting multiple modalities (e.g., visual and auditory) simultaneously (Bornhofen & Mcdonald, 2008; Haskins et al., 2012). Once participants demonstrate some comfort and/or success in discriminating emotions, the SLP can fine-tune emotional perception skills by training participants to *interpret* situational cues (e.g., interpret a speaker's emotional demeanor, body language, or tone of voice) (Haskins et al., 2012).

Two general strategies, errorless learning and self-instruction training, are often used to facilitate the learning process and improve emotion perception skill among individuals with TBI. Descriptions and examples of how these strategies might be used are provided in Table 10–8. Use of checklists and observation forms, like that provided in Appendix 10–6, can also be used in activities where participants are shown clips and asked to identify intention.

The best way to develop social communication skills, such as listening, and social emotional perception skills is through distributed and massed practice. The SLP should spend adequate time discussing, planning, and role-playing socially relevant scenarios and provide individuals with adequate opportunities to practice newly learned skills in natural settings through homework assignment (Keohane & Prince, 2017). Too, the SLP can make videos and include participants and/or communication partners in the feedback or review process to promote self-monitoring skills and enhance retention of learned material or skills.

## Step 4: Refine and Plan for Transfer

In the final sessions of social communication training, participants are to review information and techniques previously taught, revise application of techniques, and plan for ongoing practice (Behn et al., 2012; Togher, 2014, 2015; Togher, McDonald, Code, & Grant, 2004; Togher et al., 2013, 2016; ). In this step (Refine and Plan for Transfer), the SLP should engage clients in more intensive conversational practice (Togher, 2014) wherein participants respond to examples from pre-training literature with the use

**Table 10–8.** Learning Strategies for Training Emotion Perception

| Strategy | Definition/Goal | Example Application |
|---|---|---|
| Errorless Learning | • Involves closely guided instruction with repeated rehearsal and practice of newly learned information.<br>• The goal is to *not* allow the client(s) to make a mistake on which he or she may perseverate repeatedly. | • Participants are specifically instructed to respond only when *certain* of an answer. They are not to make guesses when they are unsure of an answer.<br>• E.g., if an individual is asked to identify an audiovisual emotion, but are not entirely sure whether the speaker portrays sadness or anger, the clinician should inform the client of the correct answer (e.g., anger) and replay the video clip. |
| Self-Instruction Training | • Involves equipping the individual with procedural steps that are to be verbalized as they complete a task.<br>• The goal is to learn the acronym, "WALTER" (or WALT, a shorted version): (1) **W**hat am I deciding about?; (2) What do I **A**lready know about it?; (3) What do I need to **L**ook/**L**isten for? (4) **T**ry out my answer; (5) **E**valuate how it went (6) **R**eward myself for having a go | • The acronym "WALTER" is first used by the therapist, and eventually the participant as a strategic approach to emotion discrimination tasks.<br>• The participant is trained to use these self-guiding statements to intensify attention to discriminating emotions in a step-by-step manner, and to self-correct errors when they occur. |

*Sources:* Data from Haskins et al., 2012, p. 115 and Bornhofen & McDonald, 2008, p. 104.

of newly learned techniques (Togher et al., 2004). Concurrently, the clinician should provide feedback with extensive review of guiding principles to assist individuals with brain injury and their communication partner(s) in monitoring performance and individual contributions to interactions. In a group setting, this can be facilitated through small group activities; dyads can take turns role-playing a conversational exchange, and feedback can be provided through group discussion.

The goal is for individuals to approach interactions with improved awareness of how *both* participants in a conversation contribute to the interactional exchange (Togher, 2014). Put another way, the participants should have established emotion perception skills, as well as monitoring techniques, which enable them to be more self-aware of their verbal and nonverbal behaviors, as well as the behavior of others. With this awareness, and feedback provided by the SLP and group members, the individual learns to make the necessary adjustments to facilitate more appropriate, effective, and enjoyable interactions. Practice should continue to extend into daily conversations through homework assignments and/or community outings. For example, the SLP might take group members on an outing to a coffee shop to observe or practice interactional skills. In this way, the client(s) can continue to refine and transfer conversational skills in more natural, real-world environments. During home application and throughout final training sessions, the SLP should encourage individuals to plan for ongoing practice. This may involve setting up a schedule to periodically revisit handouts and information learned in therapy, or incorporating use of external supports or reminders (e.g., visuals with strategies posted on a wall, diaries, written organizers) in environments where discourse commonly takes place.

## References

American Speech-Language-Hearing Association. (2003). *Evaluating and treating communication and cognitive disorders: Approaches to referral and collaboration for speech-language pathology and clinical neuropsychology* [Technical report]. Retrieved from http://www.asha.org/policy

Bayley, M., Tate, R., Douglas, J., Turkstra, L., Ponsford, J., Stergiou-Kita, M., . . . INGOG Expert Panel. (2014). INCOG guidelines for cognitive rehabilitation following traumatic brain injury: Methods and overview. *Journal of Head Trauma Rehabilitation, 29*(4), 290–306.

Behn, N., Togher, L., Power, E., & Heard, R. (2012). Evaluating communication training for paid carers of people with traumatic brain injury. *Brain Injury, 26*(13–14), 1702–1715.

Bergquist, T. F., & Jacket, M. P. (1993). Programme methodology: Awareness and goal setting with the traumatically brain injured. *Brain Injury 7*, 275–282.

Bornhofen, C., & McDonald, S. (2008). Comparing strategies for treating emotion perception deficits in traumatic brain injury. *Journal of Head Trauma Rehabilitation, 23*(2), 103–115.

Braden, C. (2014). Communication and social skills training. In S. McDonald, L. Togher, & C. Code (Eds.), *Social and communication disorders following traumatic brain injury* (2nd ed., pp. 307–335). Hove, East Sussex, UK: Psychology Press.

Dahlberg, C., Cusick, C., Hawley, L., Newman, J., Morey, C., Harrison-Felix, C. L., & Whiteneck, G. G. (2007). Treatment efficacy of social communication skills training after traumatic brain injury: A randomized treatment and deferred treatment controlled trial. *Archives of Physical Medicine and Rehabilitation, 88*(12), 1561–1573.

Ezrachi, O., Ben-Yishay, Y., & Kay, T. DiUer, L., & Rattock, J. (1991). Predicting employment in traumatic brain injury following neuropsychological rehabilitation. *Journal of Head Trauma Rehabilitation, 6,* 71–84.

Finch, E., Copley, A., Cornwell, P., & Kelly, C. (2016). Systematic review of behavioral interventions targeting social communication difficulties after traumatic brain injury. *Archives of Physical Medicine and Rehabilitation, 97*(8), 1352–1365.

Flashman, L. A., Amador, X., & McAllister, T. W. (1998). Lack of awareness of deficits in traumatic brain injury. *Seminars in Clinical Neuropsychiatry 3,* 201–210.

Flashman, L., & Mcallister, T. (2002). Lack of awareness and its impact in traumatic brain injury. *NeuroRehabilitation, 17*(4), 285–296.

Haskins, E. C., Shapiro-Rosenbaum, A., Dams-O'Connor, K., Eberle, R., Cicerone, K., & Langenbahn, D. (2012). Rehabilitation of impairments of social communication. In L. E. Trexler (Ed.), *Cognitive rehabilitation manual: Translating evidence-based recommendations into practice* (pp. 110–119). Reston, VA: American Congress of Rehabilitation Medicine.

Kagan, A., Winckel, J., Black, S., Duchan, J. F., Simmons-Mackie, N., & Square, P. (2004). A set of observational measures for rating support and participation in conversation between adults with aphasia and their conversation partners. *Topics in Stroke Rehabilitation, 11*(1), 67–83.

Keohane, C., & Prince, L. (2017). Communication. In R. Winson, B. A. Wilson, & A. Bateman

(Eds.), *The brain injury rehabilitation workbook* (pp. 139–166). New York, NY: Guilford Press.

MacDonald, S., & Wiseman-Hakes, C. (2010). Knowledge translation in ABI rehabilitation: A model for consolidating and applying the evidence for cognitive-communication interventions. *Brain Injury, 24*(3), 486–508.

Prigatano, G. P., Altman, I. M., & O'Brien, K. P. (1990). Behavioral limitations that brain injured patients tend to underestimate. *Clinical Neuropsychologist, 4*, 163–176.

Self-Study Modules. (2015). Retrieved from http://www.tbistafftraining.info/Home_SELF _STUDY.htm

Sohlberg, M. M., & Mateer, C. A. (2001). *Cognitive rehabilitation: An integrative neuropsychological approach.* New York, NY: Guilford Press.

Struchen, M. A. (n.d.). *Social communication and traumatic brain injury (TBI): A guide for professionals.* Retrieved from http://www.tbi community.org/resources/publications/pro fessional_education_social_comm.pdf

Struchen, M. A. (2014). Social communication interventions. In M. Sherer & A. M. Sander (Eds.), *Handbook on the neuropsychology of traumatic brain injury* (pp. 173–190). New York, NY: Springer.

Togher, L. (2014). Training communication partners of people with TBI: Communication really is a two-way process. In S. McDonald, L. Togher, & C. Code (Eds.), *Social and communication disorders following traumatic brain injury* (2nd ed., pp. 336–360). Hove, East Sussex, UK: Psychology Press.

Togher, L. (2015). *TBI Express partner training.* Retrieved from http://www.nchn.org.au/ a2k/docs/telehealthhandouts/handoutahtele healthtbiexpress10032015.pdf

Togher, L., Hand, L., & Code, C. (1997). Measuring service encounters in the traumatic brain injury population. *Aphasiology, 11*(4/5), 491–504.

Togher, L., McDonald, S., Code, C., & Grant, S. (2004). Training communication partners of people with traumatic brain injury: A randomised controlled trial. *Aphasiology, 18*(4), 313–335.

Togher, L., McDonald, S., Tate, R., Power, E., & Rietdijk, R. (2009). Training communication partners of people with traumatic brain injury: Reporting the protocol for a clinical trial. *Brain Impairment, 10*(2), 188–204.

Togher, L., McDonald, S., Tate, R., Power, E., & Rietdijk, R. (2010). *TBI Express: For people with TBI and their everyday conversational partners.* Sydney: Australian Society for the Study of Brain Impairment (ASSBI).

Togher, L., McDonald, S., Tate, R., Power, E., & Rietdijk, R. (2013). Training communication partners of people with severe traumatic brain injury improves everyday conversations: A multicenter single-blind clinical trial. *Journal of Rehabilitation Medicine, 45*, 637–645.

Togher, L., McDonald, S., Tate, R., Power, E., & Rietdijk, R. (2014). *TBI Express partner training.* Retrieved from http://sydney.edu .au/health-sciences/tbi-express/index.shtml

Togher, L., McDonald, S., Tate, R., Rietdijk, R., & Power, E. (2016). The effectiveness of social communication partner training for adults with severe chronic TBI and their families using a measure of perceived communication ability. *NeuroRehabilitation, 38*(3), 243–255.

Togher, L., Power, E., Tate, R., McDonald, S., & Rietdijk, R. (2010). Measuring the social interactions of people with traumatic brain injury and their communication partners: The Adapted Kagan Scales. *Aphasiology, 24*(6–8), 914–927.

Togher, L., Wiseman-Hakes, C., Douglas, J., Stergiou-Kita, M., Ponsford, J., Teasell, R., . . . Turkstra, L. S. (2014). INCOG recommendations for management of cognition following traumatic brain injury, Part iv: Cognitive communication. *Journal of Head Trauma Rehabilitation, 29*(4), 353–368.

Ylvisaker, M., Feeny, T. J., & Urbanczyk, B. (1993). Developing a positive communication culture for rehabilitation: Communication training for staff and family embers. In C. J. Durgin, N. D. Schmidt, & L. J. Fryer (Eds.), *Staff development and clinical intervention in brain injury rehabilitation* (pp. 57–81). Gaithersburg, MD: Aspen.

Ylvisaker, M., Sellars, M., & Edelman, L. (1998). Rehabilitation after traumatic brain injury in preschoolers. In M. Ylvisaker (Ed.), *Traumatic brain injury rehabilitation: Children and adolescents* (2nd ed., pp. 303–329). Newton, MA: Butterworth-Heinemann.

Ylvisaker, M., Turkstra, L. S., & Coelho, C. (2005). Behavioral and social interventions for individuals with traumatic brain injury: A summary of the research with clinical implications. *Seminars in Speech and Language, 26*(4), 256–267.

APPENDIX 10–1

## Self-Observation:  Social Communication

Client: _____

| Date/Time | Conversation:<br>What was the topic?<br>Who did I talk to?<br>Where was I? | How was my *turn-taking?*<br>Rate and describe[1] | How was my *eye contact?*<br>Rate and describe[1] | Is there anything I would do differently (or remember for next time)? |
|---|---|---|---|---|
| | | | | |
| | | | | |
| | | | | |
| | | | | |

1 = Good/Fair/Poor

# Self-Reflection: Social Communication

Client: _____

|  | KNOWLEDGE | | ATTRIBUTE | EMOTION | IMPACT | | |
|---|---|---|---|---|---|---|---|
|  | *What are my strengths?* | *What are my challenges?* | *What is causing difficulty in this area?* | *How do I feel about this?* | *How does this impact me in my daily life?* | *What things help?* | *What things make it more challenging?* |
| Topic Selection |  |  |  |  |  |  |  |
| Initiation |  |  |  |  |  |  |  |
| Nonverbal Communication (facial expressions and body language) |  |  |  |  |  |  |  |
| Organization |  |  |  |  |  |  |  |
| Turn-taking |  |  |  |  |  |  |  |

# Adapted Kagan Scales

| A. Acknowledging Competence | |
|---|---|
| **Natural adult talk appropriate to context** | • Feel and flow of natural adult conversation appropriate to context,<br>  ○ e.g., social chat vs. interview; respectful approach to verification (verifying that the conversation partner has understood rather than verifying that adult with brain injury knows what they want to say; not oververifying)<br>• Not patronizing (loudness, tone of voice, rate, enunciation)<br>• Appropriate emotional tone/use of humor<br>• Uses collaborative talk (rather than teaching/testing)<br>• Establishes equal leadership roles in the conversation<br>• Uses true questions rather than testing questions |
| **Sensitivity to partner** | • Incorrect/unclear responses handled respectfully by giving correct information in a non-punitive manner<br>• Sensitive to TBI's attempts to engage in conversation, confirms partner's contribution<br>• Encourage when appropriate, shows enthusiasm for partner's contribution<br>• Acknowledge competence when adult with brain injury is frustrated, e.g., "I know you know what you want to say," acknowledges difficulties<br>• "Listening attitude," demonstrates active listening (e.g., acknowledging, back-channeling)<br>• Takes on communicative burden as appropriate/making adult with brain injury feel comfortable<br>• Communicates respect for other person's concerns, perspectives and abilities<br>• Questions in a non-demanding, supportive manner<br>• Takes appropriate conversational turns |
| **Score MSC** *Acknow* **Comp:** | <br>  \|___\|___\|___\|___\|___\|___\|___\|___\|<br>  **0**  0.5  **1**  1.5  **2**  2.5  **3**  3.5  **4**<br>Not supportive    Basic skill in support    Highly skilled support |

| A. Acknowledging Competence Anchors | | |
|---|---|---|
| NONE | 0 | Competence of person with TBI **not acknowledged**. Patronizing. |
| | 1 | **Minimally acknowledges** competence of person with TBI. |
| BASIC | 2 | Basic level of skill. **Some acknowledgment** of the competence of person with TBI. |
| | 3 | **Mostly acknowledges** the competence of person with TBI. |
| HIGHLY | 4 | Interactionally outstanding. **Full acknowledgment** of the competence of the person with TBI. |

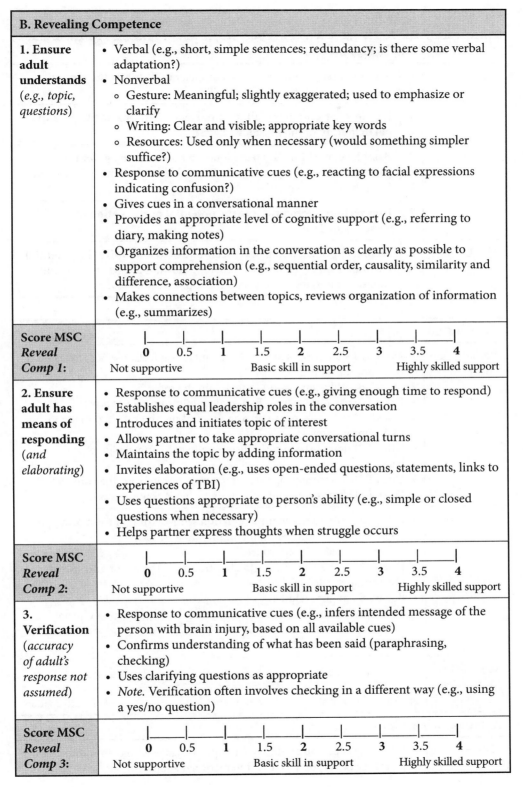

| B. Revealing Competence | |
|---|---|
| **1. Ensure adult understands** (*e.g., topic, questions*) | • Verbal (e.g., short, simple sentences; redundancy; is there some verbal adaptation?)<br>• Nonverbal<br>  ○ Gesture: Meaningful; slightly exaggerated; used to emphasize or clarify<br>  ○ Writing: Clear and visible; appropriate key words<br>  ○ Resources: Used only when necessary (would something simpler suffice?)<br>• Response to communicative cues (e.g., reacting to facial expressions indicating confusion?)<br>• Gives cues in a conversational manner<br>• Provides an appropriate level of cognitive support (e.g., referring to diary, making notes)<br>• Organizes information in the conversation as clearly as possible to support comprehension (e.g., sequential order, causality, similarity and difference, association)<br>• Makes connections between topics, reviews organization of information (e.g., summarizes) |
| **Score MSC Reveal Comp 1:** | \|____\|____\|____\|____\|____\|____\|____\|____\|<br>0   0.5   1   1.5   2   2.5   3   3.5   4<br>Not supportive     Basic skill in support     Highly skilled support |
| **2. Ensure adult has means of responding** (*and elaborating*) | • Response to communicative cues (e.g., giving enough time to respond)<br>• Establishes equal leadership roles in the conversation<br>• Introduces and initiates topic of interest<br>• Allows partner to take appropriate conversational turns<br>• Maintains the topic by adding information<br>• Invites elaboration (e.g., uses open-ended questions, statements, links to experiences of TBI)<br>• Uses questions appropriate to person's ability (e.g., simple or closed questions when necessary)<br>• Helps partner express thoughts when struggle occurs |
| **Score MSC Reveal Comp 2:** | \|____\|____\|____\|____\|____\|____\|____\|____\|<br>0   0.5   1   1.5   2   2.5   3   3.5   4<br>Not supportive     Basic skill in support     Highly skilled support |
| **3. Verification** (*accuracy of adult's response not assumed*) | • Response to communicative cues (e.g., infers intended message of the person with brain injury, based on all available cues)<br>• Confirms understanding of what has been said (paraphrasing, checking)<br>• Uses clarifying questions as appropriate<br>• *Note.* Verification often involves checking in a different way (e.g., using a yes/no question) |
| **Score MSC Reveal Comp 3:** | \|____\|____\|____\|____\|____\|____\|____\|____\|<br>0   0.5   1   1.5   2   2.5   3   3.5   4<br>Not supportive     Basic skill in support     Highly skilled support |

*continues*

| B. Revealing Competence Anchors | | |
|---|---|---|
| NONE | 0 | **No use of techniques** to reveal competence. **Inhibits the potential participation** of the person with TBI. |
| | 1 | **Low level of skill** in revealing competence. **Minimizes the potential participation** of the person with TBI. |
| SOME | 2 | **Basic level of skill**. Uses techniques to **maintain the potential participation** of the person with TBI. Able to get some information from the person with TBI. |
| | 3 | **Uses techniques to promote the potential participation** of the person with TBI. |
| FULL | 4 | Technically outstanding. **Uses techniques to maximize the potential participation** of the person with TBI. May not always succeed, but applies techniques flexibly and in a sophisticated way. |

| A. Interaction | |
|---|---|
| **Verbal/ vocal** | • Does TBI share responsibility for maintaining feel/flow of conversation (incl: appropriate affect)?<br>• Does TBI add information to maintain the topic?<br>• Does TBI ask questions of ECP which follow up on the topic?<br>• Does TBI use appropriate turn-taking (taking their turn, passing turn to ECP appropriately)?<br>• Does TBI demonstrate active listening (e.g., acknowledging, back-channeling)?<br>• Does TBI choose appropriate topics and questions for the context?<br>• Does TBI show communicative intent even if content is poor? |
| **Nonverbal** | • Does TBI initiate/maintain interaction with CP or make use of supports offered by CP to initiate/maintain interaction?<br>• Is TBI pragmatically appropriate?<br>• Does TBI ever acknowledge the frustration of the CP or acknowledge their competence/skill?<br>• Behaviors might include:<br>  ○ Appropriate eye contact, use of gesture, body posture, and facial expression, use of writing or drawing in any form, use of resource material |
| **Score MPC Interaction:** | \|___\|___\|___\|___\|___\|___\|___\|___\|<br>**0**   0.5   **1**   1.5   **2**   2.5   **3**   3.5   **4**<br>No participation at all     Some participation     Full participation |
| **A. Interaction Anchors** | |
| NONE   0 | **No participation at all**. No attempt to engage with communication partner or respond to their interactional attempts. |

| | 1 | Person with TBI beginning to take **occasional responsibility for sharing the conversational interaction**, in order to achieve the purpose of the task. |
|---|---|---|
| SOME | 2 | Person with TBI making **clear attempts to share the conversational interaction some of the time**, in order to achieve the purpose of the task. |
| | 3 | Person with TBI **taking increased responsibility most of the time** for sharing the conversational interaction, in order to achieve the purpose of the task. |
| FULL | 4 | Person with TBI has **full and appropriate participation**. Takes responsibility for sharing the conversational interaction, in order to achieve the purpose of the task. |

| **B. Transaction** |
|---|
| **Verbal/ vocal and Nonverbal** | <ul><li>Does TBI maintain exchange of information, opinions and feelings with CP, by sharing details or by inviting CP to share details (i.e., is there good content and more than intent alone)?</li><li>Does TBI present information in an organized way?</li><li>Does TBI provide an appropriate amount of information?</li><li>Does TBI ask clarifying questions when necessary?</li><li>Does TBI ever initiate transaction?<ul><li>Introducing or referring back to a previous topic</li><li>Spontaneously using a compensatory technique</li></ul></li><li>Does content of transaction appear to be accurate (depending on context and purpose of rating, rater would have more/less access to means of verification of information)?</li><li>Does TBI use support offered by CP for purpose of transaction? E.g., referring to a list/diary, using the organization of the conversation provided by CP (e.g., responding to closed choice questions)</li></ul> |

| **Score MPC** *Transaction*: | |_____|_____|_____|_____|_____|_____|_____|_____| <br> 0    0.5    1    1.5    2    2.5    3    3.5    4 <br> No participation at all    Some participation    Full participation |
|---|---|

| **B. Transaction Anchors** | | |
|---|---|---|
| NONE | 0 | **No evidence** of person with TBI **conveying content**, in order to achieve the purpose of the task. |
| | 1 | Person with TBI **occasionally conveying content**, in order to achieve the purpose of the task. |
| SOME | 2 | Person with TBI is **conveying some content**, in order to achieve the purpose of the task. |
| | 3 | Person with TBI is **conveying content most of the time**, in order to achieve the purpose of the task. |
| FULL | 4 | Person with TBI **consistently conveys content** in order to achieve the purpose of the task. |

*Source:* Togher, Power, Tate, McDonald, & Rietdijk (2010). Copyright © Taylor and Francis. Used with permission.

# Communication and Neuropsychological Assessment for Individual with TBI

| Measure | Description |
|---|---|
| *Scales of Cognitive Ability for Traumatic Brain Injury* (SCATBI) | A measure of cognitive and linguistic skills, involving five subtests assessing areas of underlying impairment (Perception/ Discrimination, Orientation, Organization, Recall, and Reasoning). |
| *Functional Assessment of Verbal Reasoning and Executive Strategies* (FAVRES) | A measure of cognitive-communication difficulties assessing the ability to participate in functional communication contexts, involving four complex verbal reasoning tasks that simulate everyday situations and require processing of text and discourse. |
| *Wechsler Adult Intelligence Scale®—Third Edition* (WAIS III) | Provides measures of premorbid ability, verbal reasoning, working memory, and information processing speed. |
| *Wechsler Memory Scale®—Third Edition* (WMS III) | A measure of ability for new learning. |
| *Wisconsin Card Sorting Test®* (WCST) | A measure of executive functioning and reasoning. |
| *Controlled Oral Word Association Test* (CFL) | A measure of executive functioning, flexibility, and inhibition. |
| *The Trail Making Test A and B* (TMT A and B) | A measure of attention focusing and shifting, and cognitive flexibility. |
| *Rey Figure* | A measure of planning and nonverbal memory. |

*Source*: Togher, McDonald, Tate, Power, & Rietjikik (2009, p. 193).

# Positive Communication Strategies for Communication Partner Training

| Strategy | Aim | Components | Examples/Application |
|---|---|---|---|
| Collaboration: *"We are doing this together, as a cooperative project"* | Focuses on techniques that help conversations to be a collaborative, more equal and organized process. It also helps communicative partners provide structure and support to the person with TBI for their conversations. | • Collaborative intent: *"We're doing this together"* <br><br> • Cognitive support: *"What can help make this easier?"* <br><br> • Emotional support: *"I'm with you, it's OK"* <br><br> • Positive question style: *I'm interested in what you have to say'* <br><br> • Collaborative turn-taking: *"I'm interested in sharing conversation"* | Collaborative intent: <br> • Partner shares information; does not just demand it <br> • Partner uses collaborative talk (e.g., "Let's try to remember the day we . . .", "I enjoy thinking about these things with you.") <br> • Partner confirms partner's contributions ("That's right, that was next.") <br><br> Cognitive Support: <br> • Partner gives information when needed (within statements or questions) <br> • Partner makes available memory and organization supports (e.g., photos, memory book, gestures) <br> • Partner gives cues in a conversational manner <br> • Partner responds to errors by giving correct information in a non-threatening, non-punitive manner <br><br> Emotional Support: <br> • Partner respects others' concerns <br> • Partner explicitly acknowledges difficulty of the task (e.g., "It's hard to put all these things in order, isn't it?") <br><br> Positive question style: <br> • See *"Asking Questions"* below |

*continues*

**Appendix 10–5.** *continued*

| Strategy | Aim | Components | Examples/Application |
|---|---|---|---|
| Collaboration *continued* | | | Collaborative turn-taking:<br><br>• Partner takes appropriate conversational turns<br>• Partner avoids speaking for the individual<br>• Partner helps individual express thoughts when struggle occurs (word finding difficulties) |
| Elaboration:<br>*"I am going to help you organize and extend your thoughts"* | Focuses on the concept of keeping conversations going by exploring techniques that help to organize and link topics, with use of both questions and comments. This strategy assists communication partners to scaffold conversations for the person with TBI without taking over the conversation. | • Elaboration of topics: *"We'll choose topics which keep things going—in this conversation and into the future"*<br><br>• Elaboration of organization: *"I'll help organize the conversation so we can talk in more detail"* | Elaboration of topics:<br><br>• Partner introduces and initiates topics of interest that can go further<br>• Partner maintains the topic for many turns (e.g., repeats partner; affirms partner's contribution; adds information; asks open questions; reviews topic; expresses interest; if necessary, corrects partner in nonthreatening manner)<br>• Partner invite elaboration (e.g., "I wonder what happened . . .")<br><br>Elaboration of organization:<br><br>• Partner tries to organize information clearly<br>  o sequential order (e.g., "First, we . . ., then we . . .")<br>  o physical causality (e.g., "It looks broken because you dropped it"),<br>  o psychological causality (e.g., "You ran because you were scared")<br>  o similarity and difference (e.g., "Yes, they are similar because . . .")<br>  o analogy and association (e.g., "That reminds me of . . . because . . .") |

| Strategy | Aim | Components | Examples/Application |
|---|---|---|---|
| Elaboration: *continued* | | | Elaboration of organization: *continued*<br>• Partner makes connections when topics change<br>• Partner makes connection among day-to-day conversational themes<br>• Partner reviews organization of information |
| Asking Questions: *"What can I ask to help you contribute?"* | Explores the use of appropriate and helpful questions to start and keep conversations going. For the communication partners, this strategy addresses how to avoid negative or "testing" questions and instead focus on a positive questioning style. Explores the role of questions in conversation. | • Positive questioning style<br>• Negative or "testing" questions (e.g., questions that the partner already knows that answer to) | • When questions are used, they are used in a non-demanding and supportive manner ("What do you need to do that?")<br>• Partner uses specific questions that include cues, if necessary (e.g., "Did we go swimming next?" versus "What did we do next?"<br>• Using questions that promote good conversation<br>  ○ Open ended<br>• True questions (about events where partner was not present, feelings, and opinions versus testing questions that asker already knows the answer to) |

*Sources:* Adapted from TBI Express group training program (Mann et al., 2015, p. 1108; Togher, 2014; 2015; Togher, McDonald, Tate, et al., 2009, 2013, 2016; Togher, Power, Tate, et al., 2010; Ylvisaker, Sellars, & Edelman, 1998, pp. 310–311; Ylvisaker, Jacobs, & Feeney, 2003).

# Form to Use for Identifying
# Communicative Behaviors/Intentions

| Identifying Communicative Behaviors and Intentions | |
|---|---|
| Name: _____ | Date: _____ |
| **Communicative:** Intentions | **Number (#) of times observed** |
| Asking for information |卌 |
| Complimenting | || |
| Giving information | |||| |
| | |
| | |
| | |
| | |
| | |
| | |
| | |
| | |
| | |

# Index

**Note:** Page numbers in **bold** reference non-text material.